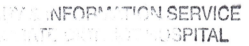

Recent Advances in

Surgery
25

Recent Advances in Surgery 24
Edited by I. Taylor & C. D. Johnson

ISBN 0-443-070660

ISSN 0143 8395

Recent Advances in

Surgery
25

Edited by

C. D. Johnson MChir FRCS
Reader and Consultant Surgeon, University Surgical Unit, Southampton
General Hospital, Southampton, UK

I. Taylor MD ChM FRCS
David Patey Professor of Surgery, Royal Free and University College London
Medical School, University College London, London, UK

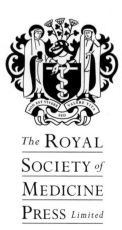

The ROYAL
SOCIETY *of*
MEDICINE
PRESS *Limited*

1 Wimpole Street, London W1G 0AE, UK
207 E Westminster Road, Lake Forest, IL 60045, USA
http://www.rsm.ac.uk

British Library Cataloguing in Publication Data
A catalogue record for this book is available from the British Library
ISBN 1-85315-508-X
ISSN 0143 8395

Commissioning editor - Peter Richardson
Editorial assistant - Gabrielle Lowis
Production by GM & BA Haddock, Midlothian, UK
Printed in Great Britain by Bell & Bain, Glasgow, UK

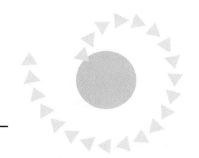

Contents

Contributors

A.G. Acheson MB BCh FRCS
Specialist Registrar in General Surgery, Department of Surgery, Queen's
Medical Centre, Nottingham, UK

Tan Arulampalam FRCS
Department of Surgery and Institute of Nuclear Medicine, Royal Free and
University College Medical School, Middlesex Hospital, London, UK

Jonathan D. Beard BSc ChM FRCS
Consultant Vascular Surgeon, Sheffield Vascular Institute, Northern General
Hospital, Sheffield, UK

Ian J. Beckingham MD FRCS
Senior Lecturer, Department of Surgery, Queen's Medical Centre,
Nottingham, UK

Douglas M.G. Bowley FRCS
Fellow in Trauma Surgery, Trauma Unit, Johannesburg Hospital,
Johannesburg, Republic of South Africa; Specialist Registar in General
Surgery, Ministry of Defence, UK; and Honorary Lecturer, Department of
Surgery, University of the Witwatersrand Medical School, Johannesburg,
Republic of South Africa

Rachel M. Bright-Thomas MA BM BCh MD FRCS
Specialist Registrar in General Surgery, North West Thames Deanery, Ealing
Hospital NHS Trust, Southall, Middlesex, UK

Arun Chaturvedi MBBS MS MAMS
Professor of Surgical Oncology, Department of Surgical Oncology, King
George's Medical College, Lucknow, India

J. Michael Dixon MD FRCS FRCSEd
Consultant Surgeon and Senior Lecturer, Academic Office, Edinburgh Breast
Unit, Western General Hospital, Edinburgh, UK

Michael Douek MD FRCS
Lecturer in Surgery, Royal Free and University College London Medical School, University College London, London, UK

Peter A. Gaines MRCP FRCR
Consultant Vascular Radiologist, Sheffield Vascular Institute, Northern General Hospital, Sheffield, UK

Andrew D. Gilliam MBChB MRCS
Research Registrar, Department of Surgery, Queen's Medical Centre, Nottingham, UK

N. Griffin MB ChB MRCS
Research Registrar in General Surgery, Department of Surgery, Queen's Medical Centre, Nottingham, UK

K.G. Harding MB ChB MRCGP FRCS
Professor of Rehabilitation Medicine (Wound Healing) Wound Healing Research Unit, Cardiff Medicentre, Heath Park, Cardiff, UK

D.J. Leaper MD ChM FRCS FACS
Professor of Surgery, Professorial Unit of Surgery, University Hospital of North Tees, Stockton-on-Tees, Cleveland, UK

N.C. Misra MBBS MS FRCS FICS FACS FAMS
Professor of Siurgery (Oncology), Head of Department of Surgery (Ex), King George's Medical College, Director Lucknow Cancer Centre, Lucknow, India

Sanjeev Misra MBBS MS MCh FICSMAMS
Assistant Professor, Department of Surgical Oncology, King George's Medical College, Lucknow, India

John R.T. Monson MD FRCS FRCSI FACS FRCPSGlas(Hon)
Professor of Surgery and Head of Department, Academic Surgical Unit, Castle Hill Hospital, Cottingham, UK

Karen P. Nugent MA MS FRCS
Senior Lecturer/Honorary Consultant, University Surgical Unit, University of Southampton, Southampton General Hospital, Southampton, UK

Ayo Oshowo MS FRCS(Gen)
Specialist Registrar, Department of Surgery, Royal Free and University College London Medical School, University College London, London, UK

C.J. Phillips BSc MSc PhD
Reader in Health Economics, Centre for Health Economics and Policy Studies, School of Health Science, University of Wales, Swansea

J.N. Primrose MD FRCS
Professor of Surgery, University of Southampton and Honorary Consultant Surgeon, Southampton University Hospitals NHS Trust, Southampton, UK

James M. Ryan MCh FRCS DMCC FFAEM (Hons)
Leonard Cheshire Professor, Leonard Cheshire Centre of Conflict Recovery, Department of Surgery, University College London, UK

J.H. Scholefield MB ChB FRCS ChM
Professor of Surgery, Queen's Medical Centre, Nottingham, UK

Meheshinder Singh MBBS MMed(S'pore) FRCS(Edin) FRCSI
Colorectal Clinical Fellow, Academic Surgical Unit, Castle Hill Hospital, Cottingham, UK

Mike Stroud BSc MD FRCP
Senior Lecturer in Medicine and Nutrition, Honorary Consultant Gastroenterologist, University of Southampton, Southampton General Hospital, UK

Malvena E. Stuart Taylor BSc(Hons) FRCA
Consultant Anaesthetist and Lead Consultant for the Acute Pain Service, Southampton Universities Hospitals NHS Trust, Shackleton Department of Anaesthetics, University of Southampton, UK

Irving Taylor MD ChM FRCS
David Patey Professor of Surgery, Head of Department of Surgery, Royal Free and University College London Medical School, University College London, London, UK

Susan A. Watson PhD
Professor, Cancer Studies Unit, University of Nottingham, Queen's Medical Centre, Nottingham, UK

Douglas M.G. Bowley James M. Ryan

1

Resuscitation and trauma surgery

In 1990, about 5 million people died as a result of injury world-wide. For people under 35 years of age, injury is now the leading cause of death.[1] It is estimated that by the year 2020, injuries from road traffic accidents will be the third most common cause of disability world-wide and 8.4 million people will die every year from injury. Around one-third of these deaths will be due to haemorrhagic shock and, therefore, could potentially be avoided by appropriate surgical intervention.[2] This chapter reviews advances in the last 10 years in peri-operative and non-operative management of the trauma patient, and in a number of specific surgical approaches.

RESUSCITATION AFTER MAJOR TRAUMA

PREHOSPITAL CARE

The question of whether to attempt to stabilise a trauma patient with advanced life support (ALS) techniques or transfer the patient direct to hospital without interventions at the scene has been much debated. In the UK, paramedic interventions have been reported to result in an additional 12 min at the scene when intravenous cannulation is attempted.[3] In contrast, in a 3-year review from the US, Johnson *et al.*[4] reported an average total scene time of less than 10 min for patients with critical injuries.

A meta-analysis of four cohort studies showed an increased ($P = 0.03$) risk of death in patients attended by paramedics. The risk of death after paramedic

Mr Douglas M.G. Bowley FRCS, Department of Surgery, University of Witwatersrand Medical School, 7 York Road, Parktown 2193, Johannesburg, Republic of South Africa

Prof. James M. Ryan MCh FRCS DMCC FFAEM (Hons), Leonard Cheshire Professor, Leonard Cheshire Centre of Conflict Recovery, Department of Surgery, University College London, 4 Taviton Street, London WC1H 0BT, UK (for correspondence)

care was especially high in patients with bleeding injuries (relative risk = 4.60; 95% CI = 1.07–20.0).[3]

A recent analysis reviewed 174 reports on prehospital ALS *versus* basic life support measures with immediate transfer to hospital (the so-called 'scoop and run' policy). These aggregated data failed to demonstrate a benefit for on-site ALS provided to trauma patients and supported the scoop and run approach.[5]

However, while short scene times are commendable, they are not the whole story. The overall organisation of prehospital services has an impact on outcomes after trauma. Mock *et al.*[6] studied the patterns of trauma mortality in three countries with different socio-economic status. With similar injury patterns, mortality decreased with increased per-capita income, mainly due to prehospital deaths.

Key point 1

- Scoop and run: when appropriate prehospital care should involve basic life support measures on scene and rapid transport to hospital.

FLUID RESUSCITATION

An awareness of the experimental and clinical evidence that fluid administration before surgical control of haemorrhage may actually worsen bleeding and increase mortality after penetrating injury has led members of the Cochrane Injuries Group to describe current resuscitation practice as 'potentially harmful and at best experimental'.[7]

After securing the airway and ensuring adequate oxygenation and ventilation, ATLS® protocols have shifted their emphasis away from immediate fluid resuscitation to stress the importance of surgical control of haemorrhage along with transfusion with intravenous fluids.

Intravenous fluids have been shown to inhibit platelet aggregation, dilute clotting factors, modulate the physical properties of thrombus and cause increases in blood pressure that can mechanically disrupt clot.[7] Animal models have demonstrated reductions in mortality with resuscitation to a mean arterial pressure (MAP) of 40 mmHg *versus* more normal MAP (80 mmHg).[8] In a study of hypotensive patients with penetrating injuries in Houston, significantly more patients survived when they were randomised to a policy of fluid resuscitation delayed until haemorrhage had been controlled compared with immediate fluid administration.[44] The methodology of this study has been criticised,[7] and the concept of delayed administration of fluids may not be universally applicable. Permissive hypotension may not be beneficial after blunt trauma, for the elderly or for those with co-morbid illness, for patients with head or spinal injuries or for those patients whose prehospital time is likely to be prolonged.

More recent animals studies have found that moderately resuscitated animals survive better than animals that receive either less aggressive or more aggressive resuscitation, confirming the potential benefit of controlled fluid resuscitation in the setting of injured patients with a site of on-going bleeding.[9] Controlled infusion of fluids after massive initial blood loss may restore sufficient tissue perfusion and oxygen delivery to prevent irreversible ischaemia. This form of graded resuscitation is an attractive concept, but the over-riding priority remains timely surgical intervention.

Key point 2

- Minimal fluid resuscitation is likely to be beneficial in selected cases. Always avoid over-transfusion.

Crystalloid *versus* colloid

The relative benefits of administering crystalloid or colloid fluids have received much attention. In a systematic review of randomised controlled trials comparing colloid and crystalloid resuscitation in critically ill trauma patients, the relative risk of death with colloid was 1.3 (95% CI = 0.95–1.77).[10] The results of a second similar review were even more discouraging with a relative risk of death with colloid of 2.6 (95% CI = 1.1–5.9).[11] Several reasons have been advanced to explain these findings, but they are consistent with the hypothesis that expansion of the circulating volume in trauma patients with on-going bleeding is harmful.[7]

Hypertonic saline

Hypertonic saline (3–7.5% formulations), with or without added colloid, can effectively improve haemodynamics and oxygen transport when given in volumes substantially less than standard crystalloids.[12] A number of trials have been reported, with survival advantages being suggested for subgroups of patients with severe head injuries or hypotensive patients requiring surgery. However, combining the data into a meta-analysis did not reveal a significant increase in survival with the use of hypertonic saline.[13] Hypertonic saline may improve microcirculatory haemodynamics and provide a measure of immuno-logical protection.

Blood transfusion and haemoglobin-based oxygen carriers

Although the availability of blood for transfusion is known to be a major determinant of outcome after injury,[14] packed red blood cell transfusions have been shown to have significant immunosuppressive potential, and transmission of fatal diseases through blood supply has been extensively documented. Packed red blood cell transfusions are an independent risk factor for postinjury infection and multiple organ failure.[15] Initially, transfusion was felt to be a surrogate for injury severity, but it has been found to be a robust and independent predictor of postoperative complications. Attitudes to transfusion have changed substantially since the early 1990s and at least one large trial has found that using a restrictive blood transfusion protocol in place of a more traditional one improved survival.[16] These findings have led to a paradigm shift with respect to blood transfusion: whereas the traditional view was that anaemia by itself was a sufficient indication for transfusion, the current consensus is that a second indication must be present in addition to a decreased haemoglobin concentration.

Key point 3

- Young trauma patients can usually tolerate a haemoglobin level of 70 g/l.

Diverse clinical experience has substantiated the feasibility of auto-transfusion in trauma.[17] Autotransfusion eliminates the infectious, allergic, and incompatibility problems of stored blood, an important concern because of the acquired immunodeficiency syndrome (AIDS). However, when large amounts of collected blood are re-infused, consumptive coagulopathy and platelet dysfunction may occur.[18] These risks may outweigh the benefits of autotransfusion in the critically injured patient who has multiple potential bleeding sites.

The ideal blood substitute provides simultaneous volume expansion and oxygen carrying capacity; it is universally compatible, free from disease and has a long shelf-life. Haemoglobin-based oxygen carriers (HBOCs) are formulated from outdated human blood cells, other animal species, or can be made using recombinant technology. So-called 'new generation' HBOCs include enzymes and antioxidants designed to modulate reperfusion injury.[19] Although enthusiasm has been somewhat tempered by the early closure of a phase III randomised trial due to excess mortality in the HBOC arm,[20] multicentre trials are on-going.

EARLY ENTERAL FEEDING

Trauma patients have increased nutritional needs and early enteral feeding has been shown to reduce postoperative septic morbidity after trauma. Following a number of randomised trials, a meta-analysis demonstrated a 2-fold decrease in infectious complications in patients treated with early enteral nutrition compared to total parenteral nutrition.[21] Enteral nutrition has been shown to promote splanchnic blood flow, maintain gastrointestinal mucosal barrier function, limit alteration in normal gut flora, blunt the catabolic response to stress and bolster immune defences. Intestinal anastomoses are not a contra-indication to enteral feeding.[22]

Enteral feeding should be started as soon as possible in trauma patients to maintain gastrointestinal mucosal function and immune competence (*i.e.* within 24–48 h after injury when possible). It may be possible to manipulate a fine-bore feeding tube beyond the pylorus, but, if not, then a feeding jejunostomy may be inserted.

Key point 4

- Early enteral feeding is likely to reduce morbidity after major trauma.

NON-OPERATIVE MANAGEMENT OF PENETRATING ABDOMINAL INJURIES

It has been apparent for many years that wounds to the abdomen do not automatically have visceral injury requiring operative repair. During the Boer War (1899–1902), the dismal results of laparotomy led Sir William MacCormac, the senior British surgeon, to advocate a non-operative strategy for penetrating abdominal wounds. In what became known as MacCormac's aphorism he wrote: 'a man wounded in the abdomen dies if he is operated on and remains alive if he is left in peace'.[23] That not all war wounds of the abdomen have significant visceral injuries was corroborated in more recent conflicts; a series of 1350 laparotomies from the Vietnam War revealed a rate of non-therapeutic laparotomy of 19.2%.[24] Experience from the Red Cross with patients whose evacuation to hospital has been delayed by several days after abdominal wounding shows that some low energy transfer wounds to the intestine will seal themselves and not lead to generalised peritonitis.[14]

A policy of selective non-operative management after stab wounds to the abdomen based almost exclusively on clinical examination has been shown to be safe and effective in reducing the number of non-therapeutic laparotomies.[26] Despite this experience, surgeons have been reluctant to extend the indications of this policy to include gunshot injuries, as the likelihood of significant visceral injury after gunshot wounds is much higher than with bladed weapons. It should be remembered that the initial physical examination of the abdomen can be misleading. In one study, more than 40% of patients with subsequently confirmed intra-abdominal injury were asymptomatic on admission.[27]

In the civilian trauma setting, Ivatury et al.[25] investigated 100 haemodynamically stable patients with penetrating wounds to the abdomen using laparoscopy; they found 43 had no peritoneal penetration.

The largest series in the literature, prospectively studied 309 patients with gunshot wounds to the anterior abdomen.[28] Overall, 106 (34%) patients were selected for conservative management. Of these, 14 (13%) had late laparotomy of which 5 were therapeutic. Abdominal complications developed in 2 of the late laparotomies. The authors concluded that, in an appropriate setting, selective conservative management of abdominal gunshot wounds is safe. However, the importance of careful serial clinical examination by an experienced surgeon in an established trauma centre was stressed.

Key point 5

- Non-operative management of abdominal injuries is feasible and practised in some centres.

OPERATIVE STRATEGIES

PRIMARY REPAIR OF COLONIC INJURY

The universally fatal results of breakdown of colonic repairs in the Second World War led to a policy of mandatory exteriorisation of colon injuries that was later credited as 'the greatest single factor in improved results'.[29] This policy arose in the context of wounds from warfare, with delays in surgery, rudimentary anaesthesia and antibiotics, lack of blood for transfusion and tenuous chains of evacuation. Nevertheless, this policy of mandatory faecal diversion led post-war surgeons, both civilian and military to consider primary repair to be unsafe, and it was not until 1979 that the first randomised trial was undertaken to question the role of mandatory faecal diversion after penetrating colonic injury.[30]

Sufficient evidence has now been produced to enable recommendations to be published supporting primary repair for the majority of penetrating colon wounds in civilian practice. Current internet-based Trauma Guidelines support primary repair for non-destructive colon wounds in the absence of peritonitis.[31] However, the numbers of patients in published studies with destructive colonic wounds requiring resection or associated factors likely to increase morbidity have been relatively small and several authors have counselled against abandoning colostomy in high-risk patients.

In a review of 27 patients with high risk colonic injuries,[32] intra-abdominal sepsis occurred in 20% of the primary repair group and there were 2/25 anastomotic leaks (8%) both of which were fatal, leading to a conclusion that there was still a place for faecal diversion in severe colon injury. Most recently, the American Association for the Surgery of Trauma (AAST) have enrolled patients with severe colonic injuries requiring resection into a prospective, multinational trial. A total of 297 patients were recruited and no significant difference in morbidity was found between matched patients undergoing primary anastomosis or diversion of the faecal stream, irrespective of associated risk factors.[33]

The significant morbidity and financial costs associated with creation and reversal of colostomy, and the destructive effect of colostomy on the patients' quality-of-life have been cited as further reasons to support the primary repair of colonic wounds.[34]

The cultural and socio-economic status of the patient is especially relevant to the population of emerging nations. This may make colostomy inappropriate. Colostomy may be poorly managed due to poor patient education, inadequate sanitary facilities and unequal access to medical care. Colostomy after trauma may adversely affect working, social and sexual interaction.[35]

Key point 6

- Primary repair of colonic injuries should be undertaken in the majority of patients.

DAMAGE CONTROL SURGERY

The traditional surgical approach to resuscitation after abdominal trauma has been based on tried and tested methods of managing penetrating injury with exploration, control of bleeding and contamination, and attempts to achieve definitive repair of damaged structures. Exsanguinating haemorrhage after severe trauma leads to the onset of a cycle of three inter-related variables: metabolic acidosis, profound hypothermia, and a clinically obvious coagulopathy. Each of these factors re-inforces the others to form 'a bloody vicious cycle', which leads to death as a consequence of an irreversible metabolic insult.[36] In the early 1980s, surgeons in the US extended their technique of abdominal packing of liver injuries to include the cold, exsanguinating, coagulopathic trauma patient.[37]

Damage control is a term used by the US Navy that describes the capacity of a ship to absorb damage and maintain mission integrity.[4] The phrase was adopted by Schwab and his co-workers in Pennsylvania, to describe the evolving concept of saving life after major trauma by deferring treatment of anatomical disruptions and focusing on restoring the patient's physiology.

Damage control is a three-phase surgical approach to an injured patient at the limit of his or her physiological reserves. Phase one is the initial surgical procedure when only the minimum is done to stop haemorrhage and limit or contain contamination. Phase two occurs in the intensive care unit where attempts are made to restore normal physiological parameters before returning the patient to the operating theatre for phase three, when definitive surgery is undertaken.

Most patients with penetrating abdominal injury require traditional management, with the damage control approach being necessary in only a few. In a busy urban trauma unit, only approximately 8% of patients undergoing laparotomy required damage control.[4] The damage control approach should be limited to those few patients who are critically unstable, with multivisceral injury and exsanguination.

During a damage control laparotomy, a full midline incision is made, haemoperitoneum is evacuated and the abdomen is packed in four quadrants. Control of haemorrhage is achieved either by direct means or by indirect means with use of packs or balloon tamponade for deep hepatic wounds. The key principle is that packing should re-approximate disrupted tissue planes. Overpacking will result in raised intra-abdominal pressure and haemodynamic compromise due to compression of the inferior vena cava, effectively producing an abdominal compartment syndrome. Underpacking is ineffective placement of packs, which fail to stop the bleeding. Packing will not control arterial bleeders, which must be controlled by other methods.

Hollow viscus injuries are controlled by tying with tapes, simple running sutures or by the use of stapling devices. Reconstruction is deferred and the closed-off loops of bowel are returned into the abdominal cavity. Vascular injuries may be treated by ligation or by placement of temporary vascular shunts. Biliary, pancreatic and urological injuries are controlled by external tube drainage with stenting.

Temporary closure of the abdominal wall may be achieved by a variety of means; however, most centres have abandoned closure of fascia or skin.[4] Vacuum-pack dressings[38] allow rapid abdominal closure and considerable expansion of intra-abdominal contents, reducing the incidence of abdominal compartment syndrome.[4]

On completion of the initial laparotomy, efforts are focused on restoring the patient's deranged physiology. The goal is adequate oxygen delivery at a cellular level and the priorities are optimisation of haemodynamic status, re-warming and restoration of normal coagulation parameters.[39]

The range of time between a damage control laparotomy and the planned return to theatre is wide, varying between 6–90 h, the majority being returned within 48 h. When the patient is returned to the operating room for removal of packs and completion of definitive surgical procedures, a thorough search must be made for missed injuries. Injuries missed at initial operation have been shown to be a potent cause of morbidity and death and have been described as 'the nemesis of the trauma surgeon'.[40]

Key point 7

- Damage control surgery should have a defined place in the surgeon's armamentarium.

FUTURE DIRECTIONS

RECOMBINANT FACTOR VII

Intravenous administration of recombinant activated human clotting factor VII (rFVIIa) has an established place in prevention of bleeding in haemophiliac patients undergoing surgery. In a hypothermic, coagulopathic animal model, rFVIIa reduced blood loss and restored abnormal coagulation function when used as an adjunct to damage control surgery techniques.[41] Seven massively bleeding, multitransfused, coagulopathic trauma patients have also been treated with rFVIIa after failure to achieve haemostasis with conventional means. The coagulopathic bleeding resolved in all patients, coagulation parameters improved dramatically and 4 from 7 patients survived.[42] This experience holds great promise for the use of rFVIIa and randomised, multinational trials have commenced.

Key point 8

- Recombinant factor VII may represent salvage for critically wounded patients as an adjunct to damage control.

PREVENTABLE DEATHS

Currently, there is much to improve in trauma management. Preventable morbidity and mortality must be identified by a thorough audit structure; a commitment to improvement in all aspects of trauma care is required. Awareness of the prevalence of missed injuries can make a great contribution to reducing morbidity. In a prospective study from Australia, Janjua et al.[43] found a 15% incidence of clinically significant injuries diagnosed after initial resuscitation. They concluded that a so-called tertiary survey (physical examination and review of results) would allow for the early detection of almost all clinically significant injuries.

Key point 9

- Tertiary survey will prevent much morbidity after trauma.

TRAUMA AND SOCIETY

Finally, acceptance that trauma is a world-wide problem is required at governmental and societal levels. Improvements in prehospital and emergency room care have the potential to greatly improve survival, especially in the non-industrialised world.[6] Public health strategies, education and injury-prevention legislation have a pivotal place in reducing the financial, social and human impact of trauma.

Key points for clinical practice

- Scoop and run: effective prehospital care should involve basic life support measures on scene and rapid transport to hospital.
- Minimal fluid resuscitation is likely to be beneficial in selected cases. Always avoid over-transfusion.
- Young trauma patients can usually tolerate a haemoglobin level of 70 g/l.
- Early enteral feeding is likely to reduce morbidity after major trauma.
- Non-operative management of abdominal injuries is feasible and practised in some centres.
- Primary repair of colonic injuries should be undertaken in the majority of patients.
- Damage control surgery should have a defined place in the surgeon's armamentarium.
- Recombinant factor VII may represent salvage for critically wounded patients as an adjunct to damage control.
- Tertiary survey will prevent much morbidity after trauma.

References

1. Murray CJL, Lopez AD. Mortality by cause for eight regions of the world. Global burden of disease. *Lancet* 1997; **349**: 1269–1276.
2. Murray CJL, Lopez AD. Alternative projections of mortality and disability by cause 1990–2020: global burden of disease study. *Lancet* 1997; **349**: 1498–1504.
3. Nicholl J, Hughes S, Dixon S, Turner J, Yates D. The costs and benefits of paramedic skill in pre-hospital trauma care. *Health Technol Assess* 1998; **2**: 7.
4. Johnson J, Gracias VH, Schwab CW *et al.* Evolution in damage control for exsanguinating penetrating abdominal injury. *J Trauma* 2001; **51**: 261–271.

5. Liberman M, Mulder D, Sampalis J. Advanced or basic life support for trauma: meta-analysis and critical review of the literature. *J Trauma* 2000; **49**: 584–599.
6. Mock CN, Jurkovich GJ, nii-Amon-Kotei D, Arreola-Risa C, Maier RV. Trauma mortality patterns in three nations at different economic levels. *J Trauma* 1998; **44**: 804–812.
7. Roberts I, Evans P, Bunn F, Kwan I, Crowhurst E. Is the normalisation of blood pressure in bleeding trauma patients harmful? *Lancet* 2001; **357**: 385–387.
8. Kowalenko T, Stern S, Dronen S. Improved outcome with hypotensive resuscitation of uncontrolled haemorrhagic shock in a swine model. *J Trauma* 1992; **33**: 349–354.
9. Soucy DM, Rude M, Hsia WC, Hagedorn FN, Illner H, Shires GT. The effect of varying fluid volume and rate of resuscitation during uncontrolled haemorrhage. *J Trauma* 1999; **46**; 209–215.
10. Alderson P, Schierhout G, Roberts I, Bunn F. Colloid versus crystalloids for fluid resuscitation in critically ill patients. (Cochrane Review). In: *The Cochrane Library*, Issue 2. Oxford: Update Software, 2000.
11. Choi PT, Yip G, Quinonez LG, Cook DJ. Crystalloids vs colloid in fluid resuscitation: a systematic review. *Crit Care Med* 1999; **27**: 200–210.
12. Diedel LN, Tyberski JG, Dulchavsky SA. Effects of hypertonic saline solution and dextran on ventricular blood flow and heart-lung interaction after hemorrhagic shock. *Surgery* 1998; **124**: 642–650.
13. Wade CE, Kramer CG, Grady JJ, Fabian TC, Younes RN. Efficacy of hypertonic 7.5% saline and 60% dextran-70 in treating trauma: a meta-analysis of controlled clinical studies. *Surgery* 1997; **122**: 609–616.
14. Coupland RM. Abdominal wounds in war. *Br J Surg* 1996; **83**: 1505–1511.
15. Zallen G, Moore EE, Ciesla DJ, Brown M, Biffl WL, Silliman CC. Stored red blood cells selectively activate human neutrophils to release IL-8 and secretory PLA$_2$. *Shock* 2000; **13**: 29–33.
16. Hebert PC, Wells G, Blajchman MA *et al*. A multicenter, randomized, controlled clinical trial of transfusion requirements in critical care. Transfusion Requirements in Critical Care Investigators, Canadian Critical Care Trials Group. *N Engl J Med* 1999; **340**: 409–417.
17. Smith LA, Barker DE, Burns RP. Autotransfusion utilization in abdominal trauma. *Am J Surg* 1997; **63**: 47–49.
18. Horst MH, Dlugos S, Fath JJ, Sorensen VJ, Obeid FN, Bivins BA. Coagulopathy and intraoperative blood salvage. *J Trauma* 1992; **32**: 646–653.
19. Chang TMS. Future prospects for artificial blood. *Trends Biotechnol* 1999; **17**: 61–67.
20. Sloan EF, Koneigsburg M, Gens D. Diaspirin cross-linked hemoglobin (DCLHb) in the treatment of severe traumatic hemorrhagic shock. *JAMA* 1999; **282**: 1857–1864.
21. Moore FA, Feliciano DV, Andrassy RJ *et al*. Early enteral feeding compared with parenteral reduces postoperative septic complications: the result of a meta analysis. *Ann Surg* 1992; **216**: 172–183.
22. Kiyana T, Efram DT, Tantry U, Barbul A. Effect of nutritional route on colonic anastomotic healing in the rat. *J Gastrointest Surg* 1999; **3**: 441–446.
23. Edwards DP. The history of colonic surgery in war. *J R Army Med Corps* 1999; **145**: 107–108.
24. Hardaway III RM. Vietnam wound analysis. *J Trauma* 1978; **18**: 635–642.
25. Ivatury RR, Simon RJ, Stahl WM. A critical evaluation of laparoscopy in penetrating abdominal trauma. *J Trauma* 1993; **34**: 822–827.
26. Shorr RM, Gottlieb MM, Webb K, Ishiguro LI, Berne TV. Selective management of penetrating wounds of the abdomen: importance of the physical examination. *Arch Surg* 1988; **123**: 1141–1145.
27. Lowe RJ, Saletta JD, Read DR, Radhakrishnan J, Moss GS. Should laparotomy be mandatory or selective in gunshot wounds to the abdomen? *J Trauma* 1977; **17**: 903–907.
28. Demetriades D. Selective nonoperative management of gunshot wounds to the anterior abdomen. *Arch Surg* 1997; **132**: 178–183.
29. Ogilvie WH. Abdominal wounds in the Western Desert. *Surg Gynaecol Obstet* 1944; **78**: 225–230.
30. Stone HH, Fabian TC. Management of perforating colon trauma: randomization between primary closure and exteriorization. *Ann Surg* 1979; **190**: 430–436.
31. Cayten CG, Fabian TC, Garcia VF, Ivatury RR, Morris JA. Patient management guidelines for penetrating intraperitoneal colon injury. <www.east.org> 2000.

32. Cornwell 3rd EE, Velmahos GC, Berne TV *et al*. The fate of colonic suture lines in high risk trauma patients: a prospective analysis. *J Am Coll Surg* 1998; **187**: 58–63.

33. Demetriades D, Murray JA, Chan L *et al*. Penetrating colon injuries requiring resection: Diversion or primary anastomosis? An AAST, prospective multicenter study. *J Trauma* 2001; **50**: 765–775.

34. Bern JD, Velmahos GC, Chan LS, Asensio JA, Demetriades D. The high morbidity of colostomy closure after trauma: further support for primary repair of colon injuries. *Surgery* 1998; **123**: 157–164.

35. Naraynsingh V, Ariyanayagam D, Pooran S. Primary repair of colon injuries in a developing country. *Br J Surg* 1991; **78**: 319–320.

36. Kashuk JL, Moore EE, Millikan JS, Moore JB. Major abdominal vascular trauma: a unified approach. *J Trauma* 1982; **22**: 672–679.

37. Stone HH, Strom PR, Mullins RJ. Management of the major coagulopathy with onset during laparotomy. *Ann Surg* 1983; **197**: 532–535.

38. Barker DE, Kaufmann HJ, Smith LA, Ciraulo DL, Richartl CL, Burns PR. Vacuum pack technique of temporary abdominal closure: a 7 year experience with 112 patients. *J Trauma* 2000; **48**: 201–207.

39. Moore EE, Burch JM, Francoise RJ. Staged physiologic restoration and damage control surgery. *World J Surg* 1998; **22**: 1184–1191.

40. Scalea TM, Phillips TF, Goldstein AS *et al*. Injuries missed at operation: nemesis of the trauma surgeon. *J Trauma* 1988; **28**: 962–967.

41. Martinowitz U, Holcomb JB, Pusateri AE *et al*. Intravenous rFVIIa administered for hemorrhage control in hypothermic, coagulopathic swine with grade V liver injuries. *J Trauma* 2001; **50**: 721–729.

42. Martinowitz U, Kenet G, Segal E *et al*. Recombinant activated factor VII for adjunctive hemorrhage control in trauma. *J Trauma* 2001; **51**: 431–439.

43. Janjua KJ, Sugrue M, Deane SA. Prospective evaluation of early missed injuries and the role of the tertiary trauma survey. *J Trauma* 1998; **44**: 148–147.

44. Bickell WH, Wall MJ, Pepe PE, Mattox K. Immediate versus delayed fluid resuscitation for hypotensive patients with penetrating torso injuries. *N Engl J Med* 1994; **331**: 1105–1109.

D.J. Leaper K.G. Harding C.J. Phillips

2

Management of wounds

The surgical concept of a wound caused deliberately by a scalpel, or accidentally by a traumatic penetrating injury or laceration, has been widened to include chronic, open wounds and ulcers, healing by secondary intention. Healing in primary sutured wounds is largely predictable, but many open wounds have an underlying pathology which delays their healing. A chronic wound is hard to define, but they are far from inactive; their failure to heal probably relates to abnormalities within 'cascades' (haemostasis, inflammation, proliferation and remodelling sequences) of wound healing (Fig. 1). Many of these chronic wounds are now managed by interdisciplinary teams of physicians. This is reflected by the proliferation of active wound healing societies (*e.g.* European Tissue Repair Society, European Wound Management Association, Tissue Viability Society and Wound Care Society). Surgeons are no longer passive members of such teams and may be called on for help with debridement of wounds or for revascularisation of an ischaemic limb. In fact, many surgeons lead in leg ulcer clinics with surgical interests in venous, diabetic and pressure ulcers as well as those caused by peripheral vascular disease. In this article, we have reviewed advances in acute and chronic wound care with the experimental background, together with consideration of the economics of their implementation, as part of established clinical practice.

Key point 1
- Achieving good wound healing remains a major clinical problem.

Prof. D.J. Leaper MD ChM FRCS FACS, Professor of Surgery, Professorial Unit of Surgery, University Hospital of North Tees, Stockton-on-Tees, Cleveland TS19 8PE, UK (for correspondence)

Prof. K.G. Harding MB ChB MRCGP FRCS, Professor of Rehabilitation Medicine (Wound Healing) Wound Healing Research Unit, Cardiff Medicentre, Heath Park, Cardiff

Dr C.J. Phillips BSc MSc PhD, Reader in Health Economics, Centre for Health Economics and Policy Studies, School of Health Science, University of Wales, Swansea

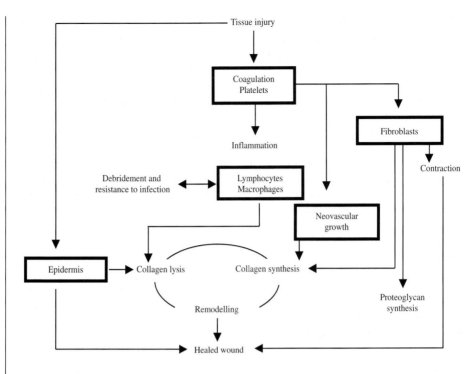

Fig. 1 Wound healing cascade adapted from Harding *et al.*[54]

CLINICAL ASPECTS OF WOUND CLOSURE IN SURGERY IN GENERAL

ABDOMINAL WALL CLOSURE

Burst abdomen reflects technical failure and, provided appropriate techniques are used for abdominal closure, its true incidence should be less than 1%. Catgut, which has little place in surgery because of its unpredictable performance, has been replaced by a range of synthetic polymers. Incisional hernia, when extending the full length of the wound and when it appears within a few weeks of surgery is also probably a technical failure, whereas late presentation (after 12 months), or small hernias, are more likely due to the 'cheese-wiring' effect of sutures or deep wound infections.

Key point 2

- Choice of sutures and techniques employed influence rate of complications.

Much of the apparent evidence to support management of this problem is based on comparative, sometimes randomised, studies which are rarely adequately powered, or alternatively on clinical experience and opinion. Two recent reviews, which do not permit an adequate meta-analysis, come down in favour of monofilament polymeric sutures of non-absorbable type (polyamide or polypropylene) or absorbable type (polydioxanone, PDS).[1,2] Absorbable sutures with a shorter period of integrity in the tissues than PDS are probably inadequate. Burst abdomen appears to be of historical interest only, but the incidence of incisional hernia is lessened using these sutures with a continuous wide bite technique. The lateral paramedian incision appears to be the gold standard,[3] although some would argue it takes longer to make, and to close; upper midline or standard paramedian incisions have more complications. The theoretical suture length:wound length of 4:1 is not validated by meta-analysis,[1] and there are varied reports of its importance. It may well simply relate to the size of each fascial suture bite.[4] Because it depends on technical factors, it may be that the complication could be considered a marker of surgical technique. Surgeons prefer sutures which handle and knot easily; the monofilament polymers are challenging to surgeons in training, but the absorbables are associated with less wound pain and fewer persistent knot sinuses.

Key point 3

- Rate of wound complications may be an indicator of surgical competence.

INCISIONAL HERNIA REPAIR

Incisional hernias follow 5–15% of laparotomy closures. A third are recognised more than 5 years postoperatively and 20% overall need repair. Failure rates of repair are high; being 40% after non-mesh repair (*e.g.* mass closure, keel repair) and 20% after mesh repair. Laparoscopic repair probably needs clinical trial evidence of efficacy, but it seems that polypropylene is the most favoured mesh. The best results appear to follow a combined mesh and fascial repair.[5]

SKIN CLOSURE (SURGERY IN GENERAL)

There is wide-spread use of subcuticular closure which gives the best cosmetic results. Which is the best suture is still not clear. Certainly silk, with its risk of entry wound stitch abscesses and subsequent skin scarring, is not acceptable. Absorbable polymers should not need removal from the wound, but we still require an adequately powered study to identify whether they have an increased risk of later wound infections or delayed healing. The alternatives, which have their advocates, also need randomised controlled trial evidence of superiority. Clips allow rapid skin closure after long operations but are expensive;[6] glues such as the cyanoacrylates[7] or fibrin sealants[8] may also have their place. Skin closure strips, which have always been useful in paediatric trauma or to close a gaping incisional wound, would be good trial comparators.

Many other aspects of skin closure also need evidence-based indications for clinical use. Whether contaminated or dirty wounds need to be left open for delayed primary closure or healing by secondary intention is unclear. Management and control of an infection source is probably more important.[9] Even the definition of wound infection is not clear or standardised, so that surveillance and studies of antibiotic prophylaxis and treatment may be flawed. Local or systemic warming is effective in reducing infection when clear definitions of infection are used. However, such defined criteria reveal a much higher wound infection rate is usually expected.[10] Whether these 'infections' actually represent a failure to heal is not clear, but certainly obesity carries a higher incidence of postoperative wound complications. There is experimental evidence that priming a surgical incision by the use of growth factors is useful[11] and this may help prevent incisional hernias.[12] Optimisation or acceleration of tensile strength has been described in colonic healing[13] and so has the use of inhibitors of metalloproteinases.[14] All these modalities may soon be tested in clinical practice. Robson and colleagues[15] discuss these to maximise healing trajectories and argue that the risk of surgical wound complications is reduced when the 'wound burden of contamination' is less, as in minimally invasive surgery.

CLINICAL ASPECTS OF CHRONIC WOUND MANAGEMENT

The multidisciplinary approach to chronic wound management has obvious advantages. The general surgeon can give support for wound debridement and delayed suture; split thickness grafts or flap closures may require plastic surgical help. A vascular surgeon provides help with revascularisation, sometimes with the help of interventional radiology, and to undertake venous surgery when indicated.[16] All this is supported by endocrinologists (diabetic ulcers), care of the elderly physicians, nurse specialists and professions allied to medicine, such as podiatrists (Table 1).

Table 1 Wound healing interventions

Dressings	Physical therapies	Biological therapies	Surgical interventions
Alginates	Hyperbaric oxygen	Cytokines	Debridement
Hydrocolloids	Lasers	Growth factors	Drainage
Hydrogels	Magnetic stimulation	Protease inhibitors	Excision
Films	Ultrasound	Cadaver skin	Skin grafting
Foams	Vacuum devices	Epidermal allograft	Revascularisation
Medicated dressings	Warming	Dermal allograft	Reconstruction

Key point 4

• Chronic wounds require professional expertise from a wide range of backgrounds.

Systematic reviews have identified many deficiencies in the evidence-base supporting practice in this field; compression bandaging in venous ulceration, surgery for venous ulceration, use of antiseptics, debridement, and surgery for pressure sores serve as examples.[17–20] Recently introduced techniques need evaluation, such as slow release antiseptic dressings and silver ion dressings. Performing adequate debridement requires education of many staff, and larva therapy needs structured evaluation to confirm its value. Vacuum-assisted chronic wound closure reduces oedema, enhances granulation tissue and controls wound exudate, but must be supported by evidence that it enhances healing as compared to other methods of wound closure. Factors which traditionally delay healing have usually been identified as secondary outcomes of wound healing studies.[15] It is unlikely that deficiencies of zinc or vitamins C and A are relevant to routine practice in the UK, but clearly immunodeficiency of any cause is likely to be relevant and may be correctable. Poor perfusion and tissue hypoxia are the most important, and sepsis relating to infection in open chronic wounds, particularly pressure sores, is often overlooked with its associated links to poor nutrition, hypo-albuminaemia and general debility.

Key point 5

- Evidence to support the use of a wide range of interventions in chronic wounds is limited.

There is promise from experimental studies and early clinical trials of advances to come. The cosmetic advantages of healing by regeneration, not repair, are obvious,[21] but surgical wounds will still need suture or other support during regeneration so that they are not vulnerable during healing. Fetal healing involves a higher level of hyaluronic acid in the extracellular matrix with less expression of platelet derived growth factor (PDGF), transforming growth factor β (TGF-β) and less influx of polymorphonuclear neutrophils.[21] There is also growing understanding of the processes of healing in ageing with the promise, in women at least, that tamoxifen and other hormones may be helpful.

GROWTH FACTORS

The clinical use of growth factors in the healing of chronic wounds has met with varied success. These growth factors are mostly derived by recombinant techniques and the uncertainty of their action in human wounds may be related to timing of administration and dose. Enhancing only one element of a healing or inflammatory cascade may be inappropriate, much like the failure to control sepsis with antibodies to specific cytokines. Combinations, sequential use, or use with inhibitors of proteases may lead to more predictable success. Nevertheless, PDGF has been shown to be useful in diabetic[22] and pressure sores,[23] epidermal growth factor (EGF) in venous ulcers,[24] fibroblast growth factor (FGF) in pressure ulcers,[25] and granulocyte-macrophage colony stimulating factor (GM-CSF) in diabetic ulcers.[26]

ARTIFICIAL ADJUNCTS

A more orchestrated method of enhancing healing in recalcitrant chronic ulcers has been shown following the application of acellular dermal matrices. These have found most use in burns management, particularly in the preparation of a burn wound to receive a split thickness graft. Alloderm is an allogeneic acellular, human dermal matrix and Integra is bovine collagen and chondroitin sulphate with a silastic membrane (which is removed once the matrix is vascularised). Keratinocytes can be rapidly grown in confluent monolayers in tissue culture, but their potential in burns has yet to be realised. Dermagraft is a non-immunogenic neonatal polyglactin mesh seeded with fibroblasts and freeze dried before reconstitution for use. It has been used in burns and diabetic ulcers.[27] Apligraf is one of a new group of living skin equivalents which incorporate live human fibroblasts in a bovine collagen 'dermis', bonded to a live stratified human squamous epithelium. Histologically, this looks very similar to skin and success has been reported in diabetic, venous and pressure ulcers.[28,29]

Key point 6

- Understanding wound biology may lead to the development and logical use of new therapies, but further development of models and markers of healing is required.

EXPERIMENTAL METHODS OF MEASUREMENT IN WOUND HEALING

By comparison to the clinical aspects of wound healing, experimental studies continue to incorporate more and more high technology with the unravelling of the complex interactions of inflammation and healing (Table 2). Clinical measurements remain crude, such as wound size planimetry; colour image analysis (*e.g.* black-yellow-red healing progression in chronic wounds); linear analogue scale assessment of exudate, smell, granulation and epithelialisation; and sequential photography to allow blinded assessments. Increasingly, they are complemented by links with vascular laboratory technology.

The use of artificial wounds continues to improve knowledge.[30] The use of simple surrogates, such as the examination of wound fluid from chronic[31] or acute[32] wounds stimulates criticism as they do not give precise sequential snapshots of healing; they are more a reflection of the haphazard mid-points of healing cascades. Table 2 gives an overview of the wide range of investigation currently being used.

ECONOMICS OF WOUND HEALING AND INTRODUCTION OF NEW TREATMENTS

The nature of the healthcare dilemma, with ever increasing demands placed on healthcare services against constraints on the resources available to meet them,

Table 2 Current experimental methodology in wound healing

Artificial wounds
Polyvinyl alcohol sponge*
Goretex tubes*
Cellstick (viscose cellular sponge and silicone lining)*
Ear chamber, cheek pouch, cornea (direct observation of healing)

Wound surrogates
Wound fluid (collected under film dressings)
Drain fluid (collected postoperatively)
Vacuum pump therapy wound fluid
Microbiological sequential analysis

Bursting and tensile wound strengths

Histochemistry

Biochemistry

Simple hydroxyproline and DNA assays	
Spectrometry	Proteomics
Zymography	PAGE HPLC ELISA
Molecular biology	DNA probes and gene sequencing
RT-PCR amplification	
Knockout gene models	
Measures of apoptosis (*e.g.* TUNEL)	

Cell culture

Viability and cell proliferation	
Collagen lattice contraction	Scarification
Biochemical analysis of supernatants	
Migration assays	
Organ culture (*e.g.* aortic ring endothelial models)	

Blood flow measurement

Trans and subcutaneous oxygen	
Laser Doppler and laser scanning	
Ultrasound	
ABPI	Vascular laboratory angiography MRA

---

*Can be also implanted in humans.

---

continues to be difficult at all levels of policy-making, decision-making, commissioning services and the provision and delivery of healthcare services. The need to ensure that limited resources are channelled into effective interventions has provided additional impetus to the drive towards evidence-based practice and coupled by claims that the way to reduce cost pressures in health care is to focus on proven quality.[33]

COSTS OF POOR HEALING

The costs associated with wound management and wound healing are substantial. For example, 6 million operations were carried out in England in Wales in 1998/99; it has been estimated that, as a result, there may be 21,000 difficult to heal surgical wounds each year, although it was acknowledged that this estimate was likely to be a significant underestimate.[34] Pressure sores reportedly cost $8.5 billion.[35] In diabetes, foot problems have been estimated to account for 25–50% of in-patient costs[36] and over 50% of bed-occupancy,[37] while it has been suggested that each hospital admission for foot ulcers costs £1451[38] and a cost to the UK NHS of £17 million.[39] In a study of Medicare claims, expenditures for lower-extremity ulcer patients were on average 3 times higher than those for Medicare patients in general ($15,309 *versus* $5226). Improving the 20-week healing rate from 31% to 40% would save Medicare $189 per episode and any wound care intervention that could prevent even a small percentage of wounds from progressing to the stage at which in-patient care was required would have favourable cost effect on the Medicare system, which spent $1.5 billion on lower-extremity ulcers in 1995.[40]

As well as the resource burden posed by wound management, the impact on the quality-of-life of patients and their families is highly significant,[41,42] and any management strategy should include patients and their carers in the decision-making process.[33]

COST-EFFECTIVE TREATMENT

However, while there is some evidence to suggest that pressure ulcers and other chronic wounds treated at home with negative pressure wound therapy close faster and reduce treatment costs compared to conventional therapies,[43] the general perspective is that the evidence-base of effective interventions and management strategies in wound healing is very thin.[33,44–46] Despite the relative paucity of evidence, a multidisciplinary approach to treatment has been advocated[47,48] and with the focus of care increasingly moving towards the community.[33]

The move in the UK to unified, cash-limited budgets within primary care will obviously assist in adopting multidisciplinary treatment strategies. GPs will have to take more responsibility for determining priorities and controlling prescribing and hospital budgets, which should act as a stimulus to develop cost-effective management. For example, the choice of relatively cheaper dressings, intended to ensure that drug budgets are not exceeded, now needs to be made within a wider context, since the administration of a more expensive dressing may well prevent even more expensive nursing visits or hospital admissions, thereby producing a net benefit in terms of the overall budget and patient outcomes.

Similarly, cost-effective management of wounds requires both a short- and long-term perspective. For example, while early amputation may appear to be less expensive in the short-term, the costs to society resulting from lengthy hospitalisation, rehabilitation, home-care and other social services support will mean that the long-term costs far exceed those of preventive, multidisciplinary approaches to wound management.[47]

The introduction of new treatments and approaches to management needs to be based on a much firmer evidence-base of both clinical and cost-

---

Key point 7

- Economic aspects of managing wound problems is a new, but important, aspect of evaluation.

effectiveness. Each of the reviews of evidence undertaken to date have highlighted the need for epidemiological studies to evaluate the extent of the problem and large multicentre trials of high methodological quality to determine both the effectiveness and efficiency of interventions.[44–46]

CONCLUSIONS

The precise control of healing in wounds seems likely but not imminent. The use of stem cells and gene therapy is exciting, in particular the use of transfection with adenoviruses and plasmids.[49] However, the gap between this experimental methodology and clinical practice is as wide as our failure to understand the difference between fetal scarless healing and healing in human adults.[15] The introduction of growth factors, inhibitors of proteases and artificial skin substitutes will demand rigorous clinical trials to demonstrate efficacy and cost-effectiveness before we can make these new treatments more widely available. In addition, whilst clinicians may understandably focus on healing as a measure of success of a new treatment, the increasing importance of economic evaluation of new therapies will influence the way in which new therapies are evaluated considerably.

Key point 8

- Re-examination of existing therapies in addition to continued development of new interventions is required to deal with the common, complex and diverse clinical area.

Against this background, there are studies of simple interventions which are clinically effective, such as warming;[10,50] but there are other time-honoured therapies, which are still anecdotal and remain to be proven by adequately powered random controlled trials, such as hyperbaric oxygen therapy.[31] Research into the clinical aspects of wound healing proceeds forward, but it is interesting to note that even making a surgical incision is not standardised! Surgeons are still investigating whether electrocautery is better than a scalpel – one recent study suggests no difference[52] and another claims electrocautery is quicker with less blood loss and less postoperative pain.[53]

Key points for clinical practice

- Achieving good wound healing remains a major clinical problem.

- Choice of sutures and techniques employed influence rate of complications.

- Rate of wound complications may be an indicator of surgical competence.

(Continued next page)

Key points for clinical practice (continued)

- Chronic wounds require professional expertise from a wide range of backgrounds.

- Evidence to support the use of a wide range of interventions in chronic wounds is limited.

- Understanding wound biology may lead to the development and logical use of new therapies, but further development of models and markers of healing is required.

- Economic aspects of managing wound problems is a new, but important, aspect of evaluation.

- Re-examination of existing therapies in addition to continued development of new interventions is required to deal with the common, complex and diverse clinical area.

References

1. Weiland DI, Curtis Bay R, Del Sordi S. Choosing the best abdominal closure by meta analysis. *Am J Surg* 1998; **176**: 666–670.
2. Hodgson NCF, Malthaner RA, Ostbye T. The search for an ideal method of abdominal fascial closure. *Ann Surg* 2000; **231**: 436–442.
3. Kendall WH, Brennan TG, Guillou PJ. Suture length to wound length ratio and integrity of midline and lateral paramedian incisions. *Br J Surg* 1991; **78**: 705–707.
4. Cengiz Y, Blomquist P, Israelsson LA. Small tissue bites and wound strength: an experimental study. *Arch Surg* 2001; **136**: 272–275.
5. Khaira HS, Lau P, Hunter Brown JH. Repair of incisional hernias. *J R Coll Surg Edinb* 2001; **46**: 39–43.
6. Chughtai T, Chen LQ, Salasidis G, Nguyen D, Tchervenkov C, Morin JF. Clips versus suture technique: is there a difference? *Can J Cardiol* 2000; **16**: 1403–1407.
7. Perron AD, Garcia JA, Parker Hayes E, Schafermeyer R. The efficacy of cyanoacrylate-derived surgical adhesive for use in the repair of lacerations during competitive athletics. *Am J Emerg Med* 2000; **18**: 261–263.
8. Clark RA. Fibrin sealant in wound repair: a systematic survey of the literature. *Expert Opin Invest Drugs* 2000; **9**: 2371–2392.
9. Jimenez MF, Marshall JC. Source control in the management of sepsis. *Intensive Care Med* 2001; **27 (Suppl 1)**: S49–S62.
10. Melling AC, Ali B, Scott EM, Leaper DJ. The effects of preoperative warming on the incidence of wound infection after clean surgery. *Lancet* 2001; **358**: 876–880.
11. Smith PD, Kuhn MA, Franz MG, Wachtel TL, Wright TE, Robson MC. Initiating the inflammatory phase of incisional healing prior to tissue injury. *J Surg Res* 2000; **92**: 11–17.
12. Franz MG, Kuhn MA, Nguyen K *et al*. Transforming growth factor beta (2) lowers the incidence of incisional hernias. *J Surg Res* 2001; **97**: 109–116.
13. Egger B, Inglin R, Zeeh J, Dirsch O, Huang Y, Buchler MW. Insulin-like growth factor I and truncated keratinocyte growth factor accelerate healing of left-sided colonic anastomoses. *Br J Surg* 2001; **88**: 90–98.
14. Syk I, Agren MS, Adawi D, Jeppsson B. Inhibition of matrix metalloproteinases enhances breaking strength of colonic anastomoses in an experimental model. *Br J Surg* 2001; **88**: 228–234.
15. Robson MC, Steed DL, Franz MG. Wound healing: biologic features and approaches to maximise healing trajectories. *Curr Prob Surg* 2001; **38**: 61–140.
16. Barwell JR, Taylor M, Deacon J *et al*. Surgical correction of isolated superficial venous reflux reduces long-term recurrence rate in chronic venous leg ulcers. *Eur J Vasc Endovasc Surg* 2000; **20**: 363–368.

17. Nelson EA. Systematic reviews of prevention of venous ulcer recurrence. *Phlebology* 2001; **16**: 20–23.
18. Lewis R, Whiting P, ter Riet G, O'Meara S, Glanville J. A rapid and systematic review of the clinical effectiveness and cost-effectiveness of debriding agents in treating surgical wounds healing by secondary intention. *Health Technol Assess* 2001; **5**: 1–131.
19. O'Meara SO, Cullum N, Majid M, Sheldon T. Systematic reviews of wound care management: (3) antimicrobial agents for chronic wounds; (4) diabetic foot ulceration. *Health Technol Assess* 2000; **4**: 1–237.
20. Schryvers OI, Stranc MF, Nance PW. Surgical treatment of pressure ulcers: 20-year experience. *Arch Phys Med Rehabil* 2000; **81**: 1556–1562.
21. Adzick NS, Lorenz P. Cells, matrix, growth factor and the surgeon: the biology of scarless fetal wound repair. *Ann Surg* 1994; **220**: 10–18.
22. Smiell JM, Wieman TJ, Steed DL, Perry PH, Sampson AR, Schwab BH. Efficacy and safety of beclapermin (recombinant human platelet-derived growth factor-BB) in patients with non healing, lower extremity diabetic ulcers: a combined analysis of four randomised studies. *Wound Repair Regen* 1999; **7**: 335–346.
23. Rees RS, Robson MC, Smiell JM, Perry BH, and the Pressure Ulcer Study Group. Beclapermin gel in the treatment of pressure ulcers. *Wound Repair Regen* 1997; **7**: 141–147.
24. Falanga V, Eaglstein WH, Bucalo B *et al*. Topical use of human recombinant epidermal growth factor (h-EGF) in venous ulcers. *J Dermatol Surg Oncol* 1992; **18**: 604–606.
25. Robson MC, Phillips LG, Laurence WT *et al*. The safety and effect of topically applied recombinant basic fibroblast growth factor on healing of chronic pressure sores. *Ann Surg* 1992; **216**: 401–408.
26. Gough A, Crapperton M, Rolando N, Foster AVM, Philpott-Howard J, Edmonds ME. Randomised placebo controlled trial of granulocyte-colony stimulating factor in diabetic foot infection. *Lancet* 1997; **350**: 845-850.
27. Pollak RA, Edington H, Jensen JL, Kroeker RD, Gentzkow GD, and the Dermagraft Diabetic Ulcer Study Group. A human dermal replacement for the treatment of diabetic foot ulcers. *Wounds* 1997; **9**: 175–183.
28. Falanga V, Margolis D, Alvarez O *et al*. Rapid healing of venous ulcers and lack of clinical rejection with an allogenic cultured human skin equivalent. *Arch Dermatol* 1998; **134**: 293–300.
29. Brem H, Balledux J, Bloom T, Kerstein M, Hollier L. Healing of diabetic foot ulcers and pressure ulcers with human skin equivalent. *Arch Surg* 2000; **135**: 627–634.
30. Gottrup F, Agren MS, Karlsmark T. Models for use in wound healing research: a survey focusing on *in vitro* and *in vivo* adult soft tissue. *Wound Repair Regen* 2000; **8**: 83–96.
31. Trengrove NJ, Bielefeldt-Ohmann H, Stacey MC. Mitogenic activity and cytokine levels in non-healing and healing chronic ulcers. *Wound Repair Regen* 2000; **8**: 13–25.
32. Baker EA, Leaper DJ. Proteinases, their inhibitors, and cytokine profiles in acute wound fluid. *Wound Repair Regen* 2000; **8**: 392–398.
33. National Institute for Clinical Excellence Technology. *National Institute for Clinical Excellence. Guidance on the use of debriding agents and specialist wound care clinics for difficult to heal surgical wounds*. Appraisal Guidance No 24, 2001
34. Marwick C. Proponents gather together to discuss practicing evidence based medicine. *JAMA* 1997; **278**: 531–532.
35. Ratliff CR, Rodeheaver GT. Pressure ulcer assessment and management. *Lippincott's Prim Care Pract* 1999; **3**: 242–258.
36. Jönsson B. Diabetes: the cost of illness and the cost of control: an estimate for Sweden 1978. *Acta Med Scand* 1983; **Suppl 671**: 19–27.
37. Levin ME. Preventing amputation in the patient with diabetes. *Diabetes Care* 1995; **18**: 1383.
38. Currie CJ, Morgan CL, Peters JB. The epidemiology and cost of inpatient care for peripheral vascular disease, infection, neuropathy and ulceration in diabetes. *Diabetes Care* 1998; **21**: 42–46.
39. Williams DRR. The size of the problem: epidemiology and economic aspects of foot problems in diabetes. In: Boulton AJM, Connor H, Cavanagh PR. (eds) *The Foot in Diabetes*. Chichester: Wiley, 1999.
40. Davies S, Gibby O, Phillips C *et al*. The health status of diabetic patients receiving

orthotic therapy. *Quality of Life Res* 2000; **9**: 233–240.

41. Brod M. Quality of life issues in diabetic patients with lower extremity ulcers and their care givers. *Quality of Life Res* 1997; **6**: 627.

42. Harrington C, Zagari MJ, Corea J, Klitenic J. A cost analysis of diabetic lower extremity ulcers. *Diabetes Care* 2000; **23**: 1333–1338.

43. Philbeck Jr TE, Whittington KT, Millsap MH *et al*. The clinical and cost effectiveness of externally applied negative pressure wound therapy in the treatment of wounds in home healthcare Medicare patients *Ostomy Wound Manage* 1999; **45**: 41–50.

44. Bradly M, Cullum N, Sheldon T. The debridement of chronic wounds: a systematic review. *Health Technol Assess* 1999; **17**.

45. Bradley M, Cullum N, Nelson EA *et al*. Systematic reviews of wound care management (2): dressings and topical agents used in the healing of chronic wounds, *Health Technol Assess* 1999; **17**.

46. Lewis R, Whiting P, ter Get G *et al*. A rapid and systematic review of the clinical and cost effectiveness of debriding agents in treating surgical wounds healing by secondary intention. *Health Technol Assess* 2001; **5**.

47. Apelqvist J. Wound healing in diabetes: outcome and costs. *Clin Podiatr Med Surg* 1998; **5**: 21–29.

48. McInnes A. Guide to assessment and management of diabetic foot wounds. *Diabetic Foot (Educ Suppl)* 2001; **4**: 19–34.

49. Yao F, Eriksson E. Gene therapy in wound repair and regeneration. *Wound Repair Regen* 2000; **8**: 443–451.

50. Scott EM, Leaper DJ, Clark M, Kelly PJ. Effects of warming therapy on pressure ulcers: a randomised trial. *J Assoc Operating Room Nurses* 2001; **73**: 921–938.

51. Davidson JD, Mustoe TA. Oxygen in wound healing: more than a nutrient. *Wound Repair Regen* 2001; **9**: 175–177.

52. Franchi M, Ghezzi F, Benedetti-Panici PL *et al*. A multi-centre collaborative study on the use of cold scalpel and electrocautery for mid-line abdominal incision. *Am J Surg* 2001; **181**: 128–132.

53. Kearns SR, Connolly EM, McNally S, McNamara DA, Deasy J. Randomised clinical trial of diathermy versus scalpel incision in elective mid-line laparotomy. *Br J Surg* 2001; **88**: 41–44.

54. Harding KG, Morris HL, Patel GK. Science, medicine, and the future; healing chronic wounds. *BMJ* 2002; **324**: 160–163.

Malvena E. Stuart Taylor

3

Postoperative pain control

For all the happiness mankind can gain
Is not in pleasure, but in rest from pain.
Dryden

Pain is probably the most common symptom that drives the patient to seek medical advice. However, once the patient arrives within the hospital system, pain is often one of the elements of care that is least well addressed.

Humane issues of good pain control are a *sine qua non* of any doctor. However, there are direct consequences upon the success of surgery and outcome of a patient if pain is not adequately controlled. What follows is an outline of key issues that need to be considered and within this subject the symptomatic control of nausea and vomiting will also be discussed since these symptoms frequently accompany pain and surgery.

PRE-EMPTIVE ANALGESIA

It is now well recognised that the central nervous system (CNS) is neuroplastic and will change structurally and functionally in response to sensory input. It also has a memory for pain. These stimuli relay via the spinal cord to the sensory cortex. Pain signals which are generated by peripheral mechanisms of tissue damage during the course of surgery can actually trigger a prolonged state of central sensitisation and hyperexcitability. Not only does this render the individual hypersensitive to sensory input, but also the duration of perception of pain is prolonged beyond the duration of tissue injury. This partly explains why the analgesic need of individuals can exceed anticipated amounts and duration. It also helps to explain the development of chronic pain states following surgery.[1] The challenge is to establish what can be done to reduce or avoid this state.

There is evidence emerging to support the concept of pre-emptive analgesia.[2] This idea is based on the concept that if one can give the patient an

Dr Malvena E. Stuart Taylor BSc(Hons) FRCA, Consultant Anaesthetist and Lead Consultant for the Acute Pain Service, Southampton Universities Hospitals NHS Trust, Shackleton Dept of Anaesthetics, Mailpoint 24, Southampton General Hospital, Tremona Road, Southampton SO16 6YD, UK

analgesic that blocks the tissue response to pain, the chain reaction of pain outlined above can be modulated. Unfortunately, there are logistic problems in designing such studies because the mechanism of pain would have to be effectively blocked for the duration of surgery **and** for the postoperative period when tissue healing is taking place. Notwithstanding this challenge, there are a number of studies which have been able to demonstrate a pre-emptive effect of analgesics using non-steroidal anti-inflammatory drugs (NSAIDs), opioids and local anaesthetic blocks.

Key point 1

- Whilst the majority of patients will exhibit similar degrees of pain for any given procedure, there is patient variability. Pain scoring and treatment tailored to individual requirements is imperative.

Key point 2

- Pre-emptive analgesia is very useful in reducing analgesic requirements during the postoperative period.

NSAIDS

This class of analgesic works by inhibiting prostaglandin production in response to tissue injury. This dampening effect will be more profound if the drug is present in the tissues prior to surgical incision and if steady state effective plasma levels of the drug are maintained. Therefore, pre-operative[3] and regular postoperative administration are needed.

In order to achieve this, several factors need to be taken into consideration.

NSAIDs as a premedicant

Generally speaking, it is not advisable to administer NSAID tablets when the patient has an empty stomach as in the pre-operative state, because there can be a local irritant effect of the tablet on the uncoated gastric mucosa. Piroxicam as Feldene Melt® is useful in this respect since it melts into the patient's saliva. Also it has a long $\beta_{1/2t}$ (40–60 h) and, therefore, will provide the therapeutic plasma levels suggested above irrespective of when it is given prior to surgery. Diclofenac, so favoured by doctors, has the disadvantage that it has a very short $\beta_{1/2t}$ (2–4 h) and, therefore, although it can be given by rectal administration, its clinical effect will wear off before the next dose is due and effective plasma levels of this drug are not maintained. In addition, the injectable form should never be used since it predisposes to cold abscess formation.

Safety profile

The disadvantage of piroxicam is that it is not one of the safest NSAIDs. Much work is being carried out to develop a safer drug because of the risk of gastrointestinal damage and renal impairment in situations of hypovolaemia or renal disease. To this end, two types of new generation drugs are worth considering. Firstly, there are single enantiomer agents such as dexketoprofen (derived from ketoprofen). Secondly, there are the highly selective COX-2 inhibitors such as celecoxib and rofecoxib. These are so specific in their action that they are alleged not to interfere with the gastric protective effect of PGI_2, with the renal artery protective effect of PGE_2 or with the platelet function of thromboxane. Also, rofecoxib in particular is licenced for use in acute pain and may be taken on an empty stomach. The Royal College of Anaesthetists has produced a very useful guide on how to use this class of drugs safely.[4]

Duration of action

Rofexocib has a relatively long $\beta_{1/2t}$ of 20 h, rendering it capable of producing long-term therapeutic plasma levels. It is worth noting that because of the absence of inhibition on platelet stickiness, it has been reported that there is an increased risk of stroke on long-term therapy though this statement has been made in the context of comparing stroke rate with that seen in patients on naproxen, an NSAID which, in the author's view, should no longer be used because of its adverse effect on the stomach and renal arterial flow.

Regular administration

There is little value in prescribing these analgesics on a *prn* basis. They need to be given early and prescribed on the regular section of the prescription chart for the duration of pain.

Key point 3

- Caution should be exercised when NSAIDs are used in vulnerable individuals, notwithstanding their excellent opioid-sparing properties.

OPIOIDS

Low dose morphine has been demonstrated to prevent the establishment of central sensitisation. That is to say that, if an opioid is given early in the tissue-damage process, less is needed to produce analgesia. If, however, pain is allowed to build up in severity and duration, much higher doses of opioid will be required to suppress it. Higher doses will predispose to more severe side-effects which are principally respiratory depression, nausea and vomiting, and constipation, all of which contribute to postoperative morbidity and even mortality. Therefore, there is an argument to use opioids pre-emptively.[5,6]

Unfortunately, if morphine derivatives are given with the premedication when there is no pain, there is an increased risk of nausea and vomiting. In practice, this can be overcome by the anaesthetist avoiding opioid premedicants and instead using an opioid of short onset of action with induction of anaesthesia (for example fentanyl, alfentanil or remifentanil). This can be supplemented later by the longer-acting morphine-type agents.

A word of caution is needed with pethidine which historically has been the opioid of choice for surgeons due to its smooth muscle effect. Unfortunately, it has two draw-backs. Firstly, it appears to be effective as an analgesic in only about 50% of the population. This effect can be seen on the labour ward where some patients just become dsyphoric, sick and out of control of their labour pain when given pethidine. Secondly, it has a relatively short $\beta_{1/2t}$. Therefore, it has to be given at least 2-hourly to provide effective pain relief and also its toxic metabolite, norpethidine, has a very long $\beta_{1/2t}$ and can accumulate to toxic levels relatively easily, triggering epileptiform-type problems.

Optimal administration of opioids

Morphine has been around for a long time. However, it continues to be used in a sub-optimal manner although several improvement strategies exist.

Prescribing intermittent doses hourly.[7] This is based on the premise that plasma analgesic levels of this drug reach a peak within 1 h (in some individuals it can be as little as 10 min). Therefore, if a patient received a dose 60 min previously, shows no signs of hypotension, respiratory depression or undue sedation and yet is in pain, they will not be thrown into narcosis by receiving another dose. The traditional 4–6-hourly regimen grossly undertreats a patient in pain. Respiratory depression usually occurs because the physiological state of the patient is not being measured or because different opioids are being given by varying routes.

If a patient is tolerating oral fluids (this includes not feeling nauseated), it is appropriate that oral morphine should be given. The problem incurred is that we do not take into account its low bioavailability (approximately 30%); we are surprised, therefore, when a patient does not derive the same analgesia from 10 mg oral morphine as from 10 mg given intramuscularly. The patient is probably only receiving the analgesic benefit of one-third of this dose. The solution is to prescribe double the dose if it is to be given by mouth. Even this underestimates the need of the patient, but it does provide a safety margin against over-administration.

PATIENT CONTROLLED ANALGESIA (PCA)

PCA has been established for many years. However, its use is often suboptimal and, if poorly applied, PCA may lead to respiratory arrest. To avoid this, patients and staff should understand the basic principles upon which the treatment is based;[8] that is to say the patient should be made familiar with its use (including the concept of locking out) before surgery and not in the misty confusion of the postanaesthetic phase.

RISK FACTORS FOR PCA

Patient selection should screen for: (i) patients who cannot physically press the hand-set (i.e. bilateral forearm injury); (ii) patients who cannot mentally understand the system; (iii) caution should be exercised with anxious patients who often frantically press the hand-set in the hope of receiving anxiolysis, but instead over-dose themselves in relation to the analgesic need of the drug – this predisposes to respiratory depression; and (iv) patients who have no wish to 'be in control'. They will not use the device effectively and, therefore, will remain in pain.

Other risk factors which predispose to respiratory depression include background infusion, old age, head injury, history of sleep apnoea, obesity, respiratory failure, concurrent sedative or opioid medication, hypovolaemia and renal failure.[9,10]

PCA morphine is associated with approximately 50% rate of postoperative nausea and vomiting (PONV).[11] Whilst it is tempting to add droperidol to the morphine, this carries the risk of increased sedation and frightening dysphoria. Additionally, patients will often administer frequent boluses to themselves in the hope of receiving more anti-emetic. As noted above, morphine in the absence of pain significantly increases the risk of respiratory depression. It is more accepted practice now to prescribe regular anti-emetic along the lines discussed below.

RESPIRATORY DEPRESSION WITH PCA

It is unwise to believe that respiratory depression or arrest cannot happen with PCA. Contrary to popular belief, the delay from intravenous administration of morphine to peak effective plasma levels varies from 5–20 min. If an individual is one of the slower responders, they can self-administer many doses before falling asleep – the plasma levels then continue to climb until respiratory arrest ensues. This could be avoided by increasing the lock-out time from the standard 5 min to 10 min. If bolus doses larger than the conventional 1 mg morphine are needed, it would indeed be prudent to increase the lock-out period to 10 min. However, current practice uses a 5 min lock-out with the proviso that diligent nursing observation of the patient on PCA is maintained.[12]

ACUTE PANCREATITIS

Pain control for acute pancreatitis can be particularly challenging. Firstly, there is significant physiological disturbance with possible sepsis. This can increase the propensity to go into respiratory failure with strong opioids. Thoracic epidural is an effective option provided systemic infection and coagulopathy are not present. An alternative is to consider PCA fentanyl due to its smooth muscle relaxant properties. However, it carries a high risk of sedation (2%).[13] Therefore, fentanyl should only be considered if the patient can be nursed in a high dependency unit. One recommended regimen is to have a 40 mcg bolus to be infused over 10 min and with provision to limit the number of boluses to 6 per hour.

Key point 4

- Patient controlled analgesia improves patient satisfaction and can improve pain control over intermittent intramuscular analgesia. However, respiratory depression is a significant risk; therefore, regular patient review is mandatory.

LOCAL ANAESTHESIA

Several studies have demonstrated a pre-emptive effect of local anaesthesia being administered in different ways.[14–16]

EPIDURAL ANALGESIA

There is no doubt that an effective epidural for intra-operative and postoperative use can significantly improve outcome following surgery.[17–21] However, there is a small risk of serious complications with this technique.

COMPLICATIONS

The estimated incidence of epidural abscess formation has been reported as approximately 1:1900 patients with in-dwelling catheters (compared with an incidence of 1:10,000 cases where no epidural catheter was placed).[22] However, there are predisposing factors such as long catheterization, and possibly immunosuppression or low dose anticoagulation with warfarin. Any patient who demonstrates signs of neurological deficit, pyrexia and back pain should be urgently investigated with MRI and, if found positive, undergo urgent decompression. It is worth noting that meningitis is uncommon as a presenting feature.

Pressure sores have also been attributed to epidural infusions. However, this should be avoidable if one avoids hypotension, sensory and motor blockade (achieved by using a mixture of weak local anaesthetic (*e.g.* 0.125% bupivicaine) and weak opioid (*e.g.* 2–4 mcg/ml fentanyl), and if the patient is turned frequently.[23,24]

Spinal haematoma, although very rare, can have disastrous consequences; therefore, careful consideration should be given to the coagulant status of the patient prior to epidural insertion and also for removal of the catheter. It has been estimated that the risk of spinal haematoma following epidural analgesia is 1:150,000 and following spinal analgesia is 1:220,000.[25] In this situation, the signs tend to be urinary retention, sharp back pain radiating in a radicular manner, and sensory and motor deficit outlasting the expected duration of the block. Urgent CT or MRI should be carried out. In order to minimize this risk, guidelines for anticoagulation should be in place in every hospital that uses epidurals.

Guidelines for coagulation control with epidural analgesia

To date, there has been no national census; however, general recommendations include:

- Whilst an epidural catheter is *in situ*, the activated partial thromboplastin ratio (APTR) should never exceed 2.5 since this is adequate for therapeutic anticoagulation and yet reduces the risk of spontaneous epidural haematoma formation.

- Unfractionated heparin should not be given within 4 h (ideally 6 h) before insertion or removal of the catheter. It can be given immediately after insertion or removal of the catheter.[26]

- Enoxaparin should not be given within 12 h before insertion or removal of the catheter. It should only be given greater than 4–6 h after either of these procedures.[27]

- Full intra-operative heparinization should be delayed for a minimum of 1 h after epidural insertion.[27]

- If an epidural catheter needs to be removed whilst a patient is on a heparin infusion, the latter should be stopped for 4 h after which an APTR should be measured. There is no firm value of maximum value for international normalized ratio (INR) or APTR for safety of insertion of epidural. Local practice has adopted a maximum ratio of 1.4 or less for epidural insertion[25] and 1.7 or less for catheter removal.

- Warfarin should not be prescribed until after the catheter has been removed due to the problems of normalizing coagulation when it is present.

Key point 5

- Epidural analgesia can be pivotal in the early mobilization of patient and early return of gut function. Such patients can be managed on general surgical wards provided nursing and medical staff are competent in their management.

ANTI-EMETICS

As with NSAIDs and opioids, anti-emetics are often not prescribed in the most effective manner because their short $\beta_{1/2t}$ (4 h) is not taken into account. Prescribing advice usually recommends a maximum of 3 doses per 24 h. Logically this gets translated into giving doses 8-hourly. From the short half-life, one can see how such drugs can become ineffective. If, instead, they are given 4-hourly for 3 doses the debilitating symptoms of nausea and vomiting can often be controlled.

In vulnerable individuals, such as those with a history of postoperative nausea and vomiting/motion sickness or in those procedures where it is vital to avoid retching (*e.g.* fundoplication, eye surgery, *etc.*), an effective solution is to prescribe two different classes of anti-emetic (*e.g.* ondansetron and cyclizine or prochlorperazine) alternating with each other every 4 h (Table 1). To reduce discomfort from multiple intramuscular injections, an intramuscular cannula such as the YCan® (Fig. 1) may be useful.

Key point 6

- More aggressive control of nausea and vomiting is needed when patients are on morphine derivatives.

Table 1 Classes of anti-emetic agents

Class	Examples	Comments/side-effects
Anticholinergics	Hyoscine	Sedation, dry mouth, visual disturbances, restlessness
Antihistamines	Cyclizine	Sedation, restlessness, dry mouth, confusion
	Cinnarizine Promethazine	
Butyrophenones	Droperidol	Sedation, hypotension, extrapyramidal signs
Dopamine agonists	Metoclopramide	Sedation, cardiovascular disturbances, dystonic reactions
	Domperidone	Does not cross blood–brain barrier; no intravenous preparation
5-HT$_3$ antagonist	Ondansetron	200 times more potent than metoclopramide via intravenous route

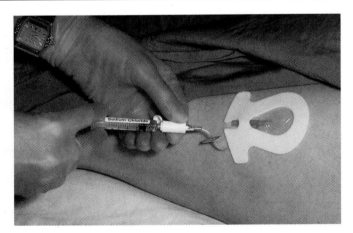

Fig. 1 The YCan® intramuscular cannula in use.

Finally, it is worth considering the likely trigger for the problem. For example, in cases of vestibular disturbance from postoperative mobilization or following ear surgery, prochlorperazine would be a logical choice; in cases of gastric distension, domperidone would be preferable as a prokinetic agent, being void of the extrapyramidal side-effects of its partner metoclopramide (Fig. 2).

NEW DRUGS

Toxic administration of bupivicaine may occur either due to inadvertent intravenous injection or due to toxic levels being administered for surgical procedures under local blockade. This is usually because the dissection

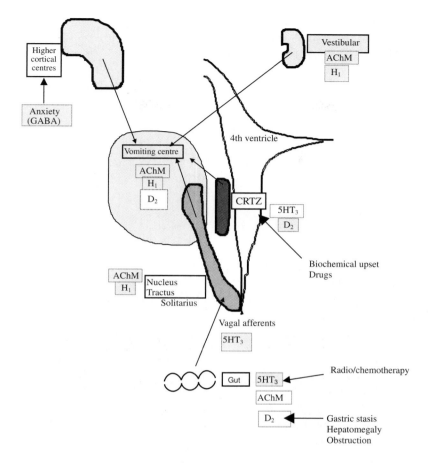

Fig. 2 Sites of action of anti-emetics. ACh, acetyl choline receptor; D_2, dopaminergic receptor; H_1, histamine receptor; $5HT_3$, 5-hydroxytryptamine receptor; CRTZ, chemoreceptor trigger zone.

becomes more extensive than anticipated at the beginning of the procedure and the maximum recommended dose of this drug based on lean body mass.

The relative toxicity of bupivicaine is 2-fold higher when given intravenously that when absorbed from injection sites, due to its high lipid solubility. Toxic levels result in sudden cardiovascular collapse, ventricular tachycardia or fibrillation and then asystole. Cardiopulmonary resuscitation would be needed until redistribution and metabolism of the drug (> 45 min).[28] To this end, there is a strong argument to change to less toxic amide-type local anaesthetic agents such as chirocaine or ropivacaine. The latter agent is probably most useful due to its reduced cardiotoxicity.[29] It has the added advantage that it is more vasoconstrictive than bupivacaine.

Oxycodone is a synthetic derivative of thebaine.[30] Its analgesic potency is approximately 1.3 times that of morphine. It has a slightly longer duration of action than morphine and does not cause histamine release. It carries the same risk of respiratory depression and nausea/vomiting. However, its value lies in the fact that it is an alternative strong opioid to consider if either the patient is

33

not responding to increasing doses of morphine or if there is a genuine anaphylactic problem with morphine and its derivatives (diamorphine, codeine, dihydrocodeine).

Remifentanil is an ultra-short-acting opioid which is only suitable for intra-operative use. Its advantage lies in the fact that its $\beta_{1/2t}$ does not increase with time ('context-sensitive half-time') and, therefore, it is useful when early extubation is useful, but where good analgesia is provided by a different agent. The classic example of this is oesophagogastrectomy with a thoracic epidural.

Key points for clinical practice

- Whilst the majority of patients will exhibit similar degrees of pain for any given procedure, there is patient variability. Pain scoring and treatment tailored to individual requirements is imperative.

- Pre-emptive analgesia is very useful in reducing analgesic requirements during the postoperative period.

- Caution should be exercised when NSAIDs are used in vulnerable individuals, notwithstanding their excellent opioid-sparing properties.

- Patient controlled analgesia improves patient satisfaction and can improve pain control over intermittent intramuscular analgesia. However, respiratory depression is a significant risk; therefore, regular patient review is mandatory.

- Epidural analgesia can be pivotal in the early mobilization of patient and early return of gut function. Such patients can be managed on general surgical wards provided nursing and medical staff are competent in their management.

- More aggressive control of nausea and vomiting is needed when patients are on morphine derivatives.

- Multimodal analgesia optimizes pain control and reduces side-effects of the individual analgesic modalities.

References

1. Macrae WA. Chronic pain after surgery. *Br J Anaesth* 2001; **87**: 88–98.
2. Woolf CJ, Chong M-S. Preemptive analgesia – treating postoperative pain by preventing the establishment of central sensitisation. *Anesth Analg* 1993; **77**: 362–379.
3. Hutchison GL, Crofts SL, Gray IG. Preoperative piroxicam for postoperative analgesia in dental surgery. *Br J Anaesth* 1990; **65**: 500–503.
4. The Royal College of Surgeons of England, College of Anaesthetists. *Commission on the Provision of Surgical Services. Report of the Working Party on Pain after Surgery.* London: Royal College of Anaesthetists, 1990.
5. Tverskoy M, Cozacov C, Ayache M *et al.* Postoperative pain after inguinal herniorraphy with different types of anaesthesia. *Anesth Analg* 1990; **70**: 29–35.
6. Kiss I, Killam M. Does opiate premedication influence postoperative analgesia? A prospective study. *Pain* 1992; **48**: 157–158.
7. Gould TH, Crosby DL, Harmer M *et al.* Policy for controlling pain after surgery: effect of sequential changes in management. *BMJ* 1992; **305**: 1187–1193.

8. White PF. Mishaps with patient-controlled analgesia. *Anesthesiology* 1987; **66**: 81–83.
9. Baxter AD. Respiratory depression with patient-controlled analgesia. *Can J Anaesth* 1994; **41**: 87–90.
10. Etches RC. Respiratory depression associated with patient-controlled analgesia: a review of eight cases. *Can J Anaesth* 1994; **41**: 125–132.
11. Tramer MR, Walder B. Efficacy and adverse effects of prophylactic antiemetics during patient-controlled analgesia therapy: a quantitative systematic review. *Anesth Analg* 1999; **88**: 1354–1361.
12. Love DR, Owen H, Ilsley AH *et al.* A comparison of variable-dose patient-controlled analgesia with fixed-dose patient-controlled analgesia. *Anesth Analg* 1996; **83**: 1060–1064.
13. Camu F, Van Aken H, Bovill JG. Postoperative analgesic effects of three demand-dose sizes of fentanyl administered by patient-controlled analgesia. *Anesth Analg* 1998; **87**: 890–895.
14. Jebels JA, Reilly JS, Gutierrez JF *et al.* The effect of preincisional infiltration of tonsils with bupivacaine on the pain following tonsillectomy under general anaesthesia. *Pain* 1991; **47**: 305–308.
15. Tuffin JR, Cuncliffe DR, Shaw SR. Do local anaesthetics injected at the time of 3rd molar removal under general anaesthesia reduce significantly postoperative analgesic requirements? *Br J Oral Maxillofac Surg* 1989; **27**: 27–32.
16. Rademaker BMP, Sih IL, Kalkman CJ *et al.* Effects of intrapleurally administered bupivacaine 0.5% on opioid analgesic requirements and endocrine response during and after cholecystectomy: a randomized double-blind controlled study. *Acta Anaesthesiol Scand* 1991; **35**: 108–121.
17. Ahn H, Bronge A, Johansson K *et al.* Effect of continuous postoperative epidural analgesia on intestinal motility. *Br J Surg* 1988; **75**: 1176–1178.
18. Lui S, Carpenter RL, Neal JM. Epidural anesthesia and analgesia. Their role in postoperative outcome. *Anesthesiology* 1995; **82**: 1474–1506.
19. Cook DW, Eaton JM, Goodwin AP. Epidural analgesia following upper abdominal surgery: United Kingdom practice. *Acta Anaesthesiol Scand* 1997; **41**: 18–24.
20. Mankikan B, Cantineau JP, Bertrand M *et al.* Improvement of diaphragmatic function by a thoracic extradural block after upper abdominal surgery. *Anesthesiology* 1998; **68**: 379–386.
21. Basse L, Hjort JD, Billesbolle P *et al.* A clinical pathway to accelerate recovery after colonic resection. *Ann Surg* 2000; **232**: 51–57.
22. Wang LP, Hauerberg J, Schmidt JF. Incidence of spinal epidural abscess after epidural analgesia: a national 1-year survey. *Anesthesiology* 1999; **91**: 1928–1936.
23. Punt CD, van Neer PA, de Lange S. Pressure sores as a possible complication of epidural analgesia. *Anesth Analg* 1991; **73**: 657–659.
24. Shah JL. Postoperative pressure sores after epidural anaesthesia. *BMJ* 2000; **321**: 941–942.
25. Vandermeulen EP, Van Aken H, Vermylen J. Anticoagulants and spinal-epidural anesthesia. *Anesth Analg* 1994; **79**: 1165–1177.
26. Wildsmith JAW, McClure JH. Anticoagulant drugs and central nerve blockade. *Anaesth* 1991; **46**: 613–614.
27. Kendell J, Checketts MR. Clotting abnormalities and central nerve blockade. *CPD Anaesthesia* 1999; **1**: 64–67.
28. Albright GA. Cardiac arrest following regional anaesthesia with etidocaine or bupivacaine. *Anesthesiology* 1979; **51**: 285–287.
29. Erichsen CJ, Vibits H, Dahl JB, Kehlet H. Wound infiltration with ropivacaine and bupivacaine for pain after inguinal herniotomy. *Acta Anaesthesiol Scand* 1995; **39**: 67–70.
30. Silvasti M, Rosenberg P, Seppala T *et al.* Comparison of analgesic efficacy of oxycodone and morphine in postoperative intravenous patient-controlled analgesia. *Acta Anaesthesiol Scand* 1998; **42**: 576–580.

Mike Stroud

4

Peri-operative nutritional support

Around 40% of surgical patients have a low body mass index (BMI) and/or a history of recent weight loss.[1] These patients have high complication and mortality rates which are often ascribed to detrimental effects of undernutrition on immunity, wound healing, gut integrity, muscle strength and psychological state.[2] It, therefore, seems logical that peri-operative nutrition would improve outcomes. This is undoubtedly true when extended intestinal failure occurs, especially as catabolic patients can die of malnutrition in 20–30 days. When feeding indications are less definite, however, studies do not always show benefit. In part, this reflects serious underlying disease in malnourished individuals, but there is also increasing recognition that nutritional needs during severe illness or injury have been misunderstood.[3] Over-feeding in particular may cause many of the metabolic and infective problems documented in some studies,[4] and this has made interpretation of all nutritional literature difficult. This chapter discusses evidence for peri-operative nutritional practice from this viewpoint.

WHAT TO FEED – COMPONENTS OF PRESCRIBED NUTRITION

Despite decades of research on the role of nutritional support in surgery, we remain uncertain about best levels of micronutrients, nitrogen and energy in feeds and the role of novel substrates and growth factors.

MICRONUTRIENTS

Vitamin and trace element deficiencies are common, yet research on micronutrient supplementation in surgery is sparse. In a recent UK survey, low

Dr Mike Stroud BSc MD FRCP, Senior Lecturer in Medicine and Nutrition, Honorary Consultant Gastroenterologist, Mailpoint 13, Southampton General Hospital, Tremona Road, Southampton SO16 6YD, UK

folate was found in 29% of 'healthy' people over 65 years of age and low vitamin C in 14%.[5] Corresponding figures for nursing home residents were 40% and 35%, respectively. Although most clinicians view the primary purpose of micronutrients as the prevention of recognised deficiency states, in reality they have multiple roles. Low levels lead to compromised function well before deficiencies are clinically evident (*e.g.* night blindness is rare but world-wide diarrhoeal illness related to low vitamin A levels probably kills thousands). Deficiencies can also occur with normal blood levels. Inadequate levels of folate, vitamin B12 or vitamin B6 impair hepatic transamination causing hyper-homocysteinaemia. This was found in 63% of a 'healthy' elderly study population yet low blood levels of the vitamins were present in only 9%.[6] In the hospitalised elderly, hyper-homocysteinaemia was present in 85%, reversible in nearly all cases by folate.

These 'functional' micronutrient deficiencies may not be immediately life-threatening but correction might help surgical outcome. Indeed, many of the detrimental effects of malnourishment are more easily attributable to micronutrient rather than macronutrient deficiencies. Vitamin and trace element provision may, therefore, underlie some of the benefits seen with peri-operative feeding and could even explain the puzzling observation that support can reduce complications after periods so short that lean body mass, nitrogen balance and plasma proteins barely alter.[7] Micronutrient deficiencies may also contribute to problems of excess feeding. The body cannot utilise protein, fat and carbohydrate fully when vitamin deficits limit metabolic processes. By the same logic, the slow recovery of appetite after expected resolution of cytokine or ileus driven anorexia, may 'protect' against intake excess. More studies on micronutrient provision in surgery are needed.

NITROGEN

Catabolism can be thought of as an evolutionary mechanism to aid survival by providing nutrients, particularly amino acids, for the acute phase response. As a consequence, high-protein feeding is generally assumed to be beneficial in catabolic patients before or after surgery. This may be untrue. High *versus* low protein feeding is known to cause increased mortality in famine victims and examination of substrate demands during severe illness provide a potential explanation. Amino acid demands not only increase to meet the needs of inflammation, immunity and repair, but relative requirements for individual amino acids alter.[8] For example, there are high demands for glutamine and arginine for the immune system, aromatic and sulphur amino acids for the acute-phase response and cysteine for glutathione maintenance. As a consequence, the composition of both dietary intake and conventional nutritional products becomes inappropriate. Excessive supply of food or standard nutritional support will then not only fail to meet needs but will provide an excess of unwanted amino acids. These free amino acids are potentially toxic and need to be 'locked up' through either oxidation to urea, a pathway with limited capacity, or the synthesis of non-acute phase peptides and proteins which require all amino acids. As a result, higher protein feeding may drive non-essential protein synthesis which can exacerbate metabolic stress and precipitate a shortage of substrates needed for acute-phase proteins, especially in sicker individuals.

This hypothesis runs against current practice. Most recommendations for protein provision range from 0.17–0.3 g nitrogen/kg/day with the advice that higher levels are used in more catabolic patients.[9] These figures were largely derived from studies of maintained nitrogen balance, but this does not necessarily equate with improved outcome. We now know from studies of growth hormone use in intensive care unit (ICU) patients, that improved nitrogen retention may be associated with increased mortality rates (perhaps not surprising if one views its effects as cutting vital nutrient supplies).[10] High protein feeding can increase nitrogen retention, but this may simply reflect high levels of free amino acids forcing synthesis of less important proteins while compromising the capacity to mount an effective response. Overall clinical thinking has cut back from the hyper-alimentation of the past, but trials of lower protein provision based on clinical outcomes are needed to decide if the cut back has been enough. Meanwhile, some authorities suggest that higher levels of protein feeding should be approached with caution.

CARBOHYDRATE AND LIPIDS

Current recommendations for non-protein energy provision range from 30–35 kcal/day with individual prescriptions based on age, sex and weight estimates of BMI with the addition of standard increments for factors such as pyrexia and metabolic stress. The Elia normogram[9] is often used but, in reality, measured energy expenditures in sick patients are frequently much lower.[3] Excluding protein provision from energy calculations is also entirely unwarranted for, unless a patient is in positive nitrogen balance, protein oxidation contributes the equivalent of at least 100% of the protein energy delivered. As a result, over-provision of energy is also frequent and, as with protein, may cause problems.

Liver abnormalities were commoner during early years of parenteral nutrition (PN) when high glucose levels were given. Hyperglycaemia is known to increase infective risks.[3] Furthermore, in a recent study of ICU patients, even minimally raised glucose levels appeared to be deleterious.[11] The study showed that keeping blood glucose under 6 mmol/l using aggressive insulin therapy reduced the mortality rate by 42% compared to using insulin only when glucose exceeded 11 mmol/l. The findings could reflect either direct benefits from insulin itself or, as seems more likely, adverse effects of minimal hyperglycaemia. The latter would have considerable implications for peri-operative feeding. In all published feeding studies, fed groups are likely to run higher glucose levels than non-fed groups especially when post-surgical insulin resistance is present. By the same logic, relative hyperglycaemia will also be seen more frequently with parenteral nutrition (PN) than with enteral nutrition (EN) since EN can rarely achieve high levels of feeding in the early postoperative period. This may account for some of the apparent advantages of EN over PN in reducing infections.

Current provision of energy in terms of carbohydrate to fat ratios vary between centres from about 70:30 to 50:50. If minimal hyperglycaemia is deleterious, a lower carbohydrate percentage would be advantageous. Excess lipid can also cause harm, however, and post-surgical patients easily become lipaemic with high-fat feeding. Fat deposition in lung and liver may then be responsible for immunosuppression and derangement of liver function. Once again, more studies are required.

Key point 1

- Immediately after surgery or in metabolically unstable patients, cautious nitrogen and energy provision may have advantages. Insulin should be used to prevent hyperglycaemia.

NOVEL SUBSTRATES

There is little space in this chapter to discuss the many new studies on novel substrates or immunonutrition. Two areas of supplementation have received particular attention – glutamine supplemented feeds and feeds containing arginine-based 'cocktails' with several potentially active components.

Glutamine is required by many biochemical processes and is in high demand during inflammation and repair. A shortage may limit immune activity, enterocyte replication and maintenance of glutathione anti-oxidant defences in ill or injured patients. Several studies in surgical patients have shown that PN containing glutamine can improve nitrogen balance. Recently, two studies have shown reductions in hospital length-of-stay of 5 or 6 days following elective postoperative glutamine supplemented PN compared with standard PN.[12,13] Powel-Tuck et al.[14] reported even greater length-of-stay reductions of 15 days in surgical patients given PN on clinical rather than defined study criteria. This outcome was shown by *post hoc* sub-group analysis, however, and no benefit from glutamine was seen in the overall study results involving much larger numbers of patients needing PN support.[14] Furthermore, only one study has reported reduced mortality when using glutamine supplemented PN feeds,[15] and overall only 30% of PN glutamine studies show clinical benefit.[16] Glutamine given enterally seems to be more definitely helpful, especially in patients with intestinal disease.[17] This is perhaps unsurprising since enterocytes have high demands for glutamine and rely quite heavily on luminal nutrients.

Most arginine-based studies have used EN feeding usually giving pre-operative oral supplementation followed by postoperative jejunostomy feeds. Several have concluded that a 'cocktail' of arginine, RNA, and omega-3 fatty acids can reduce infectious complications by around 50% in patients with GI malignancy.[18,19]. However, not all studies of arginine-based supplementation show benefit,[20] and although one study demonstrated a reduced mortality rate in ICU patients, the benefit was confined to those with low APACHE scores.[21]. This, along with other results, has raised the possibility that arginine-supplemented feeds are of no help in very sick patients. In a recent meta-analysis, Heyland et al.[22] reported that although arginine-based feeds reduced infectious complications and length-of-stay in surgical sub-groups, they did not help with overall mortality rates, ventilator days, infectious complication rates or ITU and hospital length-of-stay when sub-groups of surgery, pancreatitis, ICU, trauma and burns patients were all included. Furthermore,

Key point 2

- The evidence to support the use of glutamine- and arginine-based immunonutrition is increasing, but there are concerns regarding arginine-based feeds in critically ill patients.

an analysis of the higher quality studies suggest increased mortality rates and a trend towards increased numbers of complications in arginine treated groups, particularly in the critically ill. Therefore, it seems reasonable that the use of these feeds remains within trial settings for the present.

HOW TO FEED – ROUTE OF ADMINISTRATION

There is a widely-held belief that EN is far safer and has greater benefits than PN, but examining the literature accounting for potential overfeeding, questions these conclusions.

Although meta-analyses of elective PN in surgical patients suggest overall adverse rather than beneficial effects,[23,24] interpretation of PN studies is fraught with difficulty.[3] Older trials used very high levels of PN support and in the US Veterans Administration Trial, for example, 20% of the PN group had glucose levels greater than 16.7 mmol/l.[24] PN trials also exclude, on ethical grounds, patients with intestinal failure of a degree that warrants intravenous feeding at the time of randomization. The trials are, therefore, studies of PN given in excessive amounts to patients who do not need it. Furthermore if, during trials, patients develop prolonged ileus or have other persisting gut dysfunction, PN is often instigated. In the Veterans trial, 13% of controls received some PN treatment.[25]

The superiority of EN is frequently ascribed to maintenance of gut integrity. However, although animals show villous atrophy and increased intestinal permeability with absent luminal nutrition, complete starvation has less effect on the human gut and, while there is debate, a thorough review of the literature concluded that there was no difference to gut morphology and permeability between EN or PN feeding.[26] There are also no differences reported in bacterial translocation rates between patients fed using PN or EN prior to surgery.[27] Two recent randomised trails comparing peri-operative EN against PN also show no differences in rates of infectious and non-infectious complications, length-of-stay or mortality rates between EN and PN fed groups.[28,29] Nevertheless, a meta-analysis of EN *versus* PN feeding which included 27 studies did conclude that EN lowers risks of infection by about one-third.[30] This apparent superiority of EN may relate to levels of nutrient delivery.

As suggested above, limitations in GI tolerance after operation ensure that EN usually provides only modest levels of postoperative feeding. The majority of EN *versus* PN studies, therefore, examine differences in feeding levels as well as different routes of nutrient provision. This supposition is supported by evidence from trials in pancreatitis, in which several studies have suggested EN advantages over PN. If trials in which PN induced frank hyperglycaemia are excluded, however, no EN advantage is evident.[4]

When patients have significant gut dysfunction, EN may actually pose a risk. In a pragmatic study by Woodcock *et al.*, clinicians' assessments of GI function determined the mode of nutritional support in 562 patients. The 231 with adequate function received enteral tube feeding (ETF) while the 267 with clearly inadequate function had PN. In the remaining 64, however, adequacy of GI function was unclear, and these patients were randomised to either ETF or PN. In the randomized patients, only 22% of the ETF group received adequate nutrition compared to 75% of the PN group. There were no differences in sepsis rates between groups, but feeding-related complications were more frequent in elective and randomised ETF patients. Worryingly, they also had higher overall mortality rates in both non-randomised and randomised groups.[31]

Key point 3

- EN should be used whenever gut function is adequate and accessible, while PN is indicated in patients when the gut is inaccessible or its function is inadequate. EN is not invariably safer or of more benefit than PN and should be used very cautiously if gut function is in doubt. A combination of PN and EN can be effective and safe.

WHO AND WHEN TO FEED – INDICATIONS AND TIMING OF SUPPORT

INDICATIONS FOR FEEDING

It has been shown that undernutrition can begin to have detrimental effects on function, including surgical wound healing, when individuals lose only 5–10% body weight.[32] In catabolic surgical patients, this degree of loss can occur in only 5–10 days of starvation, even if starting from a good nutritional status. Therefore, it seems appropriate that nutrition support is considered within 5 days if a patient is completely starving. The aim should be to instigate support and meet requirements within a further 2–3 days in order to stop continuing nutritional deterioration. If patients are malnourished at the outset or gut function is clearly going to be slow to recover, feeding should be started earlier than this.

Studies of surgical patients have confirmed that this 'pre-emptive' approach is of value. In a retrospective study[34] of nearly 2500 medical and surgical patients, one-third had needed some nutritional support. In these, length-of-stay was extended by approximately 1 day for every 2 days delay in instigating nutritional therapy and costs were also increased.[33] Similarly, a recent 'Clinical Practice Improvement' study examined peri-operative nutrition in more than 1000 GI surgical patients, identifying 183 who needed nutrition support. Allowing for severity of illness, the study demonstrated that those who received early (within 48 h of operation) and sufficient support (> 60% of protein and calorie goals) stayed in hospital for 11.9 days compared to 13.3

days for patients receiving early but insufficient support, 14.6 days for sufficient but late feeding, and 14.8 days when feeding was neither early nor sufficient.[34] Corresponding costs were $34,602, $36,452, $39,883 and $38,578, respectively.

Key point 4

- Nutrition support should be considered if patients have completely starved for more than 5 days or are likely to do so and should be considered earlier in patients who already have a low BMI or a history of recent weight loss.

TIMING OF SUPPORT

Using these 'pre-emptive' feeding principles will usually confine nutrition support to the postoperative period except in patients who are already malnourished. This approach is supported by trial results which confirm that pre-operative supplementation is generally unhelpful except in high-risk groups. Despite their shortcomings, early PN trials demonstrated that 7–10 days of pre-operative feeding was of value in groups at nutritional risk based on albumin-related nutritional scores or low BMI/recent weight loss.[25] These benefits were also evident in more recent meta-analyses,[23,24] although these can be criticised since they include early, large trials in which benefit was identified on *post hoc*, sub-group analysis. Nevertheless, recent prospective trials confirm the findings with Bozzetti *et al.*,[35] for example, reporting that in 90 elective surgical patients with malignancy and more than 10% body weight loss, 10 days pre-operative and 9 days postoperative PN reduced complications rates from 57% in controls to 37%. Mortality rate may have also been reduced since no PN fed patients died while there were 5 deaths in the control group.[35]

Findings from studies of pre- and postoperative oral or ETF feeding are similar. In oral studies, postoperative sip-feeds once oral intake is tolerated show modest benefits in malnourished patients in terms of preserving body weight and decreasing infection rates and length-of-stay There is little benefit in better nourished groups, however, and the addition of pre- as well as postoperative sip-feeds is probably valueless.[36–38] Postoperative ETF is a more effective means of giving enteral nutrition allowing earlier intervention, especially if using post-pyloric feeding via a pre-or intra-operatively placed NJ tube or jejunostomy. The benefits of ETF are particularly marked in orthopaedic patients; studies of postoperative ETF in malnourished groups show reductions in complication rates, length-of-stay and even mortality rate.[39] In general surgery, results are more mixed although a recent meta-analysis of 5 randomised oral and 6 randomised ETF studies in 837 elective GI surgical patients showed that feeding within 24 h of surgery results in fewer infections and reduced length-of-stay. There was also a trend towards reduced anastamotic breakdowns although fed groups vomited more.[40]

43

Key point 5

- Keeping malnourished patients nil-by-mouth for many days after surgery is probably detrimental and routine starvation immediately prior to operation may also be harmful.

IS STARVATION NECESSARY?

A further consideration in peri-operative feeding has been raised by a recent series of studies that question the conventional wisdom of starvation immediately prior to surgery. Most surgeons restrict pre-operative GI intake to limit anaesthetic risks and peritoneal contamination, and continue restriction postoperatively to reduce anastamotic leakage and vomiting or pain from ileus. A Swedish group, however, have shown that 400 g of carbohydrate given in the few hours immediately preceding surgery by intravenous, nasogastric or oral routes will decrease post-surgical stress as measured by insulin resistance and nitrogen wasting. The same treatment can even reduce postoperative length-of-stay by approximately 20%.[41] Although explanations are speculative, it seems that glucose is altering crucial metabolic settings perhaps *via* insulin-stimulated membrane pumping. The body seems to cope better with injury when metabolically active, rather than down-regulated and perhaps this type of phenomenon is also the reason for the benefits of nutrition support having little to do with reversal of tissue wasting.[7]

CONCLUSIONS

From the above, it is clear that many questions regarding peri-operative nutrition remain unanswered and past practice may have caused problems. The greatest issue is excess feeding and even current recommendations may be too high. The problems related to excess feeding may not only make PN appear more dangerous than it really is, but may also explain why EN seems safe. Despite the difficulties, however, some key recommendations can be made.

Key points for clinical practice

- Immediately after surgery or in metabolically unstable patients, cautious nitrogen and energy provision may have advantages. Insulin should be used to prevent hyperglycaemia.

- The evidence to support the use of glutamine- and arginine-based immunonutrition is increasing, but there are concerns regarding arginine-based feeds in critically ill patients.

- EN should be used whenever gut function is adequate and accessible, while PN is indicated in patients when the gut is inaccessible or its function is inadequate. EN is not invariably safer or of more benefit than PN and should be used very cautiously if gut function is in doubt. A combination of PN and EN can be effective and safe.

Key points for clinical practice (continued)

• Nutrition support should be considered if patients have completely starved for more than 5 days or are likely to do so and should be considered earlier in patients who already have a low BMI or a history of recent weight loss.

• Keeping malnourished patients nil-by-mouth for many days after surgery is probably detrimental and routine starvation immediately prior to operation may also be harmful.

References

1. McWhirter, Pennington. Incidence and recognition of malnutrition in hospital. *BMJ* 1994; **308**: 945–948.
2. Green CJ. Existence, causes and consequences of disease related malnutrition in the hospital and the community, and the clinical and financial benefits of nutritional intervention. *Clin Nutr* 1999; **18 (Suppl 2)**: 3–38.
3. Elia M. Changing concepts of nutrient requirements in disease: implications for artificial nutrition support. *Lancet* 1995; **345**: 1279–1284.
4. Jeejeebhoy KN. Total parenteral nutrition: potion or poison? *Am J Clin Nutr* 2001; **74**:160–163.
5. Anon. *National Diet and Nutrition Survey: People Aged 65 Years and Over*. London: The Stationary Office, 1998.
6. Joosten E, van den Berg A, Riezler R *et al*. Metabolic evidence that deficiencies of vitamin B-12 (cobalamin), folate, and vitamin B-6 occur commonly in elderly people. *Am J Clin Nutr* 1993; **58**: 468–476.
7. Jeejeebhoy KN. Bulk or bounce – the object of nutritional support. *J Parenter Enter Nutr* 1988; **12**: 539–546.
8. Reeds PJ, Jahoor F. The amino acid requirements of disease. *Clin Nutr* 2001; **(Suppl 1)**: 15–22.
9. Elia M. Artificial nutrition support. *Med Int* 1990; **82**: 3392–3396.
10. Ruokonen E, Takala J. Dangers of growth hormone therapy in critically ill patients. *Ann Med* 2000; **32**: 317–322.
11. Greet Van den Berghe G, Wouters P, Weekers F *et al*. Intensive insulin therapy in critically ill patients. *N Engl J Med* 2001; **345**: 1359–1367.
12. Mertes N, Schulzki C, Goeters C *et al*. Cost containment through L-alanyl-L-glutamine supplemented total parenteral nutrition after major abdominal surgery: a prospective randomized double-blind controlled study. *Clin Nutr* 2000; **19**: 395–401.
13. Morlion BJ, Stehle P, Wachtler P *et al*. Total parenteral nutrition with glutamine dipeptide after major abdominal surgery: a randomized, double-blind, controlled study. *Ann Surg* 1998; **227**: 302–308.
14. Powell-Tuck J, Jamieson CP, Bettany GE *et al*. A double blind, randomised, controlled trial of glutamine supplementation in parenteral nutrition. *Gut* 1999; **45**: 82–88.
15. Griffiths RD, Jones C, Palmer TE. Six-month outcome of critically ill patients given glutamine-supplemented parenteral nutrition. *Nutrition* 1997; **13**: 295–302.
16. Sacks GS. Glutamine supplementation in catabolic patients. *Ann Pharmacother* 1999; **33**: 348–354.
17. Furst P, Kuhn KS. Conditionally indispensable amino acids in enteral feeds and the dipeptide concept. *Enteral Nutrition: Proceedings of the 12th Nestlé Workshop*. Karger, 2000.
18. Senkal M, Zumtobel V, Bauer KH *et al*. Outcome and cost-effectiveness of perioperative enteral immunonutrition in patients undergoing elective upper gastrointestinal tract surgery: a prospective randomized study. *Arch Surg* 1999; **134**: 1309–1316.
19. Braga M, Gianotti L, Vignali A, Cestari A, Bisagni P, Di Carlo V. Artificial nutrition after major abdominal surgery: impact of route of administration and composition of the diet. *Crit Care Med* 1998; **26**: 24–30.

20. Van Bokhorst-De Van Der Schueren MA, Quak JJ, von Blomberg-van der Flier BM *et al.* Effect of perioperative nutrition, with and without arginine supplementation, on nutritional status, immune function, postoperative morbidity, and survival in severely malnourished head and neck cancer patients. *Am J Clin Nutr* 2001; **73**: 323–332.

21. Galban C, Montejo JC, Mesejo A *et al.* An immune-enhancing enteral diet reduces mortality rate and episodes of bacteremia in septic intensive care unit patients. *Crit Care Med* 2000; **28**: 643–648.

22. Heyland *et al.* Should immunonutrition become routine in critically ill patients? A systematic review of the evidence. *JAMA* 2001; **286**: 22-29.

23. Torosian MH. Perioperative nutrition support for patients undergoing gastrointestinal surgery: critical analysis and recommendations. *World J Surg* 1999; **23**: 565–569.

24. Heyland DK, Macdonald S, Keefe L, Drover JW. Total parenteral nutrition in the critically ill patient. A meta-analysis. *JAMA* 1998; **280**: 2013–2019.

25. Veterans Affairs TPN Cooperative Study. Perioperative total parenteral nutrition in surgical patients. *N Engl J Med* 1991; **325**: 525–532.

26. Lipman TO. Grains or veins: is enteral nutrition really better than parenteral nutrition? A look at the evidence. *J Parenter Enter Nutr* 1998; **22**: 167–182.

27. Sedman PC, MacFie J, Palmer MD, Mitchell CJ, Sagar PM. Preoperative total parenteral nutrition is not associated with mucosal atrophy or bacterial translocation in humans. *Br J Surg* 1995; **82**: 1663–1667.

28. Pacelli F, Bossola M, Papa V *et al.* Enteral vs parenteral nutrition after major abdominal surgery: an even match. *Arch Surg* 2001; **136**: 933–936.

29. Braga M, Gianotti L, Gentilini O, Parisi V, Salis C, Di Carlo V. Early postoperative enteral nutrition improves gut oxygenation and reduces costs compared with total parenteral nutrition. *Crit Care Med* 2001; **29**: 242–248.

30. Braunschweig CL, Levy P, Sheean PM, Wang X. Enteral compared to parenteral nutrition: a meta-analysis. *Am J Clin Nutr* 2001; **74**: 534–542.

31. Woodcock NP, Zeigler D, Palmer MD, Buckley P, Mitchell CJ, MacFie J. Enteral versus parenteral nutrition: a pragmatic study. *Nutrition* 2001; **17**: 1–12.

32. Haydock DA, Hill GL. Impaired wound healing in surgical patients with varying degrees of malnutrition. *J Parenter Enter Nutr* 1986; **10**: 550–554.

33. Tucker HN, Miguel SG. Cost containment through nutrition intervention. *Nutr Rev* 1996; **54**: 111–121.

34. Neumayer LA, Smout RJ, Horn HG, Horn SD. Early and sufficient feeding reduces length of stay and charges in surgical patients. *J Surg Res* 2001; **95**: 73–77.

35. Bozzetti F, Gavazzi C, Miceli R *et al.* Perioperative total parenteral nutrition in malnourished, gastrointestinal cancer patients: a randomized, clinical trial. *J Parenter Enter Nutr* 2000; **24**: 7–14.

36. Rana SK, Bray J, Menzies Gow N. Short term benefits of oral post-operative dietary supplements in surgical patients. *Clin Nutr* 1992; **11**: 337–344.

37. Keele AM, Bray MJ, Emery PW, Silk DBA. Two phase randomized controlled clinical trial of post-operative oral dietary supplements in surgical patients. *Gut* 1997; **40**: 393–399.

38. MacFie J, Woodcock NP, Palmer MD, Walker A, Townsend S, Mitchell CJ. Oral dietary supplements in pre- and postoperative surgical patients: a prospective and randomised clinical trial. *Nutrition* 2000; **16**: 723–728.

39. Bastow MD, Rawlings J, Allison SP. Benefits of supplementary tube feeding after fractured neck of femur: a randomised controlled trial. *BMJ* 1983; **287**: 1589–1592.

40. Lewis SJ, Egger M, Sylvester PA, Thomas S. Early enteral feeding versus 'nil by mouth' after gastrointestinal surgery: systematic review and meta-analysis of controlled trials. *BMJ* 2001; **323**: 773–776.

41. Nygren J, Thorell A, Ljungqvist O. Preoperative oral carbohydrate nutrition: an update. *Curr Opin Clin Nutr Metab Care* 2001; **4**: 255–259.

Rachel M. Bright-Thomas

5

Genes and the surgeon

The relevance of genetics to a busy surgeon may not be immediately apparent. However, the UK Health Secretary recently outlined a £30m package of measures 'to help bring the genetics revolution into every-day medical practice' and there is a case for its increasing importance in all aspects of patient care. An understanding of genetics lies at the core of screening for many disease states, underpins our knowledge of disease biology and prognostic information, and may soon come to modulate our choice of therapy. Moreover, the field of gene therapy is rapidly unfolding as an additional weapon in our armory against vascular disease and a variety of solid tumours. Failure to recognise the importance of this area could limit the available options in the management of many 'surgical' problems.

This review will focus on the clinical application of genetic information in three commonly encountered surgical problems: solid tumours, vascular disease, and pancreatitis.

CANCER

Genetic and environmental factors interact in all aspects of tumourigenesis. Many genes are involved, including tumour suppressor genes, oncogenes, mismatch repair genes, and those encoding growth and angiogenic factors.[1] This discussion will cover recent translational research (from the laboratory to the clinic) in three of the commonest cancers: lung, colorectal and breast cancer.

SCREENING FOR GENETIC SUSCEPTIBILITY TO MALIGNANCY

It is now possible to test for genetic susceptibility to cancer in individuals deemed to be at 'high risk'. For example, Familial Adenomatous Polyposis

Ms Rachel M. Bright-Thomas MA BM BCh MD FRCS, Specialist Registrar in General Surgery, North West Thames Deanery, Ealing Hospital NHS Trust, Uxbridge Road, Southall, Middlesex UB1 3EW, UK

(FAP) is an autosomal, dominantly inherited, premalignant condition, arising as a result of a germline mutation in the *Adenomatous Polyposis Coli* (*APC*) gene. The disorder is characterised by the development of hundreds to thousands of adenomatous polyps throughout the colon and rectum of affected individuals. Without timely surgery, all patients with FAP will ultimately develop at least one colorectal carcinoma. Genetic testing is routinely used to confirm the diagnosis in an affected individual and to screen relatives within an affected pedigree.[2] This is largely because the gene responsible is fully penetrant (*i.e.* a germline mutation is invariably associated with disease).

In order to test 'at-risk' relatives, it is first necessary to establish the underlying mutation in the proband (presenting case). Once this mutation is identified, relatives can be directly tested for the same mutation and given an estimate of risk (either negligible or 100%) for the inheritance of FAP.[3] This has important clinical sequelae in that non-affected family members can be saved the physical and psychological stress of years of invasive screening procedures. At the same time, the health service makes a financial saving.[4] The identification of a mutation is also beneficial as it may increase compliance with routine clinical screening procedures. Indeed, studies have shown that the introduction of a structured genetic screening regimen and subsequent close surveillance of affected individuals significantly improves survival in FAP.[5,6]

In a similar vein, the identification of the breast and ovarian cancer susceptibility genes *BRCA 1* and *BRCA 2*,[7,8] has allowed screening for inherited mutations at these loci in families at risk of hereditary breast cancer. Carriers of *BRCA* gene mutations can be offered cancer surveillance,[9,10] chemoprevention or even prophylactic surgery.[11] Unfortunately, the benefits of any intervention are more difficult to assess than in FAP, as the penetrance of a *BRCA* mutation (likelihood that it will cause disease) is only 80%. However, on-going studies in mutation carriers should lead to improved management guidelines.

In the future, population-based screening for multiple low penetrance genes may allow the production of individualised risk profiles for cardiovascular disease, cancer and other conditions where timely prophylaxis could delay or even prevent the onset of disease. However, this is a huge undertaking and, as with all screening programmes, the clinical benefits need to be balanced against the psychological, social and economic costs.[12]

Key point 1

- It is currently possible to identify individual genetic mutations predisposing to significant disease states. In the future, population based screening for multiple low penetrance genes is likely to be widely available.

EARLY DETECTION OF ASYMPTOMATIC DISEASE

The early detection of many solid tumours could lead to a surgical cure. This requires the development of sensitive, specific, non-invasive, reproducible and cost-efficient tests that identify affected individuals at a suitable stage.

A recent study has shown that microsatellite instability (the accumulation of multiple different copies of short repeat sequences in the genome, arising through errors in DNA repair) can be seen in approximately 56% of non-small cell lung cancers (NSCLC). Of individuals with stage I tumours, 43% show the same microsatellite instability (MSI) in their plasma DNA.[13]

In colorectal cancer, it is well recognised that *APC* mutations occur at an early stage in 60–80% of sporadic tumours.[14] However, a recent study showed that 80% of individuals with *APC*-deficient colorectal carcinoma also show the same mutation in their serum.[15] This raises the possibility that simple blood tests may be able to detect a significant proportion of early stage asymptomatic lung and colon cancers.

Faecal occult blood testing is a familiar non-invasive investigation for colorectal cancer. It is now possible to detect mutations in the *k-ras* proto-oncogene in stool samples from individuals with colorectal adenomas as small as 1 cm^2. When a quantitative, reproducible assay for *k-ras* becomes available at an affordable price on a large scale, this may provide another rapid screening tool for the early detection of colorectal carcinoma.[16]

Key point 2

- The early stages of asymptomatic cancers can be detected with simple non-invasive genetic tests. This may eventually help to reduce the morbidity and mortality associated with late presentation.

GENETIC STAGING

Molecular staging at the time of cancer diagnosis, or the use of molecular markers to detect residual disease after apparently curative surgery, may enhance the sensitivity of routine staging investigations.

It is already possible to detect tumour-specific mRNA in immunohisto-chemically clear lymph nodes resected with a variety of tumours, including breast cancer.[17] The relevance of these occult micrometastases to disease-free survival is not yet clear, but it appears likely that similar investigations will be used in the future in determining the need for adjuvant therapy.

PROGNOSTIC MARKERS

Many papers have been published over the last year looking at the prognostic value of genetic factors in intestinal, lung and breast cancer. However, only a few genes have been clearly linked with altered prognosis.

Overexpression of the proto-oncogene *c-erbB2* is seen in 10–30% of breast cancers. In 1987, Slamon showed that amplification of the *c-erbB2* gene was associated with early tumour relapse after surgery.[18] Subsequent work has demonstrated that *c-erbB2* is an independent prognostic factor for node-positive breast cancers.[19]

Microsatellite instability, a marker for mismatch repair errors, has been linked to shortened disease-free survival in NSCLC,[20] but interestingly appears to confer a survival advantage in colorectal and gastric cancer.[21,22]

Thymidilate synthase and thymidine phosphorylase are enzymes necessary for DNA turnover. Overexpression of either gene has been linked to a detrimental effect on disease-free and overall survival in colorectal cancer.[23,24] k-ras mutations have also been associated with poor outcome in this tumour[25] although it is unclear whether rectal cancer may act differently if analysed independently.

Genetic markers show that loss of chromosome 17q is associated with very poor (7%) 5-year survival after pancreatic duodenectomy for ampullary adenocarcinoma. In contrast, tumours which retained this genetic material had 80% 5-year survival.[26]

Key point 3

- Knowledge of tumour aggression at a molecular level complements clinicopathological investigations when deciding on the most appropriate therapeutic intervention.

PHARMACOGENETICS

Pharmacogenetics is the study of the way in which inherited differences alter an individual's response to treatment.[27] In its simplest form, pharmacogenetics is already in regular use, with blood group analysis prior to transfusion. However, it is being increasingly studied as a way to optimise the choice of therapeutic agent and to minimise the idiosyncratic side-effects of treatment. For example, those breast cancers overexpressing c-erbB2 have been shown to respond better to doxorubicin,[28] but possibly less well to hormonal manipulation,[29] than those tumours not amplifying the gene.

Taxanes are commonly used chemotherapeutic agents. They bind to and disrupt β-tubulin (part of the cytoskeleton). However, up to one-third of NSCLCs carry β-tubulin mutations and these patients have been shown to have a poor response to paclitaxel.[30] In the future it may be worth identifying this subgroup prior to the initiation of taxane-based therapy.

Pharmacogenetics is taken to its limit in the area of pharmacogenomics, where new drugs are designed to target recognised genetic abnormalities. For example, a humanised anti-c-erbB2 antibody (Herceptin) has recently been produced. Clinical trials utilising this agent, with or without chemotherapy, have shown a survival advantage in breast cancer patients with metastatic disease overexpressing c-erbB2.[31,32]

Key point 4

- Advances in pharmacogenetics and pharmacogenomics will allow more effective, individually targeted treatment regimens, with less treatment related toxicity.

CANCER GENE THERAPY

Gene therapy attempts to correct pathological cell processes at the level of gene expression. Corrective gene therapy (replacing a defective or underexpressed gene) is only one approach to treatment. In fact, at present, cancer gene therapy is more widely used to optimise existing cytotoxic or immunological treatments.

Modulating chemotherapy

Gene-directed enzyme prodrug therapy (GDEPT) is the introduction into tumour cells of a gene whose protein product is capable of activating a non-toxic prodrug to an active cytotoxic compound. The patient is subsequently treated with the appropriate prodrug and transfected tumour cells are preferentially killed. Non-transfected normal tissue cannot activate the prodrug and remains largely unharmed. Trials of GDEPT are in progress in the treatment of metastatic colorectal cancer, where an adenoviral vector, carrying the gene for cytosine deaminase, is injected directly into hepatic metastases and the patients are subsequently treated with oral 5-fluorocytosine.[33]

Other genes can be used in the treatment of solid tumours with the aim of enhancing the therapeutic effect of cytotoxic agents. For example, the multidrug resistance gene *MDR-1* has been introduced *ex vivo* into the bone marrow or blood-derived stem cells of cancer patients, and the cells are then re-infused prior to chemotherapy with myelotoxic drugs. Phase I clinical trials are underway in breast cancer patients to see if this will minimise the bone marrow toxicity of various chemotherapeutic regimens.[34]

Genetic immunotherapy

Immunotherapy aims to boost the size and increase the specificity of the host immune response to a tumour. Non-specific immune enhancement is achieved through the introduction of genes encoding cytokines and/or allogeneic histo-compatibility antigens into tumour cells or immune effector cells. Clinical trials of immunotherapy have included the introduction of class I MHC into hepatic metastases of patients with colorectal cancer,[35] and the delivery of interleukin-2 into unresectable colorectal tumours.[36] No toxic effects have been seen and gene expression has been recorded. The therapeutic efficacy has yet to be seen.

Specific immune responses to cancer can be boosted with the use of genes encoding tumour-associated antigens. Carcinogenic embryonic antigen (CEA) is expressed on many colorectal cancers. A plasmid carrying the CEA gene has been engineered for human administration. A Phase I clinical trial of this plasmid in patients with metastatic colorectal cancer expressing CEA showed a good antibody response to CEA and no toxicity.[37]

Corrective gene therapy

Certain genetic mutations appear to be critical in the initiation or development of neoplasia. Targeting these abnormalities may impede the neoplastic process. It has been clearly shown that replacing wild-type *p53* in malignant cell lines carrying mutations of this tumour suppressor gene can suppresses the neoplastic phenotype.[38] Similarly, introducing the wild-type gene into *p53* deficient animal tumours leads to significant tumour regression[39] and enhances the effect of chemotherapy and/or radiotherapy.

Phase I trials of a retroviral vector containing wild-type *p53* have been carried out for the treatment of NSCLC where conventional therapy failed to control disease. Nine patients were treated by direct intratumoural injection. Three showed tumour regression and three showed stable disease. No significant toxic effects were noted.[40] Similar results have been seen in trials using an adenoviral vector.[41] The most recent clinical trials are considering the effect of *p53* gene therapy in combination with chemotherapy and/or radiotherapy in NSCLC.

Just as defective tumour suppressor genes can be replaced, mutant oncogenes can now be inactivated. Antisense oligodeoxynucleotides (ODNs) can be produced which are complementary to specific mRNA. These ODNs bind to and inactivate the mRNA, preventing its translation and thus blocking gene expression.[42] There is experimental evidence to show that they can suppress the growth of tumours in animal models,[43] and they are now undergoing trials in human disease.

Key point 5

- Cancer gene therapy is advancing on many fronts. Whilst it may not be the panacea that has been suggested, it looks set to enhance the action of other adjuvant treatments in a variety of tumours.

VASCULAR DISEASE

With the identification of genes encoding potent angiogenic factors, such as vascular endothelial growth factor (VEGF), new treatments for end-stage coronary artery and peripheral vascular disease have emerged.

Intra-arterial and intramuscular *VEGF* has been utilised in clinical trials of patients with critical limb ischaemia not suitable for conventional re-vascularisation. Following treatment, many patients have shown new collateral vessel formation, improvement in the ankle:brachial pressure index and even healing of ischaemic ulcers.[44,45] In diabetic patients, these treatments have also been seen to correspond with an improvement in neuropathy in the same limb.[46] This may occur via improved angiogenesis in the vasa nervorum or through a direct effect on Schwann cells.

VEGF has also been delivered directly into the coronary arteries and myocardium of individuals with end-stage coronary artery disease, and has been associated with improved perfusion, enhanced left ventricular function, improved exercise tolerance and a decrease in symptomatic angina.[47,48]

Gene therapy with angiostatic agents has been put forward as a means of impeding the development of intimal hyperplasia and re-stenosis after venous bypass grafting or angioplasty. The recent PREVENT trial introduced a specific ODN into autologous vein at the time of venous bypass grafting. This ODN bound and inhibited a crucial cell cycle transcription factor (E2F). The treatment correlated with decreased expression of cell cycle regulatory genes and was associated with fewer graft occlusions, revisions and critical stenoses.[49] Further work is awaited in this interesting area.

Key point 6

- Gene therapy may soon be able to minimise the problem of vessel re-stenosis after surgery, angioplasty or endarterectomy, and it may eventually replace invasive procedures in the management of coronary artery and peripheral vascular disease.

PANCREATIC DISEASE

The importance of genetic factors in the aetiology of some cases of pancreatitis is gradually emerging. This will hopefully elucidate some cases of so-called 'idiopathic' disease, and may help to explain why only a minority of individuals who consume excess alcohol develop pancreatitis.

Several different mutations in the cationic trypsinogen gene (PRSS1) have been clearly linked to hereditary pancreatitis and are occasionally seen in sporadic disease.[50–52] These genetic alterations stabilise trypsinogen against degradation and thus enhance the activation of pancreatic enzymes, causing irreversible pancreatic damage.

Mutations in the cystic fibrosis transmembrane conductance regulator gene (CFTR) have been demonstrated in cohorts of individuals with sporadic chronic idiopathic or alcoholic pancreatitis,[53,54] at a higher frequency than is expected in the general population including CF carriers. Within the last year, mutation in serine protease inhibitor Kazal type 1 (SPINK1; previously known as pancreatic secretory trypsin inhibitor [PTSI]) has also been linked to chronic pancreatitis.[55,56]

The implications of this knowledge are potentially far reaching. Genetic testing of individuals within families affected by hereditary pancreatitis may allow mutation carriers to consider surveillance investigation for pancreatic cancer. Now that neonatal screening for CFTR mutations is about to be instituted, affected individuals (heterozygotes) could be warned that they may be at increased risk of sporadic or alcohol-related chronic pancreatitis.

Clinical trials of gene therapy for cystic fibrosis are underway.[57,58] It has been shown that the normal human CFTR gene can be safely introduced into respiratory epithelium and that this leads to production of the normal protein and in some cases to a physiological response. however, gene therapy to

---

Key point 7

- Genetic variation may underlie disease susceptibility in pancreatitis. There is no evidence so far that behaviour modification or prophylactic gene therapy can prevent the onset of disease in 'at risk' individuals.

prevent or counter the effects of cystic fibrosis mutations in the pancreas is unlikely to become feasible in the foreseeable future.

CONCLUSIONS

With the publication of the first drafts of the entire human genome comes the potential to identify and screen multiple genes within an individual. Advances in chip technology and DNA micro-arrays[59] mean that these genetic tests will soon be performed faster and at a fraction of the present cost. A genetic revolution is at hand, and those who do not take part will surely be left behind.

Key points for clinical practice

- It is currently possible to identify individual genetic mutations predisposing to significant disease states. In the future, population based screening for multiple low penetrance genes is likely to be widely available.

- The early stages of asymptomatic cancers can be detected with simple non-invasive genetic tests. This may eventually help to reduce the morbidity and mortality associated with late presentation.

- Knowledge of tumour aggression at a molecular level complements clinicopathological investigations when deciding on the most appropriate therapeutic intervention.

- Advances in pharmacogenetics and pharmacogenomics will allow more effective, individually targeted treatment regimens, with less treatment related toxicity.

- Cancer gene therapy is advancing on many fronts. Whilst it may not be the panacea that has been suggested, it looks set to enhance the action of other adjuvant treatments in a variety of tumours.

- Gene therapy may soon be able to minimise the problem of vessel re-stenosis after surgery, angioplasty or endarterectomy, and it may eventually replace invasive procedures in the management of coronary artery and peripheral vascular disease.

- Genetic variation may underlie disease susceptibility in pancreatitis. There is no evidence so far that behaviour modification or prophylactic gene therapy can prevent the onset of disease in 'at risk' individuals.

References

1. Hanahan D, Weinberg RA. The hallmarks of cancer. *Cell* 2000; **100**: 57–70.
2. Vasen H, Bulow S and the Leeds Castle Polyposis Group. Guidelines for the surveillance and management of familial adenomatous polyposis (FAP): a world wide survey among 41 registries. *Colorectal Dis* 1999; **1**: 214–221.

3. Wong N, Lasko D, Rabelo R, Pinsky L, Gordon PH, Foulkes TW. Genetic counseling and interpretation of genetic tests in familial adenomatous polyposis and hereditary nonpolyposis colorectal cancer. *Dis Colon Rectum* 2001; **44**: 271–279.

4. Bapat B, Noorani H, Cohen Z *et al*. Cost comparison of predictive genetic testing versus conventional clinical screening for familial adenomatous polyposis. *Gut* 1999; **44**: 698–703.

5. Bulow S, Bulow C, Nielsen TF, Karlsen L, Moesgaard F. Centralized registration, prophylactic examination, and treatment results in improved prognosis in familial adenomatous polyposis. Results from the Danish Polyposis Register. *Scand J Gastroenterol* 1995; **30**: 989–993.

6. Rabelo R, Foulkes W, Gordon PH *et al*. Role of molecular diagnostic testing in familial adenomatous polyposis and hereditary nonpolyposis colorectal cancer families. *Dis Colon Rectum* 2001; **44**: 437–446.

7. Miki Y, Swensen J, Shattuck-Eidens D *et al*. A strong candidate for the breast and ovarian cancer susceptibility gene *BRCA1*. *Science* 1994; **266**: 66–71.

8. Wooster R, Bignell G, Lancaster J *et al*. Identification of the breast cancer susceptibility gene *BRCA2*. *Nature* 1995; **378**: 789–792.

9. Burke W, Daly M, Garber J *et al*. Recommendations for follow-up care of individuals with an inherited predisposition to cancer. II. BRCA1 and BRCA2. Cancer Genetics Studies Consortium. *JAMA* 1997; **277**: 997–1003.

10. Mitchell G, Trott P, Coleman Nea. Nipple fluid aspiration (NFA): a 'PAP' smear for the breast in *BRCA1/2* carriers [Abstract 1748]. *Am J Hum Genet* 1999; **65 (Suppl)**: A3111.

11. Kuschel B, Lux MP, Goecke TO, Beckmann MW. Prevention and therapy for BRCA1/2 mutation carriers and women at high risk for breast and ovarian cancer. *Eur J Cancer Prev* 2000; **9**: 139–150.

12. Goel V. Appraising organised screening programmes for testing for genetic susceptibility to cancer. *BMJ* 2001; **322**: 1174-1178.

13. Sozzi G, Musso K, Ratcliffe C, Goldstraw P, Pierotti MA, Pastorino U. Detection of microsatellite alterations in plasma DNA of non-small cell lung cancer patients: a prospect for early diagnosis. *Clin Cancer Res* 1999; **5**: 2689–2692.

14. Powell SM, Zilz N, Beazer-Barclay Y *et al*. APC mutations occur early during colorectal tumorigenesis. *Nature* 1992; **359**: 235–237.

15. Lauschke H, Caspari R, Friedl W *et al*. Detection of APC and k-ras mutations in the serum of patients with colorectal cancer. *Cancer Detect Prev* 2001; **25**: 55–61.

16. Lev Z, Kislitsin D, Rennert G, Lerner A. Utilization of k-ras mutations identified in stool DNA for the early detection of colorectal cancer. *J Cell Biochem Suppl* 2000; **34**: 35–39.

17. Noguchi S, Aihara T, Motomura K, Inaji H, Imaoka S, Koyama H. Detection of breast cancer micrometastases in axillary lymph nodes by means of reverse transcriptase-polymerase chain reaction. Comparison between MUC1 mRNA and keratin 19 mRNA amplification. *Am J Pathol* 1996; **148**: 649–656.

18. Slamon DJ, Clark GM, Wong SG, Levin WJ, Ullrich A, McGuire WL. Human breast cancer: correlation of relapse and survival with amplification of the HER-2/neu oncogene. *Science* 1987; **235**: 177–182.

19. Tsuda H, Sakamaki C, Tsugane S, Fukutomi T, Hirohashi S. A prospective study of the significance of gene and chromosome alterations as prognostic indicators of breast cancer patients with lymph node metastases. *Breast Cancer Res Treat* 1998; **48**: 21–32.

20. Zhou X, Kemp BL, Khuri FR *et al*. Prognostic implication of microsatellite alteration profiles in early-stage non-small cell lung cancer. *Clin Cancer Res* 2000; **6**: 559–565.

21. Gryfe R, Kim H, Hsieh ET *et al*. Tumor microsatellite instability and clinical outcome in young patients with colorectal cancer. *N Engl J Med* 2000; **342**: 69–77.

22. Choi SW, Choi JR, Chung YJ, Kim KM, Rhyu MG. Prognostic implications of microsatellite genotypes in gastric carcinoma. *Int J Cancer* 2000; **89**: 378–383.

23. Edler D, Kressner U, Ragnhammar P *et al*. Immunohistochemically detected thymidylate synthase in colorectal cancer: an independent prognostic factor of survival. *Clin Cancer Res* 2000; **6**: 488–492.

24. Takebayashi Y, Akiyama S, Akiba S *et al*. Clinicopathologic and prognostic significance of an angiogenic factor, thymidine phosphorylase, in human colorectal carcinoma. *J Natl Cancer Inst* 1996; **88**: 1110–1117.

25. Andreyev HJ, Norman AR, Cunningham D, Oates JR, Clarke PA. Kirsten ras mutations in patients with colorectal cancer: the multicenter 'RASCAL' study. *J Natl Cancer Inst* 1998; **90**: 675–684.

26. Scarpa A, DiPace C, Talamini G et al. Cancer of the ampulla of Vater: chromosome 17p allelic loss is associated with poor prognosis. Gut 2000; 46: 842–848.

27. Roses AD. Pharmacogenetics and the practice of medicine. Nature 2000; 405: 857–865.

28. Muss HB, Thor AD, Berry DA et al. c-erbB-2 expression and response to adjuvant therapy in women with node- positive early breast cancer. N Engl J Med 1994; 330: 1260-1266.

29. Newby JC, Johnston SR, Smith IE, Dowsett M. Expression of epidermal growth factor receptor and c-erbB2 during the development of tamoxifen resistance in human breast cancer. Clin Cancer Res 1997; 3: 1643–1651.

30. Monzo M, Rosell R, Sanchez JJ et al. Paclitaxel resistance in non-small-cell lung cancer associated with beta-tubulin gene mutations. J Clin Oncol 1999; 17: 1786–1793.

31. Cobleigh MA, Vogel CL, Tripathy D et al. Multinational study of the efficacy and safety of humanized anti-HER2 monoclonal antibody in women who have HER2-overexpressing metastatic breast cancer that has progressed after chemotherapy for metastatic disease. J Clin Oncol 1999; 17: 2639–2648.

32. Slamon DJ, Leyland-Jones B, Shak S et al. Use of chemotherapy plus a monoclonal antibody against HER2 for metastatic breast cancer that overexpresses HER2. N Engl J Med 2001; 344: 783–792.

33. Crystal RG, Hirschowitz E, Lieberman M et al. Phase I study of direct administration of a replication deficient adenovirus vector containing the E. coli cytosine deaminase gene to metastatic colon carcinoma of the liver in association with the oral administration of the pro-drug 5-fluorocytosine. Hum Gene Ther 1997; 8: 985–1001.

34. Moscow JA, Huang H, Carter C et al. Engraftment of MDR1 and NeoR gene-transduced hematopoietic cells after breast cancer chemotherapy. Blood 1999; 94: 52–61.

35. Rubin J, Galanis E, Pitot HC et al. Phase I study of immunotherapy of hepatic metastases of colorectal carcinoma by direct gene transfer of an allogeneic histocompatibility antigen, HLA-B7. Gene Ther 1997; 4: 419–425.

36. Gilly FN, Sayag-Beaujard AC, Bienvenu J et al. Gene therapy with AdV-IL2 (TG 1021) in unresectable digestive adenocarcinoma. Phase I-II study, first inclusions. Adv Exp Med Biol 1998; 451: 527–530.

37. Conry RM, Strong T, White S, Khazaeli M, LoBuglio AF, Curiel DT. Cancer Gene Ther 1997; 4: S49.

38. Baker SJ, Markowitz S, Fearon ER, Willson JK, Vogelstein B. Suppression of human colorectal carcinoma cell growth by wild-type p53. Science 1990; 249: 912–915.

39. Fujiwara T, Cai DW, Georges RN, Mukhopadhyay T, Grimm EA, Roth JA. Therapeutic effect of a retroviral wild-type p53 expression vector in an orthotopic lung cancer model [see comments]. J Natl Cancer Inst 1994; 86: 1458–1462.

40. Roth JA, Nguyen D, Lawrence DD et al. Retrovirus-mediated wild-type p53 gene transfer to tumors of patients with lung cancer [see comments]. Nat Med 1996; 2: 985–991.

41. Swisher SG, Roth JA, Nemunaitis J et al. Adenovirus-mediated p53 gene transfer in advanced non-small-cell lung cancer. J Natl Cancer Inst 1999; 91: 763–771.

42. Wagner RW. Gene inhibition using antisense oligodeoxynucleotides. Nature 1994; 372: 333–335.

43. Sacco MG, Barbieri O, Piccini D et al. In vitro and in vivo antisense-mediated growth inhibition of a mammary adenocarcinoma from MMTV-neu transgenic mice. Gene Ther 1998; 5: 388–393.

44. Baumgartner I, Pieczek A, Manor O et al. Constitutive expression of phVEGF165 after intramuscular gene transfer promotes collateral vessel development in patients with critical limb ischemia. Circulation 1998; 97: 1114–1123.

45. Baumgartner I. Lessons learned from human gene therapy in patients with chronic critical limb ischemia. J Invasive Cardiol 2001; 13: 330–332.

46. Simovic D, Isner JM, Ropper AH, Pieczek A, Weinberg DH. Improvement in chronic ischemic neuropathy after intramuscular phVEGF165 gene transfer in patients with critical limb ischemia. Arch Neurol 2001; 58: 761–768.

47. Freedman SB, Isner JM. Therapeutic angiogenesis for ischemic cardiovascular disease. J Mol Cell Cardiol 2001; 33: 379–393.

48. Symes JF, Losordo DW, Vale PR et al. Gene therapy with vascular endothelial growth factor for inoperable coronary artery disease. Ann Thorac Surg 1999; 68: 830–836; discussion 836–837.

49. Mann MJ, Whittemore AD, Donaldson MC *et al*. *Ex-vivo* gene therapy of human vascular bypass grafts with E2F decoy: the PREVENT single-centre, randomised, controlled trial. *Lancet* 1999; **354**: 1493–1498.

50. Whitcomb DC, Gorry MC, Preston RA *et al*. Hereditary pancreatitis is caused by a mutation in the cationic trypsinogen gene. *Nat Genet* 1996; **14**: 141–145.

51. Gorry MC, Gabbaizedeh D, Furey W *et al*. Mutations in the cationic trypsinogen gene are associated with recurrent acute and chronic pancreatitis. *Gastroenterology* 1997; **113**: 1063–1068.

52. Witt H, Luck W, Becker M. A signal peptide cleavage site mutation in the cationic trypsinogen gene is strongly associated with chronic pancreatitis. *Gastroenterology* 1999; **117**: 7–10.

53. Sharer N, Schwarz M, Malone G *et al*. Mutations of the cystic fibrosis gene in patients with chronic pancreatitis. *N Engl J Med* 1998; **339**: 645–652.

54. Cohn JA, Friedman KJ, Noone PG, Knowles MR, Silverman LM, Jowell PS. Relation between mutations of the cystic fibrosis gene and idiopathic pancreatitis. *N Engl J Med* 1998; **339**: 653–658.

55. Chen JM, Mercier B, Audrezet MP, Raguenes O, Quere I, Ferec C. Mutations of the pancreatic secretory trypsin inhibitor (PSTI) gene in idiopathic chronic pancreatitis. *Gastroenterology* 2001; **120**: 1061–1064.

56. Witt H, Luck W, Hennies HC *et al*. Mutations in the gene encoding the serine protease inhibitor, Kazal type 1 are associated with chronic pancreatitis. *Nat Genet* 2000; **25**: 213–216.

57. Henig NR, Aitken ML. Update on clinical trials of cystic fibrosis. *Curr Opin Pulm Med* 1997; **3**: 404–409.

58. Noone PG, Hohneker KW, Zhou Z *et al*. Safety and biological efficacy of a lipid-CFTR complex for gene transfer in the nasal epithelium of adult patients with cystic fibrosis. *Mol Ther* 2000; **1**: 105–114.

59. De Benedetti VM, Biglia N, Sismondi P, De Bortoli M. DNA chips: the future of biomarkers. *Int J Biol Markers* 2000; **15**: 1–9.

A.G. Acheson N. Griffin J.H. Scholefield

6

The role of botulinum toxin in gastrointestinal surgery

Botulinum neurotoxin is a lethal biological substance produced by the anaerobic bacterium *Clostridium botulinum*. It can cause botulism in humans which is a rare disorder characterized by a descending paralysis with prominent bulbar and associated gastrointestinal symptoms. So far, seven different neurotoxins have been recognized (A–G) but only types A, B and E are associated with botulism and serotype A is the only one commercially available that has proven therapeutic value in a variety of clinical conditions.[1]

Botulinum toxin type A is a polypeptide consisting of a heavy and light chain joined by a disulphide bond. At cholinergic nerve endings, the heavy chain binds to presynaptic receptors and is internalized. Within the neuron, the disulphide bond is cleaved releasing the light chain into the cytoplasm. These light chains bind with a number of proteins (synaptosomal associated protein [SNAP] 25, vesicle associated membrane protein [VAMP] and syntaxin); this prevents acetylcholine vesicles from fusing with the cell membrane and, as a result, its release from the neuron is impeded. The release of acetylcholine is irreversibly inhibited by botulinum toxin but the neurons do not degenerate

---

Key point 1

- Botulinum toxin can cause transient paralysis of injected smooth or skeletal muscle in the gastrointestinal tract, which lasts for approximately 3 months.

Mr A.G. Acheson MB BCh FRCS, Specialist Registrar in General Surgery, Department of Surgery, Floor E, West Block, Queen's Medical Centre, Nottingham NG7 2UH, UK (for correspondence)

Miss N. Griffin MB ChB MRCS, Research Registrar in General Surgery, Department of Surgery, Floor E, West Block, Queen's Medical Centre, Nottingham NG7 2UH, UK

Professor J.H. Scholefield \MB ChB FRCS ChM, Professor of Surgery, Floor E, West Block, Queen's Medical Centre, Nottingham NG7 2UH, UK

and function can return to affected tissue after a period of approximately 3 months when new nerve terminals have regenerated.[2]

The inhibition of acetylcholine at motor end plates causes potent skeletal neuromuscular blockade in alpha motor neurons and, for this reason, botulinum toxin was first used in 1980 as an injection into the extra-ocular muscles to treat strabismus. Smooth muscle activity can also be reduced by inhibiting acetylcholine release from parasympathetic and cholinergic postganglionic sympathetic neurons. These effects on both skeletal and smooth muscle were the underlying rationale for developing botulinum toxin as a therapeutic tool in a number of other ophthalmological, neurological and gastrointestinal conditions.[1-4] This review focuses on the therapeutic role in the gastrointestinal tract.

BOTULINUM TOXIN IN THE UPPER GASTROINTESTINAL TRACT

ACHALASIA

Achalasia is a primary oesophageal motor disorder characterized manometrically by failure of relaxation of the lower oesophageal sphincter (LOS) and by aperistalsis of the oesophageal body. It affects approximately 1 in 100,000 individuals and gives rise to symptoms of dysphagia, regurgitation, chest pain and weight loss. Oesophageal specimens in achalasia show degeneration of the myenteric plexus associated with selective loss of inhibitory neurons (nitric oxide and vasoactive intestinal peptide). This results in unopposed excitation of smooth muscle by acetylcholine and other mediators resulting in a hypertonic LOS. Traditional treatment options include pneumatic dilatation of the LOS or surgery. More recently, botulinum toxin has been used with promising results. Calcium channel blockers and nitrates have been tried, but are only recommended prior to more definitive treatment.

Surgical myotomy for achalasia was first performed by Ernest Heller in 1913. The minimally invasive approach was introduced in 1990 and was initially performed by thoracoscopy[5] and later laparoscopy.[6] Surgical myotomy improves symptoms long-term in up to 90% of cases.[7] An antireflux procedure is often performed at the same time, as there is a 10–20% risk of developing gastro-oesophageal reflux after myotomy.[8] Pneumatic dilatation is associated with long-term success rates of 70–90%. However, there is a 1–6% risk of oesophageal perforation.[9]

Efficacy and dose of botulinum toxin in achalasia

Botulinum toxin can reduce LOS pressure when injected into the LOS of piglets.[10] The same author later showed that approximately 90% of achalasia patients improved initially following botulinum toxin injection into the LOS. The response was better in patients aged over 50 years and in those with vigorous achalasia. The average duration of response was just over 1 year but approximately 60% of patients who relapsed responded to a second injection.[3,11] Others have reproduced similar results.[12-14]

When botulinum toxin was compared to saline injection, the toxin significantly reduced symptom scores.[15,16] Patients randomised to botulinum toxin or pneumatic dilatation have comparable short-term success rates but, with time, higher failure rates with botulinum toxin have been observed.[17,18] At 12 months, cumulative remission rates in one study were 70% with pneumatic dilatation compared to 32% with botulinum toxin.[18] Pneumatic dilatation causes a greater reduction in LOS pressure than botulinum toxin and this has been found to be a better predictor of response.[14,17]

> ## Key point 2
>
> * Surgery and pneumatic dilatation give better long-term results in achalasia but botulinum toxin injection into the lower oesophageal sphincter is useful in elderly and unfit patients.

Most investigators inject a dose of 80–100 U of botulinum into the LOS to achieve the desired effect. One dose ranging study looked at 3 different doses of botulinum toxin in achalasia: 50 U, 100 U with responsive patients being re-injected with an identical dose after 30 days, and 200 U. After 30 days, 82% had responded with no clear dose-related effect. At a mean follow-up of 12 months, there was a smaller relapse rate in the patients receiving the 2 x 100 U dose (17%) compared to 47% and 43% in the groups receiving 50 U and 200 U, respectively.[19] The same authors have also compared different formulations of botulinum toxin (100 U Allergan or 250 U Dysport) and noted no significant differences in the response rate or side-effect profile.[20]

Botulinum toxin has been used in patients who have either failed other treatments or subsequently developed a recurrence of their symptoms following previous myotomy or dilatation.[14,21] There appears to be little difference in response rates in these patients compared to those who have had no prior intervention. Conversely, it has been found that surgical myotomy in patients who have received prior botulinum toxin may lead to more difficult dissection and higher perforation rate.[22]

Technique for injecting and complications
During endoscopy and using sedation, the LOS is identified as a rosette, typically seen at the squamocolumnar junction. Botulinum toxin is injected through a 5 mm sclerotherapy needle into the 4 quadrants of the LOS to give a total of 80–100 U.

Side-effects from botulinum toxin occur in up to 30% of patients and include heartburn and truncal or facial rash.[14,16]

Hoffman used endoscopic ultrasonography to confirm the position of the needle tip in the muscle layer of the LOS at injection. He hypothesised that therapeutic failure to botulinum toxin was a result of inaccurate placement of the injection due to blind delivery. All patients who had this procedure remained in remission after a mean of 8.8 months.[23] Similarly, Brant showed promising results with this technique in Chagas' achalasia.[24] Further larger studies are required to see if there is any real improvement in efficacy with this technique.

Use in children

Botulinum toxin has been used in children with good short-term results.[25] However, long-term side-effects are unknown and hence it should be used with caution. Laparoscopic surgery in children with achalasia produces excellent results and many consider this as first line treatment.[26] Botulinum toxin may be useful in children following failed pneumatic dilatation or surgery.

Cost-effectiveness

Using cost minimisation analysis, the cost of various treatment options for achalasia has been calculated based on present knowledge of success rates.[27,28] It is recognised that a certain percentage of patients will require repeat botulinum toxin injections or pneumatic dilatations to maintain response and that surgery (following pneumatic dilatations) or pneumatic dilatation (following botulinum toxin) may be required. One study calculated that botulinum toxin would cost US$5033 compared to US$3608 for pneumatic dilatation. The authors found that botulinum toxin was only less costly if life expectancy was under 2 years because of the need for repeated injections. They recommended use of botulinum toxin in older patients with co-morbidity resulting in a shortened life expectancy.[27] Another study found that laparoscopic Heller myotomy with fundoplication would cost US$10,792, significantly more expensive than either botulinum toxin or pneumatic dilatation (provided perforation rate < 10%).[28]

OTHER OESOPHAGEAL DISORDERS

Diffuse oesophageal spasm is a functional disorder of unknown aetiology, mainly affecting older people. It is characterised using manometry by multiple spontaneous, non-propulsive contractions and by swallow-induced repetitive contractions of simultaneous onset, large amplitude and long duration. It gives rise to symptoms of chest pain, dysphagia and regurgitation. Prospective studies using botulinum toxin injection for diffuse oesophageal spasm (given either at the level of the gastro-oesophageal junction or at intervals along the tubular oesophagus) have shown early response rates of 70–100%.[29] Long-term response rates appear variable (40–100% after 6 months) and patients can require further repeat injections or dilatation.

Botulinum toxin has been shown to improve symptoms for up to 6 months in patients with Chagas' disease.[24]

Botulinum toxin injection into the cricopharyngeus muscle can improve dysphagia in cricopharyngeal dysfunction.[30] It has also been reported to be effective in relieving dysphagia and dysphonia following total laryngectomy when injected into the pharyngo-oesophageal region identified to be in spasm on fluoroscopy.[31]

SPHINCTER OF ODDI DYSFUNCTION

Sphincter of Oddi dysfunction can cause recurrent upper abdominal pain and is an important, but rare, cause of post-cholecystectomy symptoms. The mainstay of diagnosis is by demonstrating increased basal pressure of the sphincter by endoscopic biliary manometry, but this is difficult to perform and is not always available. Endoscopic sphincterotomy can provide successful relief of symptoms, but it is not without its problems. Complications such as bleeding, perforation and pancreatitis can occur in over 20% of patients.

Animal studies have shown that local injection of botulinum toxin into the sphincter of Oddi reduces basal sphincter pressures.[32] Botulinum toxin was first used in 1994 as an intrasphincteric injection in patients with suspected sphincter of Oddi dysfunction and caused a significant reduction in sphincter pressure.[33] A larger study of 22 patients with manometrically confirmed sphincter of Oddi dysfunction used 100 U of toxin injected into the papilla of Vater. After 6 weeks, 12 (55%) patients were symptom-free, but most developed recurrent symptoms after several months and had associated elevated sphincter pressures. These patients all had symptomatic relief following a subsequent endoscopic sphincterotomy. Of the 10 patients who did not improve clinically after botulinum toxin, 5 had normal basal sphincter pressures and these failed to improve with a later endoscopic sphincterotomy.[34]

Similarly, other small studies have shown potential benefit of botulinum toxin in patients with recurrent acute pancreatitis due to pancreatic sphincter of Oddi dysfunction or pancreas divisum.[34,35] These studies all show that botulinum toxin can cause relaxation of the sphincter of Oddi. However, abdominal pain in patients with manometrically proven sphincter dysfunction is not always due to this condition but often other associated bowel motility disorders are responsible. Therefore, this therapy may be helpful not only as an alternative to endoscopic sphincterotomy but also as a method of selecting patients who would benefit from subsequent sphincter ablation.

Key point 3

- Botulinum toxin injections can be used as an alternative treatment for sphincter of Oddi dysfunction.

BOTULINUM TOXIN IN THE LOWER GASTROINTESTINAL TRACT

ANAL FISSURE

Anal fissure or fissure-in-ano is a common benign condition that can cause severe anal pain after defaecation, bleeding and pruritus ani. It is a linear longitudinal tear in the lining of the anal canal that extends from the dentate line to the anal verge. In 90% of cases, the tear is located in the posterior midline. It is most commonly seen in young and middle aged adults, with similar frequencies in both sexes.

The majority of anal fissures are acute and self-limiting with simple conservative dietary measures. Fissures that fail to resolve after 6 weeks are defined as chronic and these usually require pharmacological or surgical intervention to promote healing.

The pathogenesis of this condition is poorly understood, but most patients with a chronic anal fissure have raised resting anal pressures caused by hypertonicity of the internal anal sphincter (IAS) and this seems to play an important role. Local ischaemia may also be important, as there is a relative hypoperfusion at the posterior commissure of the anal canal in most people.[36]

The aim of treatment is to reduce anal hypertonia, which may improve anodermal blood flow and heal the fissure. Until approximately 5 years ago, lateral internal sphincterotomy was the 'gold standard' in treatment, producing rapid symptom relief and healing rates of over 90%, but it is now less popular as disturbances in continence can occur in up to 30% of patients.[37] Pharmacological agents (nitrates, calcium antagonists and botulinum toxin) have largely replaced surgery as first line therapy for anal fissures. They reduce anal hypertonia by causing a reversible 'chemical sphincterotomy' and long-term problems with incontinence are, therefore, avoided.

Jost and Schimrigk first described botulinum toxin as an effective treatment for uncomplicated chronic anal fissures in 1993.[4]

Site, mechanism and duration of action

It remains unclear as to whether the toxin has its main effect on the striated external sphincter or the smooth muscle fibres of the internal sphincter. Jost initially described injection into the external sphincter with a resulting decrease in voluntary squeeze pressures suggesting inhibition of acetylcholine release at the neuromuscular endplate of the external striated muscle fibres. They suggested that paralysis of the IAS takes place by diffusion.

Subsequently, others have shown that injection into the IAS causes up to a 30% drop in maximum resting anal pressure with no significant change in the squeeze pressure indicating that the IAS has been significantly weakened with no effect on the external sphincter.[38–42]

In view of these conflicting studies, there is no consensus as to the optimal anatomical site for injection. The role of weakening the external sphincter is uncertain, but investigators targeting either the internal or external sphincter still report excellent healing rates of over 70%.[38,40,43]

In vitro work shows that acetylcholine can relax the IAS in rabbits and vervet monkeys, but causes contractions in the rat. In isolated human IAS, acetylcholine is mainly relaxant, but it also has contractile properties suggesting that the action of botulinum toxin on the IAS may not only be due to inhibition of acetylcholine, as this would in many cases be expected to increase anal tone, but other mechanisms may be involved.[44,45]

Botulinum toxin has a rapid onset of action and patients are often pain-free within hours of the treatment.[46] The paralysis lasts for approximately 3 months until axonal regeneration occurs.[38] This is felt to be sufficient time to allow healing of the fissure.

Key point 4

- Botulinum toxin injected into either the external or internal anal sphincter can effectively heal chronic anal fissures.

Technique for injecting

Injection is usually performed on an out-patient basis with no sedation or local anaesthetic. The patient lies in the left lateral position and most investigators inject botulinum toxin using a 25–27 gauge needle close to the fissure or at the 3- or 9-o'clock position into either the external or internal sphincter. Maria *et al.* showed that injection of the IAS away from the site of the fissure on each side of the anterior midline produced better healing rates compared with injecting each side of the posterior midline (88% *versus* 60%, $P = 0.025$).[42]

Efficacy

Many uncontrolled trials have reported botulinum toxin to be an effective treatment for chronic anal fissure.[38,43] A double blind, randomised, placebo-controlled study of botulinum versus saline injection in 30 patients reported healing rates at 2 months of 73% and 13%, respectively ($P = 0.003$). In this study following a second injection 2 months later, 100% of patients in the botulinum group had healed.[40] A follow-on, randomised study comparing botulinum with glyceryl trinitrate in 50 patients reported healing rates of 96% and 60%, respectively ($P = 0.005$),[39] although in this study glyceryl trinitrate was only given for 6 weeks as opposed to 8 weeks as previously recommended. No relapses occurred in either of these studies during an average 15 months of follow-up. However, Jost reported 8 relapses within the first 6 months in 100 patients, but still claimed a 6-month healing rate of 79%.[43]

Recent studies have shown that combining botulinum toxin with topical nitrates in those who have failed previous nitrate therapy can produce significantly better healing rates than botulinum toxin alone.[47]

Complications

Peri-anal thrombosis is rare but has been reported in up to 10% of patients following injection. This presents as severe pain about 2–3 days after the treatment and is much more common in females. Incontinence following botulinum therapy is rare ($< 7\%$) and transient as re-innervation of the musculature occurs within a few months and continence will be regained.[48]

Dose

The dose of botulinum given may be important. Maria *et al.* suggested that by increasing the dose from 15 U to 20 U was more effective in reducing resting anal pressure and in producing long-term healing.[41] Another study showed healing at 6 months after 10 U, 15 U and 21 U injection to be 83%, 78% and 90%, respectively.[49] Other investigators have shown similar healing rates with doses as low as 5 U.[46]

Repeat botulinum injection may have a role in the treatment of recurrent anal fissures and in those patients who fail to heal after the first injection. Several small studies showed greater than 50% healing rates following a second injection using a higher dose in patients with prior failure of botulinum toxin.[40–42,50] A second injection in fissures that recurred following initially successful therapy can also heal up to 70% at 3 months.[50]

CONSTIPATION

Anismus

Anismus is due to paradoxical involuntary contraction of the external anal sphincter and/or the puborectalis during defaecation. This inappropriate contraction causes the anal canal pressure to rise and commonly causes intractable constipation. The initial management of anismus involves the use of high fibre diet, laxatives and enemas. This condition is usually treated by surgery in the form of division of the puborectalis muscle, but this is associated with high rates of failure and incontinence. Subtotal colectomy and ileostomy is another unsatisfactory alternative. Biofeedback therapy has been used to treat anismus with a variable success rate, but this may not always be available.

Hallan first described local injection of botulinum toxin into the external sphincter or puborectalis muscle as a treatment for anismus. The aim is to relax the puborectalis muscle and, therefore, increase the anorectal angle making evacuation possible. The results from this small study were encouraging, but transient incontinence was reported.[51] Several subsequent small studies have confirmed these findings, but repeated injections, as expected, were necessary to maintain a clinical improvement.[52,53] Using higher doses and ensuring more accurate placement of the toxin by using transrectal ultrasound may improve the success rate.[52]

Outlet type constipation in Parkinson's disease has been successfully treated in a similar manner by injecting and weakening the puborectalis muscle.[54]

Rectocele

Patients with anterior rectoceles have reported difficulty in defaecation in up to 70% of cases. This problem is usually treated initially by conservative measures or surgery. However, the results of surgery are often disappointing and can cause incontinence.[55] Some rectoceles may be caused by paradoxical contraction of the puborectalis muscle during defaecation. Botulinum toxin has been used to treat defaecatory dysfunction in anterior rectoceles. Some 60% of patients improved symptomatically following an injection of 30 U of toxin into the puborectalis and external sphincter. The remaining patients responded after a second rescue injection of 100 U. At 18 months follow-up, there were no relapses or complications.[56]

Hirschsprung's disease

Hirschsprung's disease is a rare disorder of childhood characterised by the absence of ganglion cells in the rectum and colon. A definitive pull-through operation for this condition usually produces excellent results, but a proportion of children develop on-going obstructive symptoms and constipation probably due to the abnormal nerve supply to the internal anal sphincter. Anal myectomy can alleviate this problem, but it often leads to permanent sphincter damage and incontinence.[57] Two small reports have shown that an intrasphincteric injection of up to 60 U of botulinum toxin

Key point 5

- Botulinum toxin therapy can be used to predict how patients will respond to a more definitive irreversible surgical procedure in conditions such as anal fissure, anismus and Hirschsprung's disease.

improved symptoms in approximately 75% of these children. Transient incontinence was reported and symptoms did tend to recur within 6 months.[58] This technique may have a role in these patients either as a therapy or in predicting which patients would benefit from a myectomy prior to the surgery.

CONCLUSIONS

Botulinum toxin has been used as an innovative therapy in many gastrointestinal disorders. Although long-term results of its use in achalasia are not as promising as initially thought, it can still be recommended for elderly patients or those patients who are unfit for, have failed, or refuse surgery or dilatation. Its role in chronic anal fissures is more convincing but despite being simple to give, effective at healing with minimal side-effects, botulinum toxin has not been widely accepted in treating this condition probably as it involves injection into the sphincter complex, injection can be painful and the drug is expensive.

Further larger randomized controlled trials are needed to confirm the toxin's efficacy, optimize its dose and method of delivery before it can be universally advocated as a treatment for sphincter of Oddi dysfunction, anismus, outlet type constipation in anterior rectocele's, Parkinson's or Hirschsprung's disease.

Key points for clinical practice

- Botulinum toxin can cause transient paralysis of injected smooth or skeletal muscle in the gastrointestinal tract, which lasts for approximately 3 months.

- Surgery and pneumatic dilatation give better long-term results in achalasia but botulinum toxin injection into the lower oesophageal sphincter is useful in elderly and unfit patients.

- Botulinum toxin injections can be used as an alternative treatment for sphincter of Oddi dysfunction.

- Botulinum toxin injected into either the external or internal anal sphincter can effectively heal chronic anal fissures.

- Botulinum toxin therapy can be used to predict how patients will respond to a more definitive irreversible surgical procedure in conditions such as anal fissure, anismus and Hirschsprung's disease.

- In some conditions, repeated injections are often necessary to produce its desired sustained effect but this treatment appears to be very safe with few reported side-effects following injection.

References

1. Jankovic J, Brin MF. Therapeutic uses of botulinum toxin. *N Engl J Med* 1991; **324**: 1186–1194.

2. Munchau A, Bhatia KP. Uses of botulinum toxin injection in medicine today. *BMJ* 2000; **320**: 161–165.
3. Pasricha PJ, Ravich WJ, Hendrix TR, Sostre S, Jones B, Kalloo AN. Treatment of achalasia with intrasphincteric injection of botulinum toxin. A pilot trial. *Ann Intern Med* 1994; **121**: 590–591.
4. Jost WH, Schimrigk K. Use of botulinum toxin in anal fissure. *Dis Colon Rectum* 1993; **36**: 974.
5. Pellegrini C, Wetter LA, Patti M *et al*. Thoracoscopic esophagomyotomy. Initial experience with a new approach for the treatment of achalasia. *Ann Surg* 1992; **216**: 291–296; discussion 296–299.
6. Cushieri A, Shimi S. Laparoscopic cardiomyotomy for achalasia. *J R Coll Surg Edinb* 1991; **36**: 152–154.
7. Csendes A, Braghetto I, Henriquez A, Cortes C. Late results of a prospective randomised study comparing forceful dilatation and oesophagomyotomy in patients with achalasia. *Gut* 1989; **30**: 299–304.
8. Vantrappen G, Janssens J. To dilate or to operate? That is the question. *Gut* 1983; **24**: 1013–1019.
9. Kadakia SC, Wong RK. Pneumatic balloon dilation for esophageal achalasia. *Gastrointest Endosc Clin North Am* 2001; **11**: 325–346.
10. Pasricha PJ, Ravich WJ, Kalloo AN. Effects of intrasphincteric botulinum toxin on the lower esophageal sphincter in piglets. *Gastroenterology* 1993; **105**: 1045–1049.
11. Pasricha PJ, Rai R, Ravich WJ, Hendrix TR, Kalloo AN. Botulinum toxin for achalasia: long-term outcome and predictors of response. *Gastroenterology* 1996; **110**: 1410–1415.
12. Annese V, D'Onofrio V, Andriulli A. Botulinum toxin in long-term therapy for achalasia. *Ann Intern Med* 1998; **128**: 696.
13. Fishman VM, Parkman HP, Schiano TD *et al*. Symptomatic improvement in achalasia after botulinum toxin injection of the lower esophageal sphincter. *Am J Gastroenterol* 1996; **91**: 1724–1730.
14. Cuilliere C, Ducrotte P, Zerbib F *et al*. Achalasia: outcome of patients treated with intrasphincteric injection of botulinum toxin. *Gut* 1997; **41**: 87–92.
15. Annese V, Basciani M, Perri F *et al*. Controlled trial of botulinum toxin injection versus placebo and pneumatic dilation in achalasia. *Gastroenterology* 1996; **111**: 1418–1424.
16. Pasricha PJ, Ravich WJ, Hendrix TR, Sostre S, Jones B, Kalloo AN. Intrasphincteric botulinum toxin for the treatment of achalasia. *N Engl J Med* 1995; **332**: 774–778.
17. Schroeder P, Slaughter R, Turbey C, Morgen D, Koehler R, Richter J. Treatment of achalasia: a botulinum toxin versus pneumatic dilatation. *Am J Gastroenterol* 1995; **90**: 1571.
18. Vaezi MF, Richter JE, Wilcox CM *et al*. Botulinum toxin versus pneumatic dilatation in the treatment of achalasia: a randomised trial. *Gut* 1999; **44**: 231–239.
19. Annese V, Bassotti G, Coccia G *et al*. A multicentre randomised study of intrasphincteric botulinum toxin in patients with oesophageal achalasia. GISMAD Achalasia Study Group. *Gut* 2000; **46**: 597–600.
20. Annese V, Bassotti G, Coccia G *et al*. Comparison of two different formulations of botulinum toxin A for the treatment of oesophageal achalasia. The Gismad Achalasia Study Group. *Aliment Pharmacol Ther* 1999; **13**: 1347–1350.
21. Annese V, Basciani M, Lombardi G *et al*. Perendoscopic injection of botulinum toxin is effective in achalasia after failure of myotomy or pneumatic dilation. *Gastrointest Endosc* 1996; **44**: 461–465.
22. Horgan S, Hudda K, Eubanks T, McAllister J, Pellegrini CA. Does botulinum toxin injection make esophagomyotomy a more difficult operation? *Surg Endosc* 1999; **13**: 576–579.
23. Hoffman BJ, Knapple WL, Bhutani MS, Verne GN, Hawes RH. Treatment of achalasia by injection of botulinum toxin under endoscopic ultrasound guidance. *Gastrointest Endosc* 1997; **45**: 77–79.
24. Brant CQ, Nakao F, Ardengh JC, Nasi A, Ferrari Jr AP. Echoendoscopic evaluation of botulinum toxin intrasphincteric injections in Chagas' disease achalasia. *Dis Esophagus* 1999; **12**: 37–40.
25. Hurwitz M, Bahar RJ, Ament ME *et al*. Evaluation of the use of botulinum toxin in children with achalasia. *J Pediatr Gastroenterol Nutr* 2000; **30**: 509–514.

26. Patti MG, Albanese CT, Holcomb 3rd GW *et al.* Laparoscopic Heller myotomy and Dor fundoplication for esophageal achalasia in children. *J Pediatr Surg* 2001; **36**: 1248–1251.

27. Panaccione R, Gregor JC, Reynolds RP, Preiksaitis HG. Intrasphincteric botulinum toxin versus pneumatic dilatation for achalasia: a cost minimization analysis. *Gastrointest Endosc* 1999; **50**: 492–498.

28. Imperiale TF, O'Connor JB, Vaezi MF, Richter JE. A cost-minimization analysis of alternative treatment strategies for achalasia. *Am J Gastroenterol* 2000; **95**: 2737–2745.

29. Nebendahl JC, Brand B, Von Schrenck T, Matsui U, Thonke F, Bohnacker Sea. Effective treatment of diffuse esophageal spasm by endoscopic injection of botulinum toxin. *Gastroenterology* 1998; **114**: A240.

30. Alberty J, Oelerich M, Ludwig K, Hartmann S, Stoll W. Efficacy of botulinum toxin A for treatment of upper esophageal sphincter dysfunction. *Laryngoscope* 2000; **110**: 1151–156.

31. Crary MA, Glowasky AL. Using botulinum toxin A to improve speech and swallowing function following total laryngectomy. *Arch Otolaryngol Head Neck Surg* 1996; **122**: 760–763.

32. Sand J, Nordback I, Arvola P, Porsti I, Kalloo A, Pasricha P. Effects of botulinum toxin A on the sphincter of Oddi: an *in vivo* and *in vitro* study. *Gut* 1998; **42**: 507–510.

33. Pasricha PJ, Miskovsky EP, Kalloo AN. Intrasphincteric injection of botulinum toxin for suspected sphincter of Oddi dysfunction. *Gut* 1994; **35**: 1319–1321.

34. Wehrmann T, Seifert H, Seipp M, Lembcke B, Caspary WF. Endoscopic injection of botulinum toxin for biliary sphincter of Oddi dysfunction. *Endoscopy* 1998; **30**: 702–707.

35. Wehrmann T, Schmitt TH, Arndt A, Lembcke B, Caspary WF, Seifert H. Endoscopic injection of botulinum toxin in patients with recurrent acute pancreatitis due to pancreatic sphincter of Oddi dysfunction. *Aliment Pharmacol Ther* 2000; **14**: 1469–1477.

36. Lund JN, Binch C, McGrath J, Sparrow RA, Scholefield JH. Topographical distribution of blood supply to the anal canal. *Br J Surg* 1999; **86**: 496–498.

37. Khubchandani IT, Reed JF. Sequelae of internal sphincterotomy for chronic fissure in ano. *Br J Surg* 1989; **76**: 431–434.

38. Gui D, Cassetta E, Anastasio G, Bentivoglio AR, Maria G, Albanese A. Botulinum toxin for chronic anal fissure. *Lancet* 1994; **344**: 1127–1128.

39. Brisinda G, Maria G, Bentivoglio AR, Cassetta E, Gui D, Albanese A. A comparison of injections of botulinum toxin and topical nitroglycerin ointment for the treatment of chronic anal fissure. *N Engl J Med* 1999; **341**: 65–69.

40. Maria G, Cassetta E, Gui D, Brisinda G, Bentivoglio AR, Albanese A. A comparison of botulinum toxin and saline for the treatment of chronic anal fissure. *N Engl J Med* 1998; **338**: 217–220.

41. Maria G, Brisinda G, Bentivoglio AR, Cassetta E, Gui D, Albanese A. Botulinum toxin injections in the internal anal sphincter for the treatment of chronic anal fissure: long-term results after two different dosage regimens. *Ann Surg* 1998; **228**: 664–669.

42. Maria G, Brisinda G, Bentivoglio AR, Cassetta E, Gui D, Albanese A. Influence of botulinum toxin site of injections on healing rate in patients with chronic anal fissure. *Am J Surg* 2000; **179**: 46–50.

43. Jost WH. One hundred cases of anal fissure treated with botulin toxin: early and long-term results. *Dis Colon Rectum* 1997; **40**: 1029–1032.

44. Burleigh DE, D'Mello A, Parks AG. Responses of isolated human internal anal sphincter to drugs and electrical field stimulation. *Gastroenterology* 1979; **77**: 484–490.

45. Hasler WL. The expanding spectrum of clinical uses for botulinum toxin: healing of chronic anal fissures. *Gastroenterology* 1999; **116**: 221–223.

46. Jost WH, Schimrigk K. Therapy of anal fissure using botulin toxin. *Dis Colon Rectum* 1994; **37**: 1340.

47. Lysy J, Israelit-Yatzkan Y, Sestiery-Ittah M, Weksler-Zangen S, Keret D, Goldin E. Topical nitrates potentiate the effect of botulinum toxin in the treatment of patients with refractory anal fissure. *Gut* 2001; **48**: 221–224.

48. Jost WH, Schanne S, Mlitz H, Schimrigk K. Perianal thrombosis following injection therapy into the external anal sphincter using botulin toxin. *Dis Colon Rectum* 1995; **38**: 781.

49. Minguez M, Melo F, Espi A *et al.* Therapeutic effects of different doses of botulinum toxin in chronic anal fissure. *Dis Colon Rectum* 1999; **42**: 1016–1021.

50. Jost WH, Schrank B. Repeat botulin toxin injections in anal fissure: in patients with relapse and after insufficient effect of first treatment. *Dig Dis Sci* 1999; **44**: 1588–1589.
51. Hallan RI, Williams NS, Melling J, Waldron DJ, Womack NR, Morrison JF. Treatment of anismus in intractable constipation with botulinum A toxin. *Lancet* 1988; **2**: 714–717.
52. Maria G, Brisinda G, Bentivoglio AR, Cassetta E, Albanese A. Botulinum toxin in the treatment of outlet obstruction constipation caused by puborectalis syndrome. *Dis Colon Rectum* 2000; **43**: 376–380.
53. Shafik A, El-Sibai O. Botulin toxin in the treatment of nonrelaxing puborectalis syndrome. *Dig Surg* 1998; **15**: 347–351.
54. Albanese A, Maria G, Bentivoglio A, Brisinda G, Cassetta E, Tonali P. Botulinum toxin in the treatment of chronic constipation in Parkinson's disease. *Eur J Neurol* 1997; **4**: S81–S83.
55. Arnold MW, Stewart WR, Aguilar PS. Rectocele repair. Four years' experience. *Dis Colon Rectum* 1990; **33**: 684–687.
56. Maria G, Brisinda G, Bentivoglio AR, Albanese A, Sganga G, Castagneto M. Anterior rectocele due to obstructed defecation relieved by botulinum toxin. *Surgery* 2001; **129**: 524–529.
57. Abbas Banani S, Forootan H. Role of anorectal myectomy after failed endorectal pull-through in Hirschsprung's disease. *J Pediatr Surg* 1994; **29**: 1307–1309.
58. Minkes RK, Langer JC. A prospective study of botulinum toxin for internal anal sphincter hypertonicity in children with Hirschsprung's disease. *J Pediatr Surg* 2000; **35**: 1733–1736.

S. Misra A. Chaturvedi N.C. Misra

7

Oral carcinoma

Carcinoma of the oral cavity ranks as the twelfth most common cancer in the world and eighth most frequent in males.[1] Nearly one-third of the total cancers seen in India originate in the head and neck area compared to 5% or less in the USA. Carcinoma of the oral cavity accounts for over 30% of all head and neck cancers in India. The term oral cavity refers to lips, buccal mucosa, alveolar ridges (upper and lower gingiva) retromolar trigone, hard palate, floor of mouth and anterior two-thirds of tongue (oral or mobile tongue). As cancer of the lip behaves clinically like skin cancer, it will not be discussed further.

EPIDEMIOLOGY

World-wide, cancers of the oral cavity are common in regions where tobacco use and alcohol consumption are high. For men, the highest age-adjusted incidence rate (AAR) for cancer of the oral cavity is in France (13.4/100,000) and the lowest in Japan (0.5/100,000). For women, the highest AAR is in India (15.7/100,000) and lowest in Japan (0.2/100,000).[2] Other countries like Brazil, Puerto Rico, parts of Canada, and Czechoslovakia also have high incidence rates in men. The AAR and truncated rate of incidence in India is 3–8 times that of Oxford, UK.[3] There is not only a marked variation in the incidence and mortality rate from oral cancer between various countries but also between ethnic groups and regions of one country. Large differences in individual sites in the oral cavity is also seen, perhaps related to the difference in the practice of tobacco habits. In the west, cancer of the tongue and the floor of the mouth are the commonest subsites while in the Indian subcontinent the

Dr Sanjeev Misra MS MCh MAMS FICS, Assistant Professor, Department of Surgical Oncology, King George's Medical College, Lucknow – 226003, India (for correspondence)

Dr Arun Chaturvedi MBBS MS MAMS, Professor of Surgical Oncology, Department of Surgical Oncology, King George's Medical College, Lucknow – 226007, India

Dr N.C. Misra, MBBS MS FRCS FICS FACS FAMS, Professor of Surgery (Oncology), Director Lucknow Cancer Centre, King George's Medical College, Lucknow – 226007, India

buccal mucosa and gingiva are more often affected due to placement of the tobacco quid in the oral cavity. This cancer of the gingivo–buccal complex has been aptly described as the Indian oral cancer.

AETIOLOGY

Life-style habits and social factors have a major impact on development of oral cancer. Epidemiological studies have shown that use of alcohol, tobacco (smoked or smokeless) and betel nut is associated with a high risk of oral cancer. Other factors like infection with viruses, such as human papilloma virus (HPV) and Epstein-Barr virus, also contribute to a lesser extent. These influences occurring together can cause several fold increase in the risk of carcinogenesis.

Tobacco

The association between cancer of the oral cavity, and the use of tobacco in either the smokeless or smoked form has been demonstrated in several studies from all over the world. The risk estimates for various habits from India and Southeast Asia have shown that the highest risks are associated with the synergistic effects of smoking and chewing of tobacco.[4] Consumption of alcohol further adds to this risk.[5] A dose response relationship between tobacco chewing and the risk of oral cancer has also been shown.[6] Long-term exposure to tobacco quid, especially in the form of the night-quid, results in risk ratios as high as 63.

Smokeless tobacco is available in many forms in India where it is chewed alone, along with *pan* (betel leaf, catechu, areca nut and slaked lime) or as a commercially available *pan masala* (tobacco with areca nut, slaked lime, catechu and condiments). There is sufficient evidence to suspect that *pan masala* with tobacco is carcinogenic.[7]

Key point 1

- Oral cancer has a strong relationship to tobacco and alcohol consumption.

Alcohol

Alcohol may act as a promoter, an irritant or solvent to increase the solubility of carcinogens from tobacco leading to development of cancer. Experimental evidence suggests that alcohol suppresses the efficiency of DNA repair after exposure to nitrosamine compounds.[5]

Dietary factors

Dietary factors may also have a role in the development of oral cancer. Diets having fresh fruits and vegetables, particularly those rich in vitamin A, have a protective effect against oral cancer and precancer.[8] Iron deficiency is associated with development of Plummer-Vinson syndrome where squamous cell carcinoma (SCC) of the hypopharynx and oral cavity are frequent.

Other risk factors

A direct link between human papilloma virus (HPV) and oral cancer remains to be established. HPV can be detected in 60–90% of oral cancers;[9] however, its role in the development of cancer is uncertain as it is present in nearly 40% of normal oral cavities.[10] Poor dental hygiene and chronic irritation from ill fitting dentures or a sharp tooth have also been implicated in the genesis of oral cancer.

ORAL PRECANCER

Oral cancer is preceded in more than 70% of patients by a recognized premalignant lesion or condition. These have the same association with tobacco and alcohol as oral cancer. The risk for development of oral cancer in tobacco users with precancer is 69 times that of tobacco users who do not have precancer.[11] Identification and adequate treatment of oral precancer is thus extremely important. Oral precancer can either be a precancerous lesion or a precancerous condition.

PRECANCEROUS LESIONS

This is morphologically altered tissue in which cancer is more likely to occur than in its apparently normal counterpart. Leukoplakia, erythroplakia and palatal changes associated with reverse 'chutta' smoking are examples of precancerous lesions.

Oral leukoplakia

The condition is defined as a white patch or plaque that cannot be characterized clinically or pathologically as any other disease. The term does not carry any histological connotation. Leukoplakia may persist, regress spontaneously, recur or progress to oral cancer. Oral cancer develops in 3–6% of leukoplakias. Nodular leukoplakias have the highest risk for malignant transformation (20%) compared to homogenous leukoplakias (0.5–1.7%). Increase in nodularity and thickness, ulceration, rolled margins, growths or indurated areas may represent early clinical features of malignancy. Histologically, oral leukoplakias can have hyperkeratosis, parakeratosis or acanthosis. Premalignant oral leukoplakia shows dysplasia characterized by abnormal cell orientation and proliferation. Malignant progression occurs in 10–14% of dysplasias.[12]

Erythroplakia

These red velvety plaques cannot be characterized clinically or pathologically as any other disease. Erythroplakias show moderate to severe dysplasia and have much higher risk of malignant change.[12]

PRECANCEROUS CONDITIONS

These are generalized states associated with significantly increased risk of cancer. Examples are syphilis, sideropenic dysphagia and oral submucous fibrosis (SMF). Oral lichen planus is regarded as a possibly precancerous condition. SMF is the most important precancerous condition in India.

Oral submucous fibrosis (SMF)

SMF is a high-risk precancerous condition. A strong association has been shown between SMF and chewing areca nut. SMF can affect any part of the oral mucosa. It is characterized by mucosal rigidity of varying intensity due to fibro-elastic transformation of juxta-epithelial connective tissue. Palpable fibrous bands especially over the buccal mucosa, retromolar area and rima oris are diagnostic. Mouth opening is restricted and is impossible in severe cases. SMF is not known to regress either spontaneously or with cessation of areca nut chewing. The condition can remain stationary or may become worse and spread to involve wider areas.[13]

PATHOLOGY OF ORAL CANCER

More than 90% of oral cancers are squamous cell carcinomas (SCCs), and can present as either an exophytic or ulcerative lesion or as a combination of both. Exophytic lesions are less aggressive compared to ulcerative ones. Multiple synchronous and metachronous primary SCCs can develop in the oral cavity as a consequence of field cancerisation – dysplasia affecting a wide area of the oral mucosa and upper aero-digestive tract.

There are two common variants of the classical SCC – basaloid SCC and verrucous carcinoma (VC). VC carries a more favourable prognosis and rarely metastasizes to cervical nodes. It presents as an exophytic, whitish warty, bulky, cauliflower-like growth. The basaloid variant, on the other hand, is more aggressive than even the poorly differentiated SCC and usually presents with advanced disease and distant metastasis. Sarcomatoid carcinomas are particularly lethal, rapidly growing, bulky, polypoidal cancers.

Knowledge of the mode of spread of oral cancer is important for developing a rational therapeutic approach. Local spread to adjacent structures may lead to invasion of the underlying soft tissue and muscles, bone or neurovascular structures. The mandible may be involved by infiltration through its dental sockets or dental pores on the edentulous alveolar ridge.[14] These cells proceed along the root of the tooth into the cancellous part of the mandible and then along the mandibular canal. This understanding has led to the development of mandible-sparing surgical resections. Cervical lymph nodes are the most commonly involved metastatic site. The neck has been divided into 5 nodal levels for clinical staging and treatment planning (Table 1). The oral cavity has a fairly predictable lymphatic drainage. The first echelon lymph nodes of primary SCC of the oral cavity are in the supra-omohyoid triangle of the neck (Levels I, II, III). Skip metastasis from primary carcinomas of the oral tongue have been reported and may occur in 15% of patients without involvement of the first echelon lymph nodes.[15] Spread to lymph nodes in the posterior triangle in the absence of metastasis at other levels is rare.[16] The risk of nodal metastasis from oral cancer is related to several factors – site of the primary, T stage, depth of invasion, histological grade, vascular and perineural invasion. Tumours of the tongue have the highest incidence of neck metastasis followed in descending order by tumours of the floor of the mouth, lower alveolus, buccal mucosa, upper alveolus and hard palate. For tumours of the tongue and floor of the mouth thicker tumours (≥ 2 mm) carry a higher risk (25–41%) of dissemination to regional lymph

Table 1 Nodal levels in the neck

Level I	Submental and submandibular triangle lymph nodes
Level II	Upper deep jugular lymph nodes (skull base to carotid bifurcation)
Level III	Mid deep jugular lymph nodes (carotid bifurcation to omohyoid muscle inferiorly)
Level IV	Lower jugular lymph nodes (omohyoid muscle to clavicle)
Level V	Lymph nodes in the posterior triangle

nodes than tumours < 2 mm (7.5%).[17] Increasing T stage, endophytic tumours, poor differentiation and neurovascular invasion increase the risk of lymph node metastasis and indicate a poor prognosis. Distant metastasis from primary SCC of the oral cavity at the time of initial diagnosis are exceedingly rare. The most frequent sites for distant metastasis are lungs and bones; metastases tend to occur in patients with loco-regionally advanced or recurrent disease.

CLINICAL FEATURES

The goal of evaluating a patient with oral cancer is to assess the extent of disease and to define the tumour type histologically. Patients present with a persistent ulcer or sore in the mouth, exophytic growth, loosening of teeth, ill-fitting dentures, trismus, ankyloglossia or weight loss. Pain is a late feature and is localized or may be referred to the ear. Patients with advanced disease may present with orocutaneous fistula, severe trismus and lymph node metastasis. Many patients have associated premalignant lesions. An asymptomatic lesion, with a history of tobacco and/or alcohol consumption, should raise suspicion of oral cancer and should be biopsied.

Examination assesses the extent of involvement of critical structures such as the mandible, the musculature of the floor of the mouth, and cervical nodes. The presence of trismus suggests deep invasion with involvement of pterygoid, temporalis or masseter muscle. It is important to determine whether this trismus is due to associated submucous fibrosis or malignant disease. Trismus and ankyloglossia are ominous signs indicating poor prognosis.

The clinician should evaluate any medical and nutritional problems. Common problems in patients with cancer of the oral cavity are hepatic disease, pulmonary disease and malnutrition. Dental consultation should be obtained if radiation is being planned.

Key point 2

• Oral cancer is easily detectable and has a well-defined premalignant presentation. A non-healing ulcer/growth in the oral cavity should be biopsied.

INVESTIGATIONS

BIOPSY

Biopsy of the lesion is mandatory before treatment. Often this can be done under local anaesthesia. The biopsy should be deep and encompass a portion of the tumour as well as adjacent normal appearing mucosa. Superficial biopsies are inconclusive and often yield negative results. In suspected verrucous carcinomas, where basement membrane is intact, a deep biopsy is mandatory to reach a diagnosis. Toludine blue staining can be used to target biopsies for suspicious early lesions,[18] but has a high false positivity as inflammatory and non-cancerous lesions also stain. It is not routinely recommended.

IMAGING

Investigative work up depends on the extent of the disease. Patients with early lesions do not need an extensive evaluation. An orthopantomogram (OPG) or oblique view radiograph of the mandible are cost-effective initial investigations to assess mandibular involvement. OPG provides information regarding the entire mandible, but is limited in its ability to evaluate the symphysis and lingual cortex. In lesions close to these areas, OPG may be supplemented with dental occlusal and intra-oral X-rays.

Computerised tomography (CT) of the mandible can be used in selected cases where the above imaging is inadequate. A cross-sectional representation of the entire mandible may be seen using Dentascan, a software package which reconstructs the CT image. CT gives additional information regarding the extent of mandibular involvement, malignant infiltration and cervical nodal disease.

Magnetic resonance imaging (MRI) can be used to determine soft tissue and peri-neural involvement. MRI gives excellent definition of the extent of cancer involving the tongue and may be especially useful where lesions are not visible on CT.

However, all patients do not need CT or MRI. CT is indicated in patients with trismus, lesions abutting the mandible, where marginal mandibulectomy is being planned, to evaluate the clinically negative (N0) neck, and in patients with large nodes to look for carotid artery involvement. van den Brekel et al.[19] compared the accuracy of palpation, ultrasound, ultrasound-guided fine needle cytology (FNAC), CT and MRI in the diagnosis of cervical metastasis in clinically N0 neck. The highest rate of accuracy was with ultrasound-guided FNAC (86%), followed by MRI (75%), CT (66%), ultrasound (68%) and palpation (59%). None of the imaging methods can determine occult metastatic disease in lymph nodes. Ultrasound-guided aspiration when rigorously applied is useful in the surveillance of patients with clinically N0 necks after treatment with transoral tumour excision without elective neck dissection. All patients should undergo chest X-ray.

LABORATORY INVESTIGATIONS

These are non-specific and are done to evaluate the patient's fitness for surgery and to exclude concurrent medical illness. These usually include a full blood count and renal and liver function tests.

STAGING

The UICC/AJCC[20] TNM staging system is currently followed (Table 2). Staging is defined through physical examination, diagnostic tests and biopsies.

Though used extensively, the current clinical staging system is not perfect. It ignores the depth of invasion, node fixity and level of nodal disease which are important prognostic factors. In addition, clinical examination of the neck can be inaccurate and may miss nodal metastatic disease in 16–60% patients.[21] Finally, TNM staging does not help in deciding operability in a given patient.

Table 2 AJCC/UICC* staging of oral cavity tumours

Primary			
Tis	Carcinoma *in situ*		
T1	Tumour ≤ 2 cm		
T2	Tumour > 2 cm to ≤ 4 cm		
T3	Tumour > 4 cm		
T4	Tumour invades adjacent structures (*e.g.* through cortical bone; into deep (extrinsic) muscle of tongue, maxillary sinus, skin)		
Neck			
N0	No clinically palpable nodes		
N1	Single ipsilateral node ≤ 3 cm		
N2a	Single ipsilateral node > 3 cm to 6 cm		
N2b	Multiple ipsilateral nodes ≤ 6 cm		
N2c	Bilateral or contralateral nodes ≤ 6 cm		
N3	Nodes > 6 cm		
Distant metastasis			
MX	Distant metastasis cannot be assessed		
M0	No distant metastasis		
M1	Distant metastasis		
Stage grouping			
Stage 0	Tis	N0	M0
Stage I	T1	N0	M0
Stage II	T2	N0	M0
Stage III	T3	N0	M0
	T1	N1	M0
	T2	N1	M0
	T3	N1	M0
Stage IVA	T4	N0	M0
	T4	N1	M0
	Any T	N2	M0
Stage IVB	Any T	N3	M0
Stage IVC	Any T	Any N	M1

*American Joint Committee on Cancer; Union International Contre le Cancer (International Union Against Cancer).

TREATMENT

Three major therapeutic modalities are available: surgery, radiation and chemotherapy. Surgery or radiation therapy are used alone or in combination, with or without chemotherapy. The choice of therapy depends on the site and stage of disease, the patient's physical, social and personal status, the physician's experience and skills, and the availability of treatment facilities.

Early lesions (T1, T2) can be treated effectively with either surgery or radiation as a single modality. Certain factors influence this decision. For example, in the presence of associated SMF, surgery is preferable to radiation therapy. Lesions located in the lower gingivo-buccal sulcus or involving the mandible are not treated with radiation because of proximity to bone and the risk of osteo-radionecrosis. Advanced lesions (stage III/IV) require combined modality treatment.

SURGERY

Surgery is one of the major modalities for treating oral cancer. The aim of surgical treatment is to excise the entire primary lesion three-dimensionally, with clear margins, and to treat effectively the regional lymph nodes. This ablative surgery is followed by primary reconstruction to provide rapid healing, restore function and appearance and thereby improve patient's quality-of-life.

Treatment of the primary

Generally, the choice of initial treatment for early stage oral cancer (T1 and T2) is surgery. Surgical treatment is expeditious, cost-effective, has fewer long-term sequelae and has the advantage of allowing repeated interventions in patients who develop multiple primary lesions. The disadvantage of surgery is the risk of anaesthesia, and aesthetic and functional disability. Resection can be either by a per-oral approach, upper or lower cheek flap, visor flap or mandibulotomy approach depending upon the size and location of the primary. Per-oral resection is possible in easily accessible, small lesions (usually ≤ 2 cm), without or with minimal mandibular involvement not requiring full thickness mandibular resection and with good mouth opening. Posterior, poorly accessible, large cancers requiring full thickness mandibular resection need other approaches.

Oral cancers can abut or involve the mandible. The need to resect any part of the mandible depends upon the involvement of the mandible and its proximity to the tumour. Mandibular sparing techniques like marginal mandibulectomy have gained popularity for oral cancers. Marginal mandibulectomy is indicated in cancers of the floor of the mouth or buccal mucosa in close proximity to the lower gingiva or extending onto the mandible without clinical or radiological mandibular involvement. It may also be appropriate in patients with minimal cortical mandibular invasion. Marginal mandibulectomy involves an in-continuity excision of tumour with a margin of mandible and overlying gingiva. Mandibular continuity is maintained and a much better cosmetic and functional end result is achieved. A segment of bone at least 1 cm thick must be left inferiorly. Where gross clinical and radiological involvement of the mandible is present, or in deeply infiltrating lesions of the gingivo-buccal sulcus where mandible is uninvolved, but there is paramandibular infiltration, marginal mandibulectomy should not be done as the margin of resection may pass through infiltrated paramandibular tissue.[22] Marginal mandibulectomy is also contra-indicated in patients who have received previous radiotherapy as the pattern of invasion is less predictable, healing is delayed, and there is risk of osteo-radionecrosis and fracture.

Marginal mandibulectomy should not be attempted for retromolar lesions as clearance of the pterygoid region is possible only after resecting the ascending ramus of the mandible. Results of marginal mandibulectomy for gingivo-buccal sulcus carcinomas show an overall control rate of 79%.[22] Lesions that directly invade the bone require a segmental or hemimandibulectomy. Recent dental extraction at the site of tumour opens a portal for tumour spread into the mandible and thus usually requires a segmental mandibulectomy. In tumours involving the inferior alveolar canal, an aggressive mandibulectomy from the entry of the inferior alveolar nerve to mental foramen should be performed. Mandibulectomy is seldom required for oral tongue lesions but is often required for gingivo-buccal sulcus cancers.

Resection of the posterior part of the body or ramus of mandible leaves very little aesthetic deformity. However, there is always functional compromise with segmental resection of any part of the mandible. Resection of the anterior arch results in significant functional and cosmetic deformity (Andy Gump deformity) and immediate reconstruction should be done using an osteo-myocutaneous flap or free microvascular bone graft. If immediate reconstruction is not feasible or desirable, the mandibular stirrups should be immobilized by internal, external or interdental fixation.

Large primary tumours of the tongue with involvement of the floor of the mouth not involving or approaching the mandible and not suitable for per-oral excision can be resected monobloc via a mandibulotomy approach without violating oncological principles. A paramedian mandibulotomy with mandibular swing is preferred over a midline mandibulotomy as it does not disturb the hyomandibular complex and preserves the ability to swallow.

Radical ablative surgery is followed by reconstructive surgery. Small surgical defects do not usually need reconstruction. Larger defects may be reconstructed by primary closure, skin graft, loco-regional flaps or free tissue transfer from different sites.

Key point 3

- Early stage disease (stage I/II) can be cured with either surgery or radiation alone. Choice of treatment depends on treatment centre and patient factors.

Treatment of the neck

Surgical treatment of the neck depends on nodal status in the neck. In patients with clinically positive lymph nodes, radical neck dissection (RND) is the gold standard. A modified radical neck dissection (MRND) may give better cosmetic and functional results[23] for N1 and selected N2 patients. The classical RND removes all 5 levels of cervical nodes, sternocleidomastoid (SCM), internal jugular vein (IJV) and spinal accessory nerve (SAN). MRND also involves removal of all 5 levels of cervical nodes with the modifications shown in Table 3. Type 1 MRND is preferred over type II/III MRND.[16] A supra-omohyoid neck dissection (SOHND – clearance of level I, II and III nodes with preservation of SCM, IJV and SAN) plus postoperative radiation therapy has been advocated by some authors for N1, level I disease.[24-27] However, others have strongly condemned it.[28,29] There are still no prospective randomised

Table 3 Modifications of radical neck dissection (MRND). In all types, all 5 levels of cervical nodes are removed. [SAN: spinal accessory nerve; IJV: internal jugular vein; SCM: sternocleidomastoid muscle.]

Type 1 MRND	Preservation of SAN
Type 2 MRND	Preservation of SAN and IJV
Type 3 MRND	Preservation of SAN, IJV, and SCM

trials comparing SOHND with RND in the clinically positive neck. Patients with a history of radiation therapy to the neck and clinically positive nodes should undergo a RND rather than MRND because of the diffuse nature of disease.

Occult nodal metastatic disease is present in 5–40% of oral cancers[30–32] depending on T status and grade of primary. The clinically N0 neck should be treated by SOHND if the risk of occult nodal metastasis is greater than 15–20%, in patients with a T3/T4 primary, if it is necessary to enter the neck to resect the primary, in short-necked individuals who require a bulky flap for oral reconstruction (to create space in the neck) and in patients who are unreliable for follow-up.[33] Patients with T1/T2 cancers of the gingivo-buccal complex do not require elective neck treatment,[34] while patients with T1/T2 tongue tumours and cancers of the floor of the mouth ≥2 mm thick require elective neck dissection.[17,35] In patients undergoing elective SOHND, approximately 24–31% will have histological evidence of lymph node metastasis.[24,29]

Patients who have pathologically positive neck nodes after SOHND should receive additional treatment. If detected positive on the operating table (by frozen section examination), then SOHND should be changed to RND or MRND. If positive lymph nodes are diagnosed on histopathology following surgery, patients should either undergo subsequent RND or postoperative radiotherapy.[25,27–29,35–37] The failure rate in pathologically positive, clinically N0 necks ranges from 10–24%[28] depending on the number of positive nodes and the presence of extracapsular spread (ECS). When postoperative radiation therapy is added, the failure rate drops to 0–15%.[28,29] Patients with single, positive, level I node only, without extracapsular spread, may not need additional treatment.[36,38,39] A randomized trial[40] compared SOHND with comprehensive neck dissection in patients with clinically N0 nodes. There was no difference in the regional control and overall survival rates between the two groups. However, SOHND alone is inadequate treatment for patients with pathologically confirmed or clinically positive nodes. Byers *et al.*[15] have reported skip metastasis to level IV in 15% of patients with tongue cancers, and they advocate elective levels I through IV node dissection (extended SOHND); others, however, do not agree.[41]

If the primary tumour is being treated with definitive radiation therapy, then the clinically N0 neck with a significant risk of occult metastasis should be treated electively with external beam radiation.

Another option for managing the N0 neck is observation alone. This approach may not be appropriate for necks that are thick and difficult to examine, patients who are unreliable for follow-up and in advanced cancers with a high risk of neck metastasis. Furthermore, a decrease in regional control and overall survival rates has been reported in patients not undergoing an elective neck dissection.[37,42,43] Where palpation alone is used to assess the neck, 24–57% of patients develop neck metastasis and the reported salvage rate varies from 27–82% (average 50%).[44] van den Brekel *et al.*[44] reported aggressive observation of the N0 neck using ultrasound-guided FNAC for initial staging and follow-up. They reported a high rate of neck salvage, early detection of recurrence and prognosis comparable to that reported for patients treated with elective neck dissection. This approach requires motivation, good instruction to the patient, and a well-trained ultrasonologist dedicated to do repeated examinations and aspiration of small lymph nodes. Recently, lymphatic mapping has been used in N0 oral cancer patients but this requires further studies.[45] Nodal spread can occur to both sides of the neck specially in lesions close to midline. In patients with bilateral nodal metastasis, a bilateral neck dissection with preservation of the IJV on at least one side (the less affected side) is indicated.

Key point 4

- Advanced stage disease (stage III/IV) requires combined modality treatment of radical surgery plus reconstruction followed by postoperative radiation therapy.

RADIATION THERAPY

Radiation therapy and surgery have equal success in controlling early lesions of the oral cavity. Radiation is given either as external beam, brachytherapy or a combination of both. In most instances, both external and interstitial treatment are required for maximal therapeutic effect. Radiotherapy is usually not the preferred modality of treatment for early gingivo-buccal complex cancers (T1, T2) due to the close proximity of the tumour to bone and the risk of radionecrosis. Although radiation of the oral cavity may result in organ preservation, its long-term sequelae and complications are significant. Xerostomia, tissue oedema, erythema, skin slough, ulceration, dental caries and osteo-radionecrosis make definitive radiation therapy unattractive for early oral cancer. Radiation therapy is used for early lesions of the tongue, buccal mucosa and gingivo-buccal sulcus when the patient is not medically fit or is unwilling for surgery. The total dose of definitive radiation therapy is usually 65–75 Gy to the primary and neck for clinically evident disease, and at least 50 Gy for low-risk cervical disease.

In patients with advanced lesions (T3, T4), a combination of surgery and radiation therapy provides a better chance of cure than either modality alone. Despite the theoretical advantages of delivering radiation therapy pre-operatively, the general preference is to deliver radiation after surgery because of the deleterious effects of pre-operative radiation on wound healing. Pre-operative radiation or definitive radiation therapy is used for advanced (stage III/IV) inoperable disease or where the patient is unfit or unwilling for surgery. In these patients, radiation provides effective palliation and may also help in down-staging inoperable patients to a more operable stage of disease. For   gingivo-buccal cancers, the 3-year survival for stages III and IV disease treated with radiation or surgery alone is 41% and 15%, respectively. These rates increase to 60% and 35%, respectively, when surgery is combined with postoperative radiation therapy.[46] When adjuvant radiation therapy was used for stages III and IV oral tongue tumours, loco-regional control increased from 57% to 71%.[47]

Postoperative radiation therapy to the primary site decreases local recurrence and is indicated in patients with T3/T4 primary, residual microscopic tumour or positive surgical margins or with gross residual tumour after resection.[48,49] Adjuvant radiation therapy to the neck is indicated in patients showing extracapsular spread, pathologically positive lymph nodes after SOHND and multiple positive lymph nodes after RND. Adjuvant radiation therapy to the neck also decreases local failure rate. A dose of at least 60 Gy or more to the primary site and neck, with a boost to areas at increased risk of local recurrence, is recommended for adjuvant treatment. In the clinically N0 or N1 neck, elective neck irradiation is used if treatment of the primary with radiation therapy is effective.

Key point 5

- Inoperable disease is managed by radiation therapy with or without chemotherapy.

Use of concurrent chemo-irridation has been described for advanced head and neck SCC by several authors.[50] Most of these trials have used cisplatin-based chemotherapy along with radiation to improve the loco-regional control and to prevent distant metastasis. Though the optimal dose and timing of radiation and chemotherapy is still uncertain, there is no doubt about its effectiveness compared to radiation therapy alone. However, there is significant treatment-related morbidity.[50] Pre-operative concurrent chemoradiation has also been used with gratifying results.[51]

CHEMOTHERAPY

Chemotherapy has been used in the palliative, neo-adjuvant and adjuvant settings or concurrently with radiation. Drugs most commonly used are methotrexate, 5-fluorouracil (5FU), cisplatin, bleomycin, or ifosfamide either alone or in combination. In patients with advanced or metastatic oral cancer, chemotherapy is quite effective in providing palliation. Cisplatin-based combination chemotherapy is more effective than single agent chemotherapy. Response to cisplatin and infusion 5FU occurs in two-thirds of patients with a

Key point 6

- Chemotherapy can be used as palliation for advanced or recurrent oral cancers.

complete response in 5–15%. Patients with poor performance status should not be given palliative chemotherapy but only symptomatic and supportive treatment.

The aim of using neo-adjuvant chemotherapy is to down-stage the tumour and improve the outcome in terms of survival (overall and disease-free), organ preservation and quality-of-life. It is used in patients with advanced tumours with borderline operability or inoperable disease.[52–54] Chemotherapy is very effective in verrucous carcinomas with a high and durable response.[55]

Adjuvant chemotherapy aims at improving survival. It has shown reduction in the rate of distant metastasis in high-risk patients but without any effect on overall survival and its role remains uncertain. A recent meta-analysis[56] of randomised trials evaluating the role of chemotherapy added to loco-regional treatment in head and neck SCC has been reported. The results suggest a 4% absolute survival benefit at 5 years for patients receiving chemotherapy. The greatest absolute survival benefit at 5 years was 8% for concurrent chemoradiation, 2% for neo-adjuvant chemotherapy, and 1% for adjuvant chemotherapy.

PROGNOSIS AND SURVIVAL

The stage of disease at the time of presentation is the single most important prognostic factor. Early stages (stage I/II) have 5-year survival of 31–100% while survival of advanced stages (stage III/IV) is 7–41% only depending on the site of disease.[57] Stage-for-stage, tongue cancer has poorer prognosis compared to other subsites of oral cavity.[58] Lymph node metastasis, number of lymph nodes involved, and extracapsular spread are poor prognostic factors.

Key points for clinical practice

- Oral cancer has a strong relationship to tobacco and alcohol consumption.
- Oral cancer is easily detectable and has a well-defined premalignant presentation. A non-healing ulcer/growth in the oral cavity should be biopsied.
- Early stage disease (stage I/II) can be cured with either surgery or radiation alone. Choice of treatment depends on treatment centre and patient factors.
- Advanced stage disease (stage III/IV) requires combined modality treatment of radical surgery plus reconstruction followed by postoperative radiation therapy.
- Inoperable disease is managed by radiation therapy with or without chemotherapy.
- Chemotherapy can be used as palliation for advanced or recurrent oral cancers.

References

1. Parkin DM, Pisani P, Ferlay J. Estimates of the worldwide incidence of 25 major cancers in 1990. *Int J Cancer* 1999; **80**: 827–841.
2. International Agency for Research on Cancer. *Patterns of Cancer in Five Continents.* IARC Scientific Publication 102. Lyon: International Agency for Research on Cancer, 1990; 1–160.
3. Indian Council of Medical Research, National Cancer Registry Programme. *Consolidated Report of the Population Based Cancer Registries, Incidence and Distribution of Cancer: 1990–96.* Bangalore: Indian Council of Medical Research, 2001; 20–35.
4. Jayant K, Balakrishnan V, Sanghvi LD, Jussawalla DJ. Quantification of the role of smoking and chewing tobacco in oral, pharyngeal and oesophageal cancers. *Br J Cancer* 1977; **35**: 232–235.
5. Ogden GR, Wight AJ. Aetiology of oral cancer-alcohol. *Br J Oral Maxillofac Surg* 1998; **36**: 247–251.
6. International Agency for Research on Cancer. *Tobacco Habits other than Smoking: betel quid and areca nut chewing and some related nitrosamines.* IARC Monographs on the Evaluation of Carcinogenic Risks of Chemicals to Humans, Vol. 37. Lyon: International Agency for Research on Cancer, 1986.
7. Chaudhry K. Is pan masala-containing tobacco carcinogenic? *Natl Med J India* 1999; **12**: 21–27.
8. Hirayama T. Epidemiology of cancer of the mouth. *NCI Monogr* 1982; **62**: 179–183.
9. Watts SL, Brewer EE, Fry TL. Human papillomavirus DNA types in squamous cell carcinoma of the head and neck. *Oral Surg Oral Med Oral Pathol Oral Radiol Endod* 1991; **71**: 701–707.
10. Woods KV, Shilltoe EJ, Spitz MR, Schantz SP, Adler-Storthz K. Analysis of human papillomavirus DNA in oral squamous cell carcinomas. *J Oral Pathol* 1993; **22**: 101–108.
11. Gupta PC, Bhonsle RB, Murti PR. An epidemiologic assessment of cancer risk in oral precancerous lesions in India with special reference to nodular leukoplakia. *Cancer* 1989; **63**: 2247–2252.
12. Bouquot JE. Oral leukoplakia and erythroplakia: a review and update. *Prac Periodont Aesth Dent* 1994; **6**: 9–17.
13. Sankaranarayanan R. Oral cancer in India: an epidemiologic and clinical review. *Oral Surg Oral Med Oral Pathol Oral Radiol Endod* 1990; **69**: 325–330.
14. McGregor IA, McDonald DC. Spread of squamous carcinoma to the non-irradiated edentulous mandible: a preliminary study. *Head Neck* 1987; **9**: 157–161.
15. Byers RM, Weber RS, Andrews T et al. Frequency and therapeutic implications of 'skip metastases' in the neck from squamous carcinoma of the oral tongue. *Head Neck* 1997; **19**: 14–19.
16. Shah JP, Andersen PE. Evolving role of modifications in neck dissection for oral squamous carcinoma. *Br J Oral Maxillofac Surg* 1995; **33**: 3–8.
17. Spiro RH, Huvos AG, Wong GY et al. Predictive value of tumor thickness in squamous cell carcinoma confined to the tongue and floor of the mouth. *Am J Surg* 1986; **152**: 351–353.
18. Misra NC, Chawla TN, Srivastava YC, Jaiswal MSD. Toludine blue staining test as a diagnostic tool for early oral carcinoma. *Asian J Med* 1974; **10**: 91.
19. van den Brekel MWM, Castelijins JA, Stel HV et al. Modern imaging techniques and ultrasound-guided aspiration cytology for the assessment of neck node metastases: a prospective comparative study. *Eur Arch Otorhinolaryngol* 1993; **250**: 11–17.
20. Sobin LH, Wittekind Ch. Head and neck tumours.In: *TNM Classification of Malignant Tumours*, 5th edn. New York: Wiley-Liss, 1997; 17–46.
21. Friedman M, Mafee MF, Pacella BL et al. Rationale for elective neck dissection in 1990. *Laryngoscope* 1990; **100**: 54–59.
22. Pradhan SA, Rajpal MR. Marginal mandibulectomy in the management of squamous cancer of the oral cavity. *Indian J Cancer* 1987; **24**: 167–171.
23. Khafif RA, Gelbfish GA, Asase DK, Tepper P, Attie JN. Modified radical neck dissection in cancer of the mouth pharynx, and larynx. *Head Neck* 1990; **12**: 476–482.
24. Spiro RH, Morgan GJ, Strong EW, Shah JP. Supraomohyoid neck dissection. *Am J Surg* 1996; **172**: 650–653.

25. Traynor SJ, Cohen JI, Gray J, Andersen PE, Everts EC. Selective neck dissection and the management of the node-positive neck. *Am J Surg* 1996; **172**: 654–657.
26. Majoufre C, Faucher A, Laroche C *et al*. Supraomohyoid neck dissection in cancer of the oral cavity. *Am J Surg* 1999; **178**: 72–77.
27. Kolli VR, Datta RV, Orner JB, Hicks WL, Loree TR. The role of supraomohyoid neck dissection in patients with positive nodes. *Arch Otolaryngol Head Neck Surg* 2000; **126**: 413–416.
28. Byers RM. Modified neck dissection: a study of 967 cases from 1970–1980. *Am J Surg* 1985; **150**: 414–421.
29. Spiro JD, Spiro RH, Shah JP, Sessions RB, Strong EW. Critical assessment of supraomohyoid neck dissection. *Am J Surg* 1988; **156**: 286–289.
30. Cunningham MJ, Johnson JT, Myers EN *et al*. Cervical lymph node metastasis after local excision of early squamous cell carcinoma of the oral cavity. *Am J Surg* 1986; **152**: 361–366.
31. Shah JP, Candela FC, Poddar AK. The patterns of cervical lymph node metastases from squamous carcinoma of the oral cavity. *Cancer* 1990; **66**: 109–113.
32. Dhawan IK, Verma K, Khazanchi RK *et al*. Carcinoma of the buccal mucosa: incidence of regional lymph node involvement. *Indian J Cancer* 1993; **30**: 176–180.
33. Medina JE, Byers RM. Supraomohyoid neck dissection: rationale, indications, and surgical technique. *Head Neck* 1989; **11**: 111–122.
34. Bloom ND, Spiro RH. Carcinoma of the cheek mucosa: a retrospective analysis. *Am J Surg* 1980; **140**: 556–560.
35. Fakih AR, Rao RS, Borges AM, Patel AR. Elective versus therapeutic neck dissection in early carcinoma of the oral tongue: a prospective randomized study. *Am J Surg* 1989; **158**: 309–313.
36. Kowalski LP, Magrin J, Waksman G *et al*. Supraomohyoid neck dissection in the treatment of head and neck tumors. *Arch Otolaryngol Head Neck Surg* 1993; **119**: 958–963.
37. Kligerman J, Lima RA, Soares JR *et al*. Supraomohyoid neck dissection in the treatment of T1/T2 squamous cell carcinoma of oral cavity. *Am J Surg* 1994; **168**: 391–394.
38. Kerrebijn JD, Freeman JL, Gullane PJ. Supraomohyoid neck dissection: is it diagnostic or therapeutic? *Head Neck* 1999; **21**: 39–41.
39. Manni JJ, van den Hoogen FJ. Supraomohyoid neck dissection with frozen section biopsy as a staging procedure in the clinically node-negative neck in carcinoma of the oral cavity. *Am J Surg* 1991; **62**: 373–376.
40. Brazilian Head and Neck Cancer Study Group. Results of a prospective trial on elective modified radical classical vs supraomohyoid neck dissection in the management of oral squamous carcinoma. *Am J Surg* 1998; **176**: 422–427.
41. Khafif A, Lopez-Garza JR, Madina JE. Is dissection of level IV necessary in patients with T1-T3 N0 tongue cancer? *Laryngoscope* 2001; **111**: 1088–1090.
42. Yuen APW, Wei WI, Wong YM, Tang KC. Elective neck dissection versus observation in the treatment of early oral tongue carcinoma. *Head Neck* 1997; **19**: 583–588.
43. Haddadin KJ, Soutar DS, Oliver RJ *et al*. Improved survival for patients with clinically T1/T2, N0 tongue tumor undergoing a prophylactic neck dissection. *Head Neck* 1999; **21**: 517–525.
44. van den Brekel MW, Castelijns JA, Reitsma LC *et al*. Outcome of observing the N0 neck using ultrasonographic-guided cytology for follow up. *Arch Otolaryngol Head Neck Surg* 1999; **125**: 153–156.
45. Pitman KT, Johnson JT, Edington H *et al*. Lymphatic mapping with isosulfan blue dye in squamous cell carcinoma of the head and neck. *Arch Otolaryngol Head Neck Surg* 1998; **124**: 790–793.
46. Nair MK, Sankaranarayanan R, Padmanabhan TK. Evaluation of the role of radiotherapy in the management of carcinoma of the buccal mucosa. *Cancer* 1988; **61**: 1326–1331.
47. Franceschi D, Gupta R, Spiro RH, Shah JP. Improved survival in the treatment of squamous carcinoma of oral tongue. *Am J Surg* 1993; **166**: 360–365.
48. Vikram B, Strong EW, Shah JP, Spiro RH. Failure at the primary site following multimodality treatment in advanced head and neck cancer. *Head Neck* 1984; **6**: 720–723.
49. Zelefsky MJ, Harrison LB, Fass DE *et al*. Post-operative radiation therapy for squamous cell carcinomas of the oral cavity and oropharynx: impact of therapy on patients with positive surgical margins. *Int J Radiat Oncol Biol Phys* 1993; **25**: 17–21.
50. Vokes EE, Haraf DJ, Kies MS. The use of concurrent chemotherapy and radiotherapy for locoregionally advanced head and neck cancer. *Semin Oncol* 2000; **27**: 34–38.

51. Kirita T, Ohgi K, Shimooka H *et al*. Preoperative concurrent chemoradiotherapy plus radical surgery for advanced squamous cell carcinoma of the oral cavity: an analysis of long term results. *Oral Oncol* 1999; **35**: 597–606.

52. Misra NC, Bhattacharya S, Chaturvedi A *et al*. Therapeutic implication and effect of induction chemotherapy (IC) in advanced (T3 & T4) oral cancer: prospective study of 66 patients. *J Cancer Res Clin Oncol* 1990; **116**: 687.

53. Misra NC, Chaturvedi A, Bhattacharya S. Neoadjuvant therapy followed by radical surgery and reconstruction in advanced T3 and T4 oral cancer. In: Varma AK. (ed) *Oral Oncology*. New Delhi: Macmillan India, 1994; 327–328.

54. Misra NC, Chaturvedi A, Misra S *et al*. Multi-modal therapy with special reference to neo-adjuvant chemotherapy (NAC) in advanced T3 and T4 oral cancer in India. *Jpn J Cancer Chemother* 1997; **24**: 150.

55. Chaturvedi A, Misra NC, Kumar R *et al*. Primary chemotherapy in verrucous squamous cell carcinoma (VSCC) of oral cavity – a prospective study. *Proceedings of Fifth International Cancer Congress on Anti-Cancer Chemotherapy, Paris* 1995; 281.

56. Pignon JP, Bourhis J, Domenge C, Designe L. Chemotherapy added to locoregional treatment for head and neck squamous-cell carcinoma: three meta-analyses of updated individual data. *Lancet* 2000; **355**: 949–955.

57. Rao DN, Shroff PD, Chattopadhyay G, Dinshaw KA. Survival analysis of 5595 head and neck cancers –results of conventional treatment in a high-risk population. *Br J Cancer* 1998; **77**: 1514–1518.

58. Zelefsky MJ, Harrison LB, Fass DE *et al*. Postoperative radiotherapy for oral cavity cancers: impact of anatomic subsite on treatment outcome. *Head Neck* 1990; **12**: 470-475.

A.D. Gilliam S.A. Watson I.J. Beckingham

8

Current developments in the non-surgical management of pancreatic cancer

Pancreatic cancer is the fifth leading cause of cancer death in the Western world, making up 6% of all cancer deaths,[1,2] with an overall 5-year survival of only 0.4%.[3,4] Outside specialist units, resection rates vary from 2.6–7%.[5,6] Patients unsuitable for surgical resection have locally invasive or metastatic spread and median survival in these patients is approximately 4 months, with limited treatment options.[7] Available treatments for these patients include chemotherapy, radiotherapy and a growing range of treatments based on tumour biology.

CHEMOTHERAPY

Systemic chemotherapy is a generally unsuccessful treatment modality for advanced pancreatic cancer.[8] 5-Fluorouracil (5-FU) has been the standard chemotherapy used in the UK over recent years, with evidence suggesting a small survival advantage and improvements in quality-of-life in a proportion

---

Key point 1
- Systemic chemotherapy is generally unsuccessful for treatment of advanced pancreatic cancer.

Mr Andrew D. Gilliam MBChB MRCS, Research Registrar, Section of Surgery (Gastrointestinal Surgery), Floor E, West Block, Queen's Medical Centre, Nottingham NG7 2UH, UK

Prof. Susan A. Watson PhD, Cancer Studies Unit, D Floor, West Block, Queen's Medical Centre, Nottingham NG7 2UH, UK (for correspondence)

Mr Ian J. Beckingham MD FRCS, Senior Lecturer, Section of Surgery (Gastrointestinal Surgery), Floor E, West Block, Queen's Medical Centre, Nottingham NG7 2UH, UK

of patients with pancreatic cancer. 5-FU is administered using a variety of doses and schedules; the response rate rarely exceeds 20% and no consistent effect on disease-related symptoms or survival has been demonstrated.

Gemcitabine is a novel nucleoside analogue that exerts its action by inhibiting DNA synthesis with a wide spectrum of antitumour activity against a variety of solid tumours including pancreatic cancer.[9] Gemcitabine is licensed as a first line treatment of adult patients with locally advanced or metastatic adenocarcinoma of the pancreas and as a second line treatment of patients with 5-FU refractory pancreatic cancer. It is able to produce a clinical response rate of 24% with improvement of the median survival of treated patients from 4.4 to 5.6 months when compared to 5-FU.[10] As with all chemotherapy, gemcitabine is associated with potentially life-threatening side-effects in an already debilitated group of patients. In the Burris trial,[11] 26% of patients treated with gemcitabine had grade 3 or 4 neutropenia compared with 5% in the 5-FU group. The role of gemcitabine in the treatment of pancreatic cancer in comparison with other agents including combination regimens is being investigated in 11 on-going randomised controlled trials and 24 phase II trials.

In the UK, the National Institute for Clinical Excellence (NICE) recently published its economic evaluation of gemcitabine as first line therapy for pancreatic cancer based on the clinical effectiveness data[12] from the single randomised controlled trial by Burris et al.[11] For first line treatment, estimates for cost per life-year gained ranged from approximately £7200 to £18,700 depending on the 5-FU regimen used. These figures are very sensitive to reduced estimates of survival benefit over the comparators. Cost-effectiveness evidence, therefore, suggests that gemcitabine provides a reasonable alternative for the first-line treatment of pancreatic cancer, but this conclusion is based on the results from a single clinical trial.

Key point 2

- The National Institute for Clinical Excellence has recently approved the use of gemcitabine as first line chemotherapy for pancreatic cancer.

Of 6000 patients diagnosed with pancreatic cancer each year, at least 80% (4800 patients) have locally advanced or metastatic disease. Assuming that 25–35% of those will be offered chemotherapy and half of these patients are treated, the total number of patients eligible to receive gemcitabine would be in the range 600–840 patients per year. The incremental cost of gemcitabine treatment ranges between £1360 and £3550 per patient depending on the type of the 5-FU regimen used. If gemcitabine were to be made available for NHS use, based on the estimated number of patients above, the total additional cost to the NHS is estimated to be between £816,000 and £3 million per annum. This conservative estimate only includes the direct costs to the NHS such as drug costs and utilization of services.

RADIOTHERAPY

Pancreatic cancer is relatively 'radioresistant'.[13] Irradiation is made more difficult by the deep location of the pancreas and its proximity to areas that are sensitive to radiation (intestine, spinal cord, liver, kidneys).

A recent large randomised control trial of adjuvant chemoradiotherapy for patients with resectable pancreatic cancer showed no 2-year survival benefit in

Key point 3

- Radiotherapy alone, or in combination with chemotherapy, is of little clinical benefit for patients suffering from pancreatic cancer.

the postoperative setting.[14] Another recent trial failed to demonstrate prolongation of median survival for patients with localized pancreatic cancer treated with gemcitabine-based chemoradiation.[15]

BIOLOGICAL THERAPY

Detailed examination of the molecular make-up of pancreatic cancer has led scientists and clinicians to develop novel therapeutic approaches many of which have already entered clinical trials. We are currently in the 'molecular age', with rapid progress being made in gene and molecular technology. These new techniques have the potential to inhibit the neoplastic process in the pancreas and reduce disease progression.

The rapid development of knowledge of pancreatic cancer tumour biology is narrowing the gap between science and clinical practice. These new modalities of treatment have been described as biological therapy.

Key point 4

- Many new modalities of treatment targeting different neoplastic characteristics of cells, described as biological therapy, are entering clinical trials.

SIGNAL TRANSDUCTION INHIBITORS

A number of agents are being developed that inhibit aberrant signal transduction in neoplastic cells. BMS-214662,[16–18] SCH 66336,[19] and R115777[20,21] are oral benzodiazepine-based and quinolone inhibitors of farnesyl transferase. These agents, therefore, inhibit the first step in post-translational modification of ras proteins (monomeric GTPases), resulting in loss of the ras signal transduction cascade. Most pancreatic adenocarcinomas

(> 70%) contain mutations in k-ras[22] that effectively 'switch on' a continuous intracellular signal for cell cycle progression. This leads to uncontrolled cell division.

Sixty-three patients with advanced pancreatic carcinoma were randomized to treatment with oral SCH 66336 daily (n = 33) or gemcitabine (n = 30). The median overall survival for SCH 66336 was 3.3 months compared to 4.4 months for gemcitabine. In the patients treated with SCH 66336, two partial responses and six cases of disease stability were seen with fewer incidences of haematological toxicity and GI side-effects compared with gemcitabine. SCH 66336 is now being evaluated in combination with gemcitabine in patients with advanced pancreatic cancer.[19]

MATRIX METALLOPROTEINASE (MMP) INHIBITORS

Metalloproteinases are a group of proteolytic enzymes which degrade different substrates within the extracellular matrix. An imbalance between MMPs and tissue-specific inhibitors leads to matrix degradation and tumour invasion.[23]

Several broad-spectrum synthetic MMP inhibitors have been developed. A recent study has reported evidence of a dose response for marimastat in patients with advanced pancreatic cancer. The 1-year survival rate for patients receiving marimastat (25 mg) was similar to that of patients receiving gemcitabine.[24]

Selective non-hydroxamate MMP inhibitors that spare sheddases (related metalloproteinases) are being developed that have potential for pancreatic carcinoma treatment. Sheddase inhibition is hypothesized to play a major role in the dose-limiting arthritis noted for hydroxamate-based MMP inhibitors. For example, in a recent phase I study, BMS-275291 was well tolerated with no dose-limiting arthritis with plasma concentrations sufficient to produce sustained MMP-2 and MMP-9 inhibition in cancer patients.[25–27]

Neovastat[28] targets two angiogenesis processes: the VEGF signalling pathway and MMPs. Neovastat, which also stimulates angiostatin expression in experimental glioblastoma, has demonstrated antimetastatic properties in experimental tumour models and has no dose-limiting toxicity in phase I/II trials.

COX-2 INHIBITION

The isoform of cyclo-oxygenase (COX), COX-2, is involved in the inflammatory response and is induced by several growth factors, cytokines and tumour promoters. Following activation of oncogenes such as ras and src, COX-2 enhances proliferation, reduces apoptosis and increases angiogenesis.[29]

Selective COX-2 inhibitors, such as rofecoxib and celecoxib, have been used in clinical trials to reduce neoplastic growth, most notably in familial adenomatous polyposis.

The expression of COX-2 in human pancreatic neoplasms and the effect of COX inhibitors on the growth of human pancreatic carcinoma cells was investigated immunohistochemically in 42 human pancreatic duct cell carcinomas and in 29 intraductal papillary mucinous tumours (IPMT [adenomas, 19; carcinomas, 10]) of the pancreas.[29] The growth of four human pancreatic carcinoma cell lines also was evaluated in the presence of COX inhibitors. Marked COX-2 expression was observed in 57% (24 of 42) of ductal adenocarcinomas, in 58% (11 of 19) of adenomas, and in 70% (7 of 10) of adenocarcinomas of IPMTs. All four pancreatic cancer cell lines expressed COX-2 protein weakly or strongly, and the inhibitory effect of aspirin on cell growth was correlated with the expression of COX-2. COX inhibitors may, therefore, be worthy of investigation as therapeutic and preventative agents for pancreatic carcinomas.

IMMUNOTHERAPY

Immunotherapy involves active or passive stimulation of the immune system against cancer cells, their growth factors and growth factor receptors.

Antibodies and T-cells have the potential to recognise tumour antigens identified by modern genetic techniques.[30] It may be possible to use the host immune system to target activity against antigens such as ras protein[31] or the MUC 1 tumour antigens[32] found in virtually all pancreatic cancers.

Pancreatic cancer escapes immune recognition by producing anti-inflammatory mediators and by failure to express MHC–tumour antigen complexes. Clinically, effective immunotherapy, therefore, requires high tumour antigen specificity and good antigen delivery. Purified peptide and carbohydrate molecules, for example, can generate a potent antitumour response.

Mixed leukocyte cyto-implant (MLC) is a natural cytokine pump which reverses the anti-inflammatory activity of the tumour. It can be delivered by fine needle intratumoural injection using endoscopic ultrasound guidance.[33] In eight patients with advanced pancreatic cancer treated with the implant, there were two partial responses and one minor response.

Tumour B-cell hybrid vaccines are specific tumour antigen presenting cells that facilitate CD4 T-cell recognition of the tumour antigen. The clinical efficacy of the combination of these two treatments was investigated in a study involving 28 patients with advanced pancreatic cancer and synergistic antitumour activity was demonstrated.[34]

Passive immunotherapy with monoclonal antibodies

Both epidermal growth factor receptor (EGF-R) signaling mechanisms and VEGF-mediated angiogenesis have been used as targets for passive immunotherapy with monoclonal antibodies specifically for human pancreatic carcinoma treatment.

The anti-VEGF antibody HumV833 recently completed phase I clinical trials in patients with variety of tumours and was found to be well-tolerated and tumour-specific on PET scanning.[35]

In phase II studies of anti-epidermal growth factor receptor (EGFR) antibody Cetuximab (IMC-C225), promising activity was observed in *in vivo* studies[36] and in patients with advanced pancreatic carcinoma when used in combination with gemcitabine.[37] Of patients screened for the study, 89% tested positive for EGFR expression; 41 patients were enrolled into the study. After two courses of therapy, 5 (12%) patients achieved a partial response and 16 (39%) patients had stable disease. The median time to progression was 16 weeks, compared with 9 weeks for patients treated with gemcitabine alone in studies in the literature.

Chimeric monoclonal antibody Nd2 (c-Nd2), produced against purified mucin derived from pancreatic cancer, has been used in clinical trials for pancreatic carcinoma immunotherapy. This treatment has been shown to induce antibody-dependent cell-mediated cytotoxicity (ADCC). Cytotoxicities to Nd2-positive tumour cells during culture with c-Nd2 were significantly higher than with no antibody.

Reduced tumour marker levels in sera such as CA19-9 and SPan-1 have been observed after intravenous injection of c-Nd2 in some pancreatic cancer patients.[38]

Cytokine immune modulation

Attempted stimulation of a patient's immune response against tumour cells using cytokine immune modulation is not new; however, it has been recently used to enhance the antitumour efficacy of monoclonal antibody therapy.

IFN-γ, for example, is a lymphokine produced by T-lymphocytes in response to antigen exposure. Its immunomodulatory activity includes stimulation of natural killer cells, lymphokine-activated killer cells, stimulation of ADCC and enhancement of HLA Class II expression. Co-stimulation of natural killer (NK) cells with IL-12 and Herceptin-coated HER2-positive cancer cells lead to the secretion of large amounts of IFN-γ and other cytokines. IFN-γ treatment profoundly inhibited pancreatic cancer growth *in vitro*.[39]

Active specific immunotherapy

Active immunotherapy aims to activate a component of the immune system such as lymphocytes or antibodies against tumour-associated antigens presented by the tumour or tumour growth factors.

β-hCG belongs to a superfamily of human growth factors, and may play a role in cancer progression by modifying angiogenesis, stimulating growth and invasion, and orchestrating immunosuppression. Immunization of patients with pancreatic cancer with Avicine™, a vaccine composed of synthetic peptides derived from β-hCG conjugated to diphtheria toxin (DT), has been investigated in a phase II trial.[40] Patients were randomized to Avicine alone or Avicine plus gemcitabine. A total of 83% of patients developed β-hCG antibodies and antibody titres were decreased in the gemcitabine plus Avicine group, compared to Avicine alone. No unexpected adverse experiences were recorded in either treatment group. There was no significant difference in overall survival between the groups.

Antibody-directed enzyme-prodrug therapy (ADEPT)

This utilizes the dual specificity of antibody–enzyme conjugates for the targeted activation of an inert prodrug to generate high local drug concentrations of the active agents. This enables therapeutic concentrations of drug in the tumour with lower toxicity that may be of future use in pancreatic carcinoma. No studies in this tumour have been reported to date.

Adoptive immunotherapy

The concept of adoptive immunotherapy is that sensitized lymphocytes or dendritic cells are infused into pancreatic cancer patients. Lymphokine-activated killer (LAK) cells, autolymphocyte therapy (ALT), and tumour-infiltrating lymphocytes (TIL) have been most often studied, usually in haematological malignancies.

Dendritic cells from autotransfusion of patients with pancreatic carcinoma did not show quantitative or qualitative alterations and were able to present soluble antigen making them potentially suitable for adoptive immunotherapy.[41]

A study of adoptive immunotherapy using intraportal infusion of LAK cells after curative resection and intra-operative radiation therapy (IORT) in patients with advanced metastatic pancreatic cancer used controls that underwent tumour resection and IORT. The treatment group also underwent intraportal infusion of LAK cells combined with recombinant interleukin 2 (rIL-2). Overall survival was not statistically different between the groups; however, there were more patients (4) alive 3 years after operation in the test group (36% *versus* zero), and the incidence of liver metastases in the treatment group was lower (3 of 12 *versus* 10 of 15). LAK cell therapy influenced survival positively in multivariate analysis.[42]

HORMONAL MANIPULATION

Anti-androgen and oestrogen therapy

The growth of pancreatic adenocarcinoma may be under the control of the sex steroid hormones.[43] Oestrogen and androgen receptors have been demonstrated in pancreatic malignant tissue.

A prospective, randomised, double-blind placebo controlled trial of the anti-androgen flutamide was performed in 49 patients with pancreatic carcinoma;[44] 24 patients received flutamide and 25 received placebo. Median survival for all patients was 8 months in the flutamide group compared with 4 months in the placebo group. After exclusion of disease progression or death within the first 6 weeks, median survival was 12 months compared with 5 months, respectively. Blockade of androgen receptors requires further investigation as a new treatment approach.

Somatostatin analogues

Somatostatin analogues including octreotide, lanreotide and vapreotide have been used in numerous preclinical studies and have provided contradictory effects on the growth of ductal pancreatic adenocarcinoma. Monotherapy did not result in a prolongation of survival. In 15–20% of patients, however, tumour progression was halted for several months accompanied by a significant improvement of clinical condition without notable side-effects.[45] Somatostatin analogues used in combination with tamoxifen,[46] in patients with unresectable and resected ductal adenocarcinoma of the pancreas, apparently increased survival when compared to historical controls.

Antigastrin therapy

Gastrin is a trophic hormone in the gastrointestinal tract. It has been shown to promote the growth of normal gastrointestinal mucosa, and gastrointestinal cancers including pancreatic carcinoma.[47]

Gastrin stimulates the growth of pancreatic cancer by endocrine, autocrine and paracrine mechanisms by release of amidated gastrin and its precursor forms, which feed back to their own individual cell and neighbouring cells.

Definite expression of CCK2/gastrin receptor, progastrin, glycine-extended gastrin and amidated gastrin was observed in 95%, 91%, 55% and 23%, respectively, of sections from patients with pancreatic cancer.[48]

The potent trophic precursor forms of gastrin bind to a number of receptor isoforms, some of which may be tumour-specific. As some of the growth effects have not been ascribed to a known receptor subtype, complete receptor blockade is impossible. Antigastrin antibodies, which bind both amidated and glycine-extended forms of gastrin before they have an opportunity to bind to these receptor isoforms, inhibit the proliferative effect of glycine-extended gastrin in pancreatic cancer cell lines.[49]

G17DT (Gastrimmune) is an immunogen which raises antibodies directed against the amidated and glycine extended forms (serum and tumour-associated form) of gastrin-17. It consists of the nine amino acid fragment of G17 linked to the carrier molecule, diphtheria toxoid (DT) via a peptide spacer. The immunogen is successful in raising neutralising antibodies with the G17 sequence as the B-cell epitope. The peptide spacer allows the gastrin moiety to be spatially orientated in such a way that B-cells recognise the whole sequence. The antibodies raised are univalent and, therefore, do not induce complement fixation. Furthermore, as the antibodies induced are directed against the amino terminus of G17, the normal functions of G34, smaller C-terminal fragments of gastrin and CCK remain unimpeded.[50]

In a recently reported study,[51] G17DT was administered to 40 patients with advanced pancreatic carcinoma. An abdominal CT and chest X-ray were performed at 24 weeks to assess disease progression. Of 36 patients, 32 (89%) patients mounted an antibody response; 13 (35%) of the patients were jaundiced at screening. Antibody response was not affected by age, surgery, or raised serum bilirubin. An immunoassay confirmed that antibodies raised by these patients to G17 were effective at displacing iodinated gastrin from CCK2 receptors. G17DT was well tolerated – only one patient developed a sterile injection site abscess that settled following aspiration. There were no systemic side-effects. At week 8, 17 of 28 patients (61%) had stable weight (less than 5% change) and 4 of 28 (14%) gained weight (greater than 5% increase). At 24 weeks, 3 of 16 patients (19%) had radiologically stable disease.

The G17-DT group had a 150% longer median survival compared to a historical control group (297 days *versus* 108 days) but it would be invalid to perform statistical analysis on the two groups. Phase III trials are on-going.

GENE THERAPY

Cancer results from activation of oncogenes or inactivation of tumour-suppressor genes. The objective of gene therapy is the down-regulation of oncogenes or the restoration of tumour-suppressor genes. The therapeutic gene has to be delivered into the target cell population genome with high efficiency, specificity and safety. Gene transfer is most commonly performed

---

Key point 5

- The future use of biological therapies in combination with new chemotherapeutic agents offers new promising strategies for pancreatic carcinoma treatment.

> **Key point 6**
>
> • Active recruitment of patients into the many clinical trials of new therapies is encouraged.

by viral vectors[52] or by a liposomal technique[53] in which the target gene is delivered into cells by fusing with cell membranes. Viral vectors can be administered intratumourally, topically,[54] intraperitoneally,[55] intravenously,[56] and intra-arterially.[57]

Genetic prodrug activation therapy is a type of gene therapy in which differences in transcription between normal and malignant cells are exploited. 'Suicide genes' are introduced into neoplastic cells that convert a non-toxic prodrug into a highly cytotoxic agent at the tumour site.[58,59]

Antisense therapy involves production of complementary strands of small segments of a target mRNA that modify gene expression at a translational level. Phase II trials of such therapy have already been performed in patients with pancreatic cancer with promising results.[60]

A further discussion of these approaches is included in Chapter 5 on *Genes and the surgeon* by Bright-Thomas.

CONCLUSIONS

Novel, non-surgical therapeutic strategies are promising but require further evaluation. The molecular age is bringing better understanding and a multitude of new treatment methods for this disease. It is desirable that patients with pancreatic cancer be recruited into the many clinical trials of these new agents. A nihilistic attitude to the disease is no longer appropriate.

> **Key points for clinical practice**
>
> • Systemic chemotherapy is generally unsuccessful for treatment of advanced pancreatic cancer.
>
> • The National Institute for Clinical Excellence has recently approved the use of gemcitabine as first line chemotherapy for pancreatic cancer.
>
> • Radiotherapy alone, or in combination with chemotherapy, is of little clinical benefit for patients suffering from pancreatic cancer.
>
> • Many new modalities of treatment targeting different neoplastic characteristics of cells, described as biological therapy, are entering clinical trials.
>
> • The future use of biological therapies in combination with new chemotherapeutic agents offers new promising strategies for pancreatic carcinoma treatment.
>
> • Active recruitment of patients into the many clinical trials of new therapies is encouraged.

References

1. Parkin DM, Muir CS, Whelan SL et al. Cancer Incidence in Five Continents, vol VI. IARC Scientific Publ. No. 120. Lyon: International Agency for Research on Cancer, 1992.
2. Fernandez E, Lavecchia C, Porta M et al. Trends in pancreatic cancer mortality in Europe, 1995–89. Int J Cancer 1994; 57: 786–792.
3. Gudjonson B. Cancer of the pancreas. Fifty years of surgery. Cancer 1987; 9: 2284–2303.
4. Office of Population Censuses and Surveys. Mortality Statistics. Cause: Review of the Registrar General on Deaths by Cause, Sex and Age, in England and Wales. Series DH2, No. 19. London: HMSO, 1992.
5. Carter DC. Cancer of the pancreas. Gut 1990; 31: 494–496.
6. Fontham ETH, Correa P. Epidemiology of pancreatic cancer. Surg Clin North Am 1989; 69: 551–567.
7. Boyle P, Hsieh CC, Maisonneuve P et al. Epidemiology of pancreas cancer. Int J Pancreat 1989; 5: 327–346.
8. Brennan MF, Kinsella TJ, Casper ES. Cancer of the pancreas. In: De Vita Jr VT, Hellman S, Rosenburg SA. (eds) Cancer: Principles and Practice of Oncology, vol 3, 4th edn. Philadelphia, PA: Lippincott, 1993; 849–882.
9. Carmichael J. Clinical response benefit in patients with advanced pancreatic cancer. Role of gemcitabine. Digestion 1997; 58: 503–507.
10. Hidalgo M, Castellano D, Paz-Ares L et al. Phase I–II study of gemcitabine and fluorouracil as a continuous infusion in patients with pancreatic cancer. J Clin Oncol 1999; 17: 585–592.
11. Burris HA, Moore MJ, Anderson J et al. Improvements in survival and clinical benefit with gemcitabine as first-line therapy for patients with advanced pancreatic cancer: a randomised trial. J Clin Oncol 1997; 15: 2403–2413.
12. National Institute for Clinical Excellence. Gemcitabine for the treatment of pancreatic cancer. May 2001 <http://www.nice.org.uk/article.asp?a=16790>.
13. Houry S, Mariani P, Schlienger M, Huguier M. Intraoperative radiotherapy in cancers of the pancreas and in recurrent colorectal cancers. Ann Chir 1996; 50: 438–444
14. Neoptolemos JP, Dunn JA, Stocken DD, Almond J, Link K, Beger H et al. Influence of resection margins on survival for patients with pancreatic cancer treated by adjuvant chemoradiation and/or chemotherapy in the ESPAC-1 randomized controlled trial. Lancet 2001; 358: 1576–1585.
15. Crane CH, Janjan NA, Evans DB, Wolff RA, Ballo MT, Milas L et al. Toxicity and efficacy of concurrent gemcitabine and radiotherapy for locally advanced pancreatic cancer. Int J Pancreatol 2001; 29: 9–18.
16. Voi M, Tabernero J, Cooper MR, Marimon I, Van Vreckem A et al. A phase I study of the farnesyl transferase (FT) inhibitor BMS-214662 administered as a weekly 1-hour infusion in patients (pts) with advanced solid tumors: clinical findings. J Clin Oncol 2001; 20: Abstract 312.
17. Kim KB, Shin DM, Summey CC, Kurie JM, Fossella FV et al. Phase I study of farnesyl transferase inhibitor, BMS-214662, in solid tumors. J Clin Oncol 2001; 20; Abstract 313.
18. Bailey HH, Marnocha R, Arzoomanian R, Alberti D, Binger K et al. Phase I trial of weekly paclitaxel and BMS-214662 in patients with advanced solid tumors. J Clin Oncol 2001; 20: Abstract 314.
19. Lersch C, Van Cutsem E, Amado R, Ehninger G, Heike M et al. Randomized phase II study of SCH 66336 and gemcitabine in the treatment of metastatic adenocarcinoma of the pancreas. J Clin Oncol 2001; 20: Abstract 608.
20. Holden SN, Eckhardt SG, Fisher S, Persky M, Miluke C et al. A phase I pharmacokinetic (PK) and biological study of the farnesyl transferase inhibitor (FTI) R115777 and capecitabine in patients (pts) with advanced solid malignancies. J Clin Oncol 2001; 20: Abstract 316.
21. Nakagawa K, Yamamoto N, Nishio K, Ohashi Y, End D et al. A phase I, pharmacokinetic (PK) and pharmacodynamic (PD) study of the farnesyl transferase inhibitor (FTI) R115777 in Japanese patients with advanced non-hematological malignancies. J Clin Oncol 2001; 20: Abstract 317.
22. Manu M, Buckels J, Bramhall S. Molecular technology and pancreatic cancer. Br J Surg 2000; 87: 840–853.
23. Gress TM, Muller-Pillasch F, Lerch MM, Fries H et al. Expression and in situ localization of genes coding for extracellular matrix proteins and extracellular matrix degrading proteases in pancreatic cancer. Int J Cancer 1995; 62: 407—413.

24. Bramhall SR, Rosemurgy A, Brown PD, Bowry C, Buckels JA, Marimastat Pancreatic Cancer Study Group. Marimastat as first-line therapy for patients with unresectable pancreatic cancer: a randomized trial. *J Clin Oncol* 2001; **19**: 3447–3455.

25. Gupta E, Huang M, Mao Y, Patel R *et al*. Pharmacokinetic (PK) evaluation of BMS-275291, a matrix metalloproteinase (MMP) inhibitor, in cancer patients. *J Clin Oncol* 2001; **20**: Abstract 301.

26. Daniels R, Gupta E, Kollia G, Huang M *et al*. Safety and pharmacokinetics of BMS-275291, a novel matrix metalloproteinase inhibitor in healthy subjects. *J Clin Oncol* 2001; **20**: Abstract 395.

27. Hurwitz H, Humphrey J, Williams K, Ness E *et al*. A phase I trial of BMS-275291: a novel, non-hydroxamate, sheddase-sparing matrix metalloproteinase inhibitor (MMPI) with no dose-limiting arthritis. *J Clin Oncol* 2001; **20**: Abstract 387.

28. Franqois B, Champagne P, Evans WK, Jean L *et al*. Phase I/II trials on the safety, tolerability and efficacy of Æ-941 (Neovastat) in patients with solid tumors. *J Clin Oncol* 2001; **20**: Abstract 2861.

29. Kokawa A, Kondo H, Gotoda T *et al*. Increased expression of cyclooxygenase-2 in human pancreatic neoplasms and potential for chemoprevention by cyclooxygenase inhibitors. *Cancer* 2001; **91**: 333–338.

30. Jung S, Schluesener HJ. Human T lymphocytes recognize a peptide of single point-mutated, oncogenic ras proteins. *J Exp Med* 1991; **173**: 273–276.

31. Fossum B, Gedde-Dahl III T, Breivik J *et al*. p21-ras-peptide-specific, T-cell responses in a patient with colorectal cancer. CD4+ and CD8+ T cells recognize a peptide corresponding to a common mutation (13Gly->Asp). *Int J Cancer* 1994; **56**: 40–45.

32. Monges GM, Mathoulin-Portier MP, Acres RB, Houvenaeghel GF, Giovannini MF, Seitz JF *et al*. Differential MUC 1 expression in normal and neoplastic human pancreatic tissue. An immunohistochemical study of 60 samples. *Am J Clin Pathol* 1999; **112**: 635–640.

33. Chang KJ, Nguyen PT, Thompson JA, Kurosaki TT *et al*. Phase I clinical trial of allogeneic mixed lymphocyte culture (cytoimplant) delivered by endoscopic ultrasound-guided fine-needle injection in patients with advanced pancreatic carcinoma. *Cancer* 2000; **88**: 1325–1335.

34. Moviglia G, Iraola N, Hisserodt J *et al*. Combination immunotherapy for pancreatic cancer. *J Clin Oncol* 2001; **20**: Abstract 1052.

35. Jayson GC, Mulatero C, Ranson M, Zweit J, Hastings D *et al*. Anti-VEGF antibody HuMV833: an EORTC Biological Treatment Development Group phase I toxicity, pharmacokinetic and pharmacodynamic study. *J Clin Oncol* 2001; **20**: 14.

36. Bruns CJ, Harbison MT, Davis DW, Portera CA *et al*. Epidermal growth factor receptor blockade with C225 plus gemcitabine results in regression of human pancreatic carcinoma growing orthotopically in nude mice by antiangiogenic mechanisms. *Clin Cancer Res* 2000; **6**: 1936–1948.

37. Abbruzzese JL, Rosenberg A, Xiong O, LoBuglio A, Schmidt W *et al*. Phase II study of anti-epidermal growth factor receptor (EGFR) antibody Cetuximab (IMC-C225) in combination with gemcitabine in patients with advanced pancreatic cancer. *J Clin Oncol* 2001; **20**: Abstract 518.

38. Sawada T, Nishihara T, Yamashita Y, Tamamori Y *et al*. Targeting immunotherapy by chimeric monoclonal antibody Nd2 directed against pancreatic cancer mucin. *J Clin Oncol* 2001; **20**: Abstract 1100.

39. Detjen KM, Farwig K, Welzel M, Wiedenmann B *et al*. Interferon gamma inhibits growth of human pancreatic carcinoma cells via caspase-1 dependent induction of apoptosis. *Gut* 2001; **49**: 251–262.

40. Iversen P, Marshall J, Blanke C, Yoshihara P *et al*. Active specific immunotherapy with a β-hCG peptide vaccine in patients with pancreatic cancer. *J Clin Oncol* 2001; **20**: Abstract 1083.

41. Piemonti L, Monti P, Zerbi A, Balzano G *et al*. Generation and functional characterisation of dendritic cells from patients with pancreatic carcinoma with special regard to clinical applicability. *Cancer Immunol Immunother* 2000; **49**: 544–550.

42. Kobari M, Egawa S, Shibuya K, Sunamura M *et al*. Effect of intraportal adoptive immunotherapy on liver metastases after resection of pancreatic cancer. *Br J Surg* 2000; **87**: 43–48.

43. Targarona EM, Pons MD, Gonzalez G, Boix L *et al*. Is exocrine pancreatic cancer a hormone-dependent tumor? A study of the existence of sex hormone receptors in normal and neoplastic pancreas. *Hepatogastroenterology* 1991; **38**: 165–169.

44. Greenway BA. Effect of flutamide on survival in patients with pancreatic cancer: results of a prospective, randomised, double blind, placebo-controlled trial. *BMJ* 1998; **316**: 1935–1938.

45. Sulkowski U, Buchler M, Pederzoli P, Arnold R *et al*. A phase II study of high-dose octreotide in patients with unresectable pancreatic carcinoma. *Eur J Cancer* 1999; **35**: 1805–1808.

46. Rosenberg L, Barkun AN, Denis MH, Pollak M. Low dose octreotide and tamoxifen in the treatment of adenocarcinoma of the pancreas. *Cancer* 1995; **75**: 23–28.

47. Smith IP, Hamory MW, Verderame MF, Zagon IS. Quantitative analysis of gastrin mRNA and peptide in normal and cancerous human pancreas. *Int J Mol Med* 1998; **2**: 309–315.

48. Caplin M, Savage K, Khan K *et al*. Expression and processing of gastrin in pancreatic adenocarcinoma. *Br J Surg* 2000; **87**: 1035–1041.

49. Brett B, Savage K, Michaeli D *et al*. The effect of antibodies raised against Gastrimmune on the proliferation of human pancreatic carcinoma cell lines. *Gut* 1999; **44 (Suppl 1)**: A48.

50. Watson SA, Gilliam AD. G17DT – a new weapon in the therapeutic armoury for gastrointestinal malignancy. *Exp Opin Biol Ther* 2001; **1**: 309–317

51. Gilliam AD, Henwood M, Watson SA, Rowlands BJ *et al*. G17DT – a study to determine the safety, tolerance and antibody response in patients with advanced pancreatic carcinoma. *Gastroenterology* 2001; **120**: Abstract 1350.

52. Heise C, Sampson-Johannes A, Williams A *et al*. ONYX-015, an E1B gene-attenuated adenovirus, causes tumor-specific cytolysis and antitumoral efficacy that can be augmented by standard chemotherapeutic agents. *Nat Med* 1997; **3**: 639–645.

53. Aoki K, Yoshida T, Matsumoto N, Ide H *et al*. Gene therapy for peritoneal dissemination of pancreatic cancer by liposome-mediated transfer of herpes simplex virus thymidine kinase gene. *Hum Gene Ther* 1997; **8**: 1105–1113.

54. Kirn H, Khuri F, Ganly I, Arseneau JC *et al*. A phase II trial of ONYX-015, a selectively replicating adenovirus, in combination with cisplatin and 5-fluorouracil in patients with recurrent head and neck cancer. *J Clin Oncol* 1999; **18**: Abstract 1505.

55. Muller CY, Coleman RL, Rogers P, Merritt JE *et al*. Phase I intraperitoneal adenoviral p53 gene transfer in ovarian cancer. *J Clin Oncol* 2001; **20**: Abstract 1025.

56. Hao D, Rowinsky EK, Smetzer LA, Ochoa L *et al*. A phase I and pharmacokinetic study of intravenous (IV) p53 gene therapy with RPR/INGN-201 in patients with advanced cancer. *J Clin Oncol* 2001; **20**: Abstract 1045.

57. Reid TR, Galanis E, Abbruzzese J, Sze D *et al*. Intra-arterial administration of a replication-selective adenovirus Ci-1042 (Onyx-015) in patients with colorectal carcinoma metastatic to the liver: safety, feasibility and biological activity. *J Clin Oncol* 2001; **20**: Abstract 549.

58. Espinosa E, Casado E, Navarro JG *et al*. Drug induced transcriptional modulation for cancer gene therapy. *J Clin Oncol* 2001; **20**: Abstract 2628.

59. Hoffman RM, Miki K, Gupta A, Xu M *et al*. Combination methioninase-gene/selenomethionine prodrug cancer gene-therapy induces Bcl-2-independent apoptosis. *J Clin Oncol* 2001; **20**: Abstract 1041.

60. Perez RP, Smith III JW, Alberts SR, Kaufman H, Posey J *et al*. Phase II trial of ISIS 2503, an antisense inhibitor of H-ras, in patients (pts) with advanced pancreatic carcinoma (CA). *J Clin Oncol* 2001, **20**: Abstract 628.

J.N. Primrose

9

Primary tumours of the liver

Treating primary liver tumours is a therapeutic challenge. Many different medical disciplines need to be involved and a high degree of clinical expertise is needed to achieve the best results for patients. Although many modalities of treatment may be applied, curative treatment almost invariably involves surgery. This being said, the results of surgical treatment of primary livers tumours are inferior to the results from treating colorectal liver metastases. However, the same general principles apply.

GENERAL PRINCIPLES OF LIVER RESECTION FOR MALIGNANCY

The results of liver resection, either partial or hepatectomy with transplant, have improved markedly in recent years. There are several reasons for the improvement in the results of resectional surgery.[1] Firstly, surgeons have a much better understanding of liver anatomy, particularly with respect to the segments.[2] All of the 8 liver segments can be resected individually without compromising the remaining liver, although in the case of segment 8 this is technically more difficult. This anatomical approach allows segments containing tumour to be removed while preserving liver substance, important in patients with primary liver disease. Secondly, the technology has greatly improved. Intra-operative ultrasound is widely used by liver surgeons to determine the anatomy during the resection. Using the ultrasound dissector, which aspirates the parenchyma and leaves the fibrous structure, including the blood vessels, intact, allows a precise anatomical dissection. The argon diathermy coagulates blood vessels effectively and can even seal holes in the side of veins. Lastly, and perhaps most important, the anaesthesia has greatly

Prof. J.N. Primrose, University Surgical Unit, F Level, Centre Block, Southampton General Hospital, Tremona Road, Southampton SO16 6YD, UK

improved and now low CVP anaesthetics are used routinely.[3] In the past, liver surgery could be a very bloody affair. As the inflow to the liver can be completely occluded by clamping the free edge of the lesser omentum, it is clear that the bleeding results from the hepatic veins, which are not commonly controlled. Previously, and in anticipation of blood loss, the anaesthetist used to fill patients with fluid and blood prior to the resection commencing. This increased the central venous pressure and made the bleeding worse. It has now been realised that if the CVP is reduced to zero or below, there will be little if any bleeding from the hepatic veins, so that now most major liver resections can be carried out without the need for blood transfusion. Liver imaging has improved markedly with spiral and multislice computed tomography (CT) and magnetic resonance imaging (MRI) improving the definition. This allows better pre-operative staging of the patient and, therefore, more appropriate surgical treatment.

Key point 1

- Major liver resections can be carried out with very low morbidity and mortality rates in specialist centres.

Whatever the liver tumour, general oncological principles apply. First, it is important that a complete resection is carried out. There is no demonstrable benefit in palliative liver resection at present; therefore, it is important to try to complete the resection with at least a centimetre clear margin.[1] When this is not possible, the long-term results are compromised. Second, extrahepatic disease whether lymph nodes, distant metastases or peritoneal involvement precludes cure at present and is a contra-indication to surgery. Last, except in the rare circumstances where transplantation is being used, there should be at least two segments of healthy liver left at the end of operation to sustain the patient whilst the liver regenerates. Anecdotally, patients with even a relatively small residual liver mass, providing it is healthy and the operation is carried out with minimal blood loss, will survive. Mortality rate increases greatly in the presence of primary liver disease or if the peri-operative blood loss has been significant.

Key point 2

- The complication rate is higher in patients with liver disease.

Pre-operative percutaneous biopsy should be avoided except in exceptional circumstances. In colorectal liver metastases, 20% of patients having a percutaneous biopsy will develop needle-track recurrence and some patients will die as a result of the biopsy alone.[4] The same findings seem to apply to hepatoma and cholangiocarcinoma. Sometimes, however, there are circumstances where

Key point 3

- Percutaneous biopsy of lesions in patients with potentially operable disease is contra-indicated due to the incidence of needle track recurrence.

biopsy is essential prior to operation. This should be done using a plugged biopsy technique through liver that will ultimately be resected.

It is clear from the above description that the treatment of a primary liver tumour should be carried out in a specialist centre, which undertakes a high volume of liver surgery and has all of the appropriate diagnostic and interventional expertise. Although it is difficult to prove a volume effect from the literature, it seems reasonable to suggest that a liver centre should be performing more than 30 major resections per year and most large centres will be performing 60–120 such cases. In these circumstances, the peri-operative mortality rate in patients without primary liver disease should be in the region of 2%, with morbidity in the region of 20%. Morbidity and mortality rates are higher in patients with primary liver disease and where central resections with bile duct reconstruction are carried out.

MALIGNANT TUMOURS OF THE LIVER

The large majority of malignant tumours of the liver are carcinomas. The most common of these are hepatoma (hepatocellular carcinoma) and cholangio-carcinoma. These will be considered in this chapter, along with gallbladder cancer, which has many similarities with cholangiocarcinoma. It is, however, important to realise that there is a variety of other tumour types which are found occasionally. These include combined hepatocellular cholangio-carcinoma, adenosquamous carcinoma and, rarely, squamous carcinoma of the bile duct, and signet ring and undifferentiated carcinoma. Bile duct cystadenocarcinoma is occasionally seen and in all probability arises from a biliary cystadenoma. There is insufficient evidence in the literature to make definitive statements regarding the management of these rare tumours. However, the same principles as outlined above should be applied and, where it is possible, a complete surgical resection should be undertaken.

HEPATOMA (HEPATOCELLULAR CARCINOMA)

Hepatoma is one of the world's most common malignancies accounting for around 1.2 million deaths per year.[5] There is a considerable geographical variation, however, with incidences in some parts of Africa and Asia in the region of 100/100,000 population per year, compared to 2–4/100,000 per year in the UK. Unfortunately, most patients with hepatoma have a background of chronic liver disease, particularly cirrhosis, which makes the management problematic in most cases. Additionally, it is difficult to evaluate the effectiveness of treatment as the survival of many patients is limited by the severity of the liver disease. Cirrhosis associated with hepatitis B or C or alcohol seems to have the highest incidence of malignant transformation.[6] Not all patients who develop hepatoma, however, have cirrhosis or an obvious risk factor for the disease. These are often referred to as sporadic cases. Investigation of these cases may sometimes reveal an abnormality such as being heterozygous for alpha-1 antitrypsin deficiency. These tumours are more often amenable to surgical treatment as the remaining liver may be relatively normal.

Diagnosis and clinical features

The symptoms of hepatoma, whether in patients with liver disease or occurring sporadically, are relatively non-specific. Many are advanced and/or large when they present. The increased use of ultrasonography, which is widely available to general practitioners, has increased the number of focal liver lesions being discovered, some of which subsequently turn out to be hepatomas. In patients with liver disease, formal screening is often undertaken usually using regular ultrasound imaging and alpha-fetoprotein (AFP) measurements. AFP is elevated in 80% of patients with hepatoma. The presence of a focal liver lesion on imaging compatible with hepatoma and an elevated AFP is virtually diagnostic. However, many patients with liver disease have modestly elevated AFP levels and, in this situation, it is the trend in the level that is of most use.

A large number of imaging modalities is used in assessing patients with suspected hepatoma. These included spiral and multislice CT and MRI. However, the gold standard is still lipiodol-enhanced CT (Fig. 1).[7] Lipiodol is an iodinated derivative of poppy seed oil, which is selectively taken up by hepatoma. It is of particular value in patients with liver disease when frequently, in addition to the focal lesion being investigated, several other foci of tumour will be demonstrated within the liver. This will normally preclude resectional surgery, although not necessarily transplantation.

In most cases, the combination of imaging outlined above and an elevated AFP level is sufficient to establish a diagnosis. Percutaneous biopsy plays no part in making a diagnosis in patients who may have surgically treatable

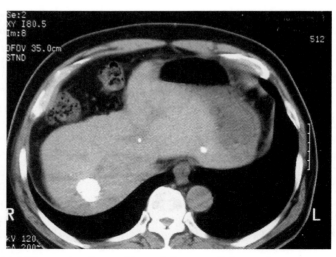

Fig. 1 Lipoidol CT scan showing multicentric hepatocellular carcinoma

disease. The difficulty arises with the indeterminate focal liver lesion and very often the diagnosis lies between a well-differentiated hepatoma, adenoma and an area of focal nodular hyperplasia. Distinguishing these conditions from each other is of importance, as whilst both hepatoma and under normal circumstances adenoma are resected focal nodular hyperplasia needs neither surgical excision nor follow-up. Current best practice is to try to establish a diagnosis on the basis of the lesion characteristic on MRI and lipiodol CT. If a diagnosis of focal nodular hyperplasia can be made with some degree of confidence, a percutaneous biopsy is warranted to confirm that the lesion is not an adenoma. In the case of a patient who is otherwise fit, adenomas should usually be excised as there is evidence that malignant transformation may occur and the lesions will commonly grow. It is, therefore, not necessary in most cases to distinguish between adenoma and a well-differentiated hepatoma. However, in patients who may not be ideally suited for resectional surgery, a percutaneous biopsy to confirm an adenoma may be occasionally necessary. Alternatively, a period of observation may settle the issue, as most hepatomas will grow in size over a period of several months.

Hepatoma in general has a poor prognosis. Many tumours rapidly invade blood vessels producing intrahepatic and extrahepatic metastases. Lymph node involvement around the hepatic artery is also common. The staging system reflects this, giving tumours which invade blood vessels a higher stage, reflecting a worse prognosis. Median survival is in the region of a year, but less than half that in patients who present with symptoms.[8] Despite this gloomy prognosis, occasional patients have prolonged survival, even in the absence of treatment.

Surgical resection

Surgical treatment is the modality which is most likely to cure a patient with a hepatoma, and this should be employed where possible. In patients with sporadic hepatoma, the liver has a normal ability to regenerate. Thus a radical resection by removal of the lobe containing the tumour is optimal. Large size is no barrier to surgical resection providing that there is no distant spread and the tumour can be completely removed. It is certainly the case that large diameter tumours have a worse prognosis than the small ones. However, even tumours weighing many kilograms can be resected with good long-term results.

Unfortunately, the vast majority of patients with hepatoma have liver disease. However, even in these patients, operative mortality rates of 4% (double that for colorectal metastases) and 5-year survivals of 30% may be achieved in very experienced centres in Japan.[9] In general terms, surgical resection should be contemplated in Childs-Pugh A patients and, occasionally, for Childs-Pugh B if the operation would be a very straightforward resection. The surgical strategy should be to remove the portal territory of the segments

Key point 4

- Hepatoma has a poor outlook overall with a median survival of 6 months in symptomatic patients. The liver disease which most commonly accompanies the tumour also severely limits survival.

involved with the tumour alone and with a 1 cm margin. Retention of functioning liver mass is essential as the ability of the liver to regenerate is largely absent in patients with cirrhosis. Patients with multifocal hepatoma (more than 2 nodules) are seldom suitable for resectional surgery although transplantation may be an option.

Liver transplantation

The use of transplantation to treat hepatoma is controversial. Patients with malignancy have less favourable outcomes after transplantation than when transplantation is performed for benign conditions. Organ availability remains a major problem such that not all patients with a benign indication for liver transplantation will receive an organ.

There is no randomised comparison of transplantation versus resection in patients with liver disease and hepatoma. However, some comparative studies are available. The summary of these studies is that the outlook for patients following transplantation is actually better than after resectional surgery providing that the tumour nodules are 3 cm or less in diameter and 3 or less in number.[10] The reason for this favourable outcome probably relates to the liver disease. The life expectancy of patients with hepatoma is often determined by the liver disease itself and this is effectively treated by the transplant. Indeed, hepatoma is sometimes diagnosed for the first time in patients who have a transplant performed for other reasons. The sensible conclusion should, therefore, be that in a patient who has an indication for liver transplantation, the presence of up to 3 nodules less than 3 cm in diameter, which may be compatible with hepatoma, but without evidence of distant spread, should not be a contra-indication for transplantation.

Non-surgical treatments

Ablative therapies

Ablative therapies have some considerable attraction in treating patients with hepatoma and liver disease. The intervention is less major than resectional surgery and the loss of functioning liver can be minimised. By contrast, however, the portal territory affected by the tumour cannot be satisfactorily ablated and spread of the tumour along portal structures is well known.

Of the ablative therapies, radio frequency ablation is the most promising. This technique uses radio frequency energy to produce tissue heat and necrosis. The device can be used percutaneously. The diameter of the tissue destruction is limited to a relatively short distance from the electrode, but manufacturers have overcome this by making arrays of electrodes or a single probe which has a tip out of which multiple electrodes emerge. With time, an area of tissue destruction several centimetres in diameter may be achieved. It is too soon to determine whether the use of radio frequency ablation can impact upon the long-term survival of patients with hepatoma. However, studies suggest that tumour masses can generally be ablated and hence there is hope that follow-up studies may demonstrate lasting benefit.[11,12] Complications include needle track recurrence, haemorrhage, and liver failure. The latter complication may be in part related to the thrombosis of portal and other vessels.

Percutaneous alcohol injection has been used for longer than radio frequency ablation.[11,12] It is simple and easy to perform and, surprisingly, destruction of tumours up to 3 cm can be achieved with relatively few complications. It is not clear why this treatment is effective in hepatoma when it appears ineffective in treating colorectal liver metastases of a similar size. Complications are similar to radio frequency ablation. It is still unclear whether alcohol injection alters the overall survival.

Key point 7

- Chemo-embolisation produces responses particularly in small tumours, but may not improve overall survival.

Transarterial chemo-embolisation (TACE)

TACE has become widely practiced in the treatment of inoperable hepatoma even in the absence of evidence of long-term clinical benefit. The technique uses a mixture of lipiodol with a chemotherapeutic agent such as doxorubicin which is injected directly into the hepatic artery. It is known that lipiodol alone does not induce significant tumour response. There is, however, good evidence that smaller tumour masses may disappear completely following treatment and overall there is a > 50% reduction in tumour size in about half the patients with small hepatomas.[13] The technique is much less successful in patients with larger tumours. Treating larger tumours is also associated with severe side-effects which include postembolisation syndrome, liver failure and liver abscess, presumably resulting from the infection of necrotic tumour.

Despite objective tumour responses being seen using this technique, there is little evidence that the patient's long-term survival is benefited, although most comparative studies are quite small.[14,15] There is an urgent need for a large randomised trial to compare TACE with no treatment.

Other treatments

Systemic chemotherapy is disappointing and should not be used outside clinical trials. Of non-chemotherapy treatments, one study has randomised 58 patients with advanced hepatoma to either receive subcutaneous injections of a somatostatin analogue (octreotide) or no treatment.[16] There was a significant survival benefit in the patients treated with octreotide, but the small size of the study makes it difficult to accept this result without corroboration. Again, there is the need for a randomised trial to be performed with sufficient size to settle the issue. This is particularly important because somatostatin analogues are now available in long-acting depot preparations and the toxicity is minimal.

CHOLANGIOCARCINOMA

Cholangiocarcinoma is a term that is now applied to malignant intrahepatic, perihilar and distal extrahepatic tumours of the bile ducts. There is unequivocal evidence that the incidence of this condition has been rising over the last several decades in the West and it now accounts for more deaths than hepatoma.[17] Although it was originally thought that the increase may simply reflect improved diagnostic methodologies in patients with obstructive jaundice, this appears not to be the case. The incidence is close to the mortality rate, as the outlook from this condition is very poor. There are some well-known risk factors[18] which, other than age, do not apply to the vast majority of patients who present with this condition. These include primary sclerosing cholangitis, for which the life-time risk is around 10%, chronic intrahepatic gallstones, Caroli's disease and choledochal cysts. In the East, liver flukes are important.

Around half of all cholangiocarcinomas are perihilar, these may be called Klatskin tumours.[18] Of the remainder, half are intrahepatic and half are related to the extrahepatic bile ducts. Bismuth and Castaing[19] suggested a classification of the Klatskin type tumours shown in Figure 2.

Diagnosis and clinical features

Most patients with cholangiocarcinoma arising in the perihilar or distal bile ducts present with obstructive jaundice or associated features. Patients with peripheral cholangiocarcinomas may present in a similar manner to sporadic hepatoma. In some cases, the diagnosis of cholangiocarcinoma can be made easily by ultrasonography and endoscopic retrograde cholangiopancreatography (ERCP) or magnetic resonance cholangiopancreatography (MRCP). Subsequent to this, the use of CT and MRI may be of additional value in staging the lesion; these allow more accurate staging, in particular diagnosing extrahepatic involvement in lymph nodes. MRI[20] is particularly useful in determining involvement of the portal vasculature. Patients with a cholangiocarcinoma but without a mass lesion on imaging appear to have a better prognosis. Endoscopic ultrasound is emerging as having considerable value in staging the disease.[21] It is particularly

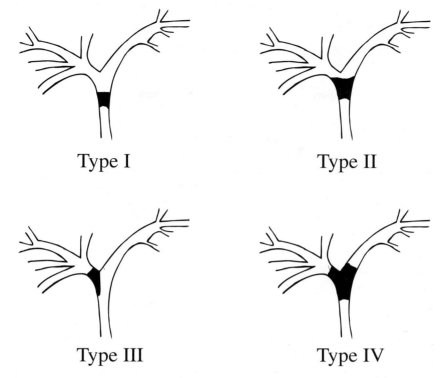

Type I Type II

Type III Type IV

Fig. 2 Classification of cholangiocarcinoma according to Bismuth et al.,[19] depending on the level of obstruction.

valuable for detecting the presence of enlarged lymph nodes and obtaining cytology in patients unsuitable for surgical treatment.

Tumour markers are of limited value. CA19-9 is elevated in cholangio-carcinoma, but it is also elevated in other causes of obstructive jaundice including those that are benign.[22] Cytology obtained at ERCP may be useful in diagnostic terms, but from experience few patients have positive cytology. Percutaneous fine needle aspiration cytology or needle biopsy are absolutely contra-indicated in patients who may be operable.

Making a specific diagnosis of a cholangiocarcinoma can be exceedingly difficult in some cases. Lymph node masses, as a result of metastases from other malignancies, are common in this region and not always easy to distinguish from cholangiocarcinoma. Additionally, benign conditions such as Mirizzi's syndrome may be surprisingly difficult to separate from malignancy even with optimal imaging. The difficulty is most extreme in patients with primary sclerosing cholangitis in which stricturing is already a feature.[22] Frank cholangiocarcinoma is a contra-indication to liver transplantation in patients with sclerosing cholangitis but, nonetheless, a significant proportion of patients transplanted for this condition turn out to have a malignancy in the excised specimen.

Surgical resection

Although most patients with cholangiocarcinoma will receive only palliative stenting, surgery is the only method of achieving cure.[23,24] The challenge for

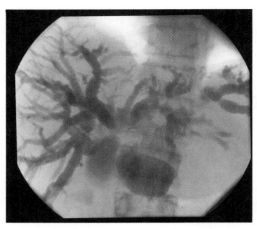

Fig. 3 Percutaneous cholangiogram showing a Bismuth Type IV cholangiocarcinoma

liver surgeons presented with this disease is considerable. The principal difficulty relates to the hilar tumour (Fig. 3) and its intimate relationship to the essential structures of the liver. Peripheral cholangiocarcinomas can be dealt with by straightforward hepatectomy as with any other liver tumour.

Controversies abound in the management of the hilar cholangiocarcinoma. A consensus of surgical opinion would be that surgical treatment is difficult and should be reserved for the fittest patients. Overt lymph node involvement on imaging or encasement of the hepatic hilar vessels are contra-indications to resectional surgery. The controversy concerning pre-operative biliary drainage remains.[25] The randomised studies, such as they are, do not provide evidence of advantage for pre-operative biliary drainage. By contrast, however, few liver surgeons are prepared to carry out major liver surgery on a patient with undrained obstructive jaundice and hence it is questionable whether the randomised trials have any particular value. Drainage of the liver from below by ERCP is optimal from a surgical point of view as the risk of tumour implantation is avoided. It is particularly important that the liver to be retained at operation should be drained. Unfortunately, cholangitis in undrained liver is quite common, particularly after an intervention like ERCP.

In tumours involving the hilum, the aim must be to achieve a tumour-free margin of at least 5 mm. Additionally, as the lymph nodes are commonly involved with micrometastases, radical resection of the lymph nodes around the hepatic artery as far as the coeliac axis and behind the duodenum should be carried out routinely.[23,24] The extent of the liver resection depends on the site of the tumour (Table 1).

For anatomical reasons, liver surgeons prefer, where possible, to perform an extended right hepatic lobectomy. The reason for this is that there is significant length of extrahepatic left bile duct. This is in marked contrast to the situation on the right. Thus there is more opportunity to achieve tumour clearance by leaving segments 2 and 3, whilst removing the rest of the liver. Obviously this is a very major procedure and techniques are being developed to reduce the chances of liver failure following the procedure. In all cases, reconstruction is made using a hepaticojejunostomy Roux-en-y.

Table 1 Extent of liver resection recommended for cholangiocarcinoma

Bismuth type	Liver resection required
Type 1	May not be necessary
Type 2	Segment 1 and all extrahepatic biliary tree
Type 3	Left or right hepatectomy, plus segment 1 and all extrahepatic biliary tree
Type 4	Extended right hepatic lobectomy (preferred option) Extended left hepatic lobectomy* Central liver resection*

*Type 4 lesions require individualised approach to obtain tumour clearance on all bile duct margins and to resect areas of vascular involvement if appropriate.

The technique of central liver resection for cholangiocarcinoma (also termed the Taj Mahal resection owing to the shape of the defect in the liver) has been described in recent years.[26] This involves removal of segments 1, 4 and 5 and the relevant bile ducts. The advantage over the extended right resection is that more functioning liver remains. By contrast, it is technically much more difficult to perform as it involves the dissection of the branches of the hepatic artery and portal vein within the right side of the liver which are intimately involved with the bile duct. The reconstruction involves the anastomosis of several bile ducts to the Roux loop, increasing the possibility of postoperative leakage. The more simple, although more destructive, extended right hepatectomy is certainly technically easier.

One of the major problems encountered from extended hepatectomy is postoperative liver failure. For this reason, interest has grown in embolising the portal vein of the liver to be removed in order to induce hypertrophy in the liver to be retained. Although this technique sounds problematic, embolisation of the right or left portal vein is associated with virtually no morbidity or systemic upset.[27] Studies following such patients with CT indicate that over the course of several weeks there is significant atrophy of the embolised liver and growth of the contralateral liver. Although objective evidence from randomised trials is lacking, many liver surgeons find this technique to be a very significant advance.

Despite aggressive surgical treatment, the outlook in the subgroup that is suitable for surgical treatment remains poor with the 5-year survival being in the region of 20%. Lymph node involvement found in the excised specimen correlates with a poor surgical outcome. By contrast, tumours with a papillary histology, and confined to the bile ducts, have a much better outlook.

Key point 9

- Resectional surgery can cure patients but the operation is technically demanding. To achieve the possibility of cure, clear tumour margins must be achieved.

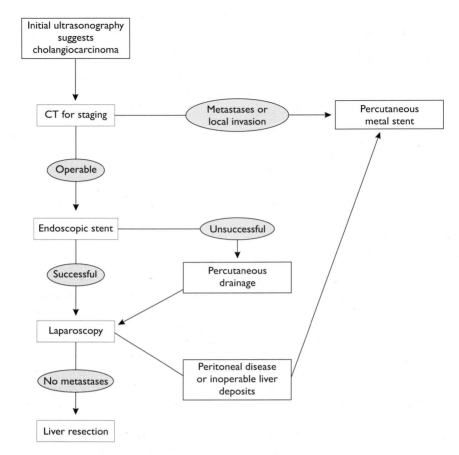

Fig. 4 Algorithm for staging and operative strategy for cholangiocarcinoma.

Liver transplantation has been attempted in patients with cholangiocarcinoma, but the results are dismal and this is now contra-indicated.

A reasonable approach to a patient who may have an operable cholangiocarcinoma is shown in Figure 4. Staging should be performed prior to stenting. Thereafter, endoscopic stenting should be employed wherever possible, draining the side of the liver to be retained. Laparoscopy at an early stage is advantageous as a proportion of patients, perhaps as many as 20%, will have unsuspected peritoneal disease which precludes further surgical treatment. In patients who will undergo an extended right resection, particular attention should be given to segments 2 and 3 of the liver. Where these are large, operation may proceed as soon as the patient is fit. If they are relatively diminutive, embolisation of the right portal vein followed by a period of a few weeks to allow the liver to hypertrophy is appropriate.

Palliative biliary decompression and stenting
The majority of patients with cholangiocarcinoma will be treated by stenting as the sole method of treatment. Stenting should not be employed prior to a decision on whether the patient is operable or not, except in extreme

circumstances, such as severe cholangitis. Most patients will have decompression performed prior to surgery despite the lack of an evidence base. Stents may be inserted endoscopically, percutaneously or using the combined approach. Which technique is used may often depend on the expertise in the centre. Certainly, it is more technically difficult to achieve adequate biliary drainage from below. This is particularly the case with hilar tumours where several stents may be necessary to adequately drain the liver. However, percutaneous drainage has the risk of seeding in the drainage track and this is of particular importance in patients who have the possibility of surgical resection. Some oncologists advocate a single fraction of radiotherapy to the drainage site to prevent local recurrence. This may not, however, prevent peritoneal dissemination.

Comparisons have been made of plastic *versus* metal stents.[28] Metal stents are cost-effective in patients who survive more than 6 months, whereas in patients surviving for less than 6 months, plastic stents are satisfactory. In the long-term, tumour growth through the mesh of metal stents may lead to further biliary obstruction, but placing a plastic stent through the lumen of the metal stent may be satisfactory. Palliative surgical drainage by anastamosing a Roux loop to the segment III duct is an effective means of palliating obstructive jaundice secondary to cholangiocarcinoma, but improvements in stent technology mean that this approach is seldom employed.

Non-surgical treatments

Cholangiocarcinoma does not respond well to other treatment modalities. In the past, chemotherapy has been relatively ineffective. More recently, it has been shown that partial responses may be achieved using gemcitabine[29] in combination, to the extent that some patients who previously were inoperable can become suitable for radical surgery. However, there is no convincing evidence that treatment with chemotherapy will improve the overall survival. Large randomised trials are needed.

There is no current evidence that external beam radiotherapy, with or without chemotherapy, improves survival. Similarly, although intraluminal brachytherapy with a irridiant implant and combined with external beam radiotherapy, may have some efficacy in treating the tumour, there is no objective evidence of increased survival.[30] Thus, all of the non-surgical approaches to cholangiocarcinoma require to be investigated in large, well designed clinical trials.

Key point 10
- Combination chemotherapy including gemcitabine may produce useful responses.

GALLBLADDER CANCER

As with cholangiocarcinoma, carcinoma of the gallbladder is increasing in frequency. Indeed, there are very many similarities between cholangiocarcinoma

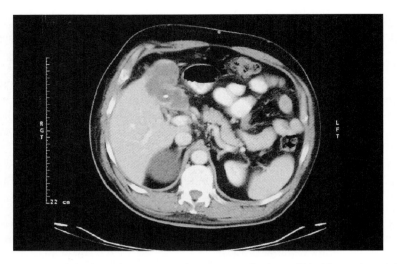

Fig. 5 CT scan of the liver showing a malignant mass in the gallbladder and a calcified gallstone

and carcinoma of the gallbladder and histologically they are similar. Unlike cholangiocarcinoma, however, the cause of gallbladder cancer is reasonably well understood. Virtually all of the patients have gallstones[31] (Fig. 5) and, in many, these have been long standing. As with cholangiocarcinoma, the overall outlook is poor.

Diagnosis and clinical features

There are several common presentations for gallbladder cancer. Some patients present with obstructive jaundice, the diagnosis being made by imaging. These patients usually have bulky, advanced and inoperable disease and there is seldom any treatment possible other than endoscopic palliation. Secondly, some patients present with gallbladder symptoms and on imaging the gallbladder appears abnormal often with a thick wall, intraluminal mass or evidence of liver invasion. It is important that such patients be recognised as having gallbladder cancer and that cholecystectomy is not attempted. The patient should be referred for specialist investigation and treatment. Lastly, and increasingly commonly, malignancy is found on histological examination of the gallbladder from a patient who has undergone laparoscopic chole-cystectomy. Although this diagnosis may come as a surprise to the surgeon, very often there were some features at operation or even in the pre-operative imaging that suggested the diagnosis. As with cholangiocarcinoma, lymph node and peritoneal metastases are common. Thus, investigation with axial imaging and laparoscopic ultrasound are particularly useful in order to stage the patient. Peritoneal involvement or extensive lymph node involvement are contra-indications to surgery whereas direct involvement of the liver substance is not particularly problematic.

Surgical treatment

Staging is crucial in the management of disease. The data suggest that patients with carcinoma confined to the mucosa may be safely treated by cholecyst-ectomy alone. However, any higher stage warrants more aggressive treatment.

Key point 11

- Patients with gallbladder cancer beyond the mucosa should have a liver resection and nodal clearance.

Specifically, patients with muscle invasive gallbladder cancer should be treated by liver resection and en-bloc lymphadenectomy of the hepatic artery nodes.[31]

Although some surgeons employ extended right hepatic lobectomy in the treatment of gallbladder cancer, most liver surgeons would favour a more conservative approach on the basis that the spread of the disease is most commonly to the peritoneum and regional lymph nodes rather than deeply into the liver substance. Thus excision of segment IV and segment V, segments which comprise the gallbladder bed, is usually sufficient, combined with the lymphadenectomy mentioned above. In performing this procedure, it is important to mobilise the duodenum and remove the retroduodenal lymph nodes, which may harbour lymph node metastases. If the tumour is well clear of the cystic duct, then excision of the extrahepatic biliary tree is not necessary. By contrast, if there is tumour in or around the cystic duct, then extrahepatic excision of the biliary tree is indicated with Roux-en-y reconstruction.

There is little doubt that, if the surface of the gallbladder is involved with tumour and the patient has undergone a laparoscopic cholecystectomy, there is an extremely high chance of peritoneal dissemination and particularly port site recurrence.[33] For this reason, it is recommended that patients in this situation should have the port sites widely excised as part of the definitive surgical treatment. However, the prognosis in these patients is probably quite poor and certainly it is better that simple cholecystectomy is avoided in the first instance. Patients with suspected gallbladder cancer should undergo evaluation and combined gallbladder and liver resection in a specialist centre.

The global outlook from gallbladder cancer is poor although this reflects the advanced stage at presentation or the preliminary surgical treatment of unrecognised gallbladder cancer. Certainly, patients with cancer confined to the mucosa have an

Key point 12

- Gallbladder cancer is almost invariably associated with gallstones. Laparoscopic cholecystectomy is contra-indicated in patients with a suspicion of malignancy.

Key point 13

- Inadvertent laparoscopic cholecystectomy in patients with incidental cancer carries a poor prognosis and the port sites should be widely excised.

excellent outlook with cholecystectomy alone. By contrast, patients with peritoneal involvement or lymph node metastases have an extremely poor outlook.

Non-surgical treatments

The situation with regard to chemotherapy in gallbladder cancer is similar to that of cholangiocarcinoma. Some newer chemotherapeutic regimens, such as those containing gemcitabine, may have some efficacy, but there is no trial evidence as yet that these regimens improve the survival. Properly performed randomised trials in this area are urgently needed. At present, there does not appear to be a convincing role for radiotherapy.

Key points for clinical practice

- Major liver resections can be carried out with very low morbidity and mortality rates in specialist centres.

- The complication rate is higher in patients with liver disease.

- Percutaneous biopsy of lesions in patients with potentially operable disease is contra-indicated due to the incidence of needle track recurrence.

- Hepatoma has a poor outlook overall with a median survival of 6 months in symptomatic patients. The liver disease which most commonly accompanies the tumour also severely limits survival.

- Surgical resection should be undertaken where possible if there are 1 or 2 nodules in a patient in Childs-Pugh A.

- Transplantation may be useful in a patient with liver disease and 3 nodules of 3 cm or less.

- Chemo-embolisation produces responses particularly in small tumours, but may not improve overall survival.

- Cholangiocarcinoma is increasing in incidence. The overall outlook is poor.

- Resectional surgery can cure patients but the operation is technically demanding. To achieve the possibility of cure, clear tumour margins must be achieved.

- Combination chemotherapy including gemcitabine may produce useful responses.

- Patients with gallbladder cancer beyond the mucosa should have a liver resection and nodal clearance.

- Gallbladder cancer is almost invariably associated with gallstones. Laparoscopic cholecystectomy is contra-indicated in patients with a suspicion of malignancy.

- Inadvertent laparoscopic cholecystectomy in patients with incidental cancer carries a poor prognosis and the port sites should be widely excised.

References

1. Scheele J, Stang R, Altendorf Hofinaun A, Paul M. Resection of colorectal liver metastases. *World J Surg* 1995; **19**: 59–71.
2. Couinaud C. Liver anatomy: portal (and suprahepatic) or biliary segmentation. *Dig Surg* 1999; **16**: 459–467.
3. Rees M, Plant G, Bygrave S. Late results justify resection for multiple hepatic metastases from colorectal cancer. *Br J Surg* 1997; **84**: 136–140.
4. John TG, Plant G, Rees M. Tumour seeding: an avoidable legacy of biopsy of colorectal liver metastases. *Gut* 1999; **44 (Suppl 1)**: A48.
5. Johnson RC. Hepatocellular carcinoma. *Hepatogastroenterology* 1997; **44**: 307–312.
6. Bain I, McMaster P. Benign and malignant liver tumours. *Surgery* 1997; **15**: 169–174.
7. Batolazzi C, Lencioni R, Caramella D *et al.* Small HCC. Detection with US, CT MRI, DSA and lipiodol–CT. *Acta Radiol* 1996; **37**: 69–74.
8. Balvie S. Hepatocellular carcinoma. *Postgrad Med J* 2000; **76**: 4–11.
9. The Liver Cancer Study Group of Japan. Primary liver cancer in Japan: clinicopathological features and results of surgical treatment. *Ann Surg* 1990; **211**: 277–287.
10. Bismuth H, Chiche L, Adam R *et al.* Liver resection versus transplantation for hepatocellular carcinoma in cirrhotic patients. *Ann Surg* 1993; **218**: 145–151.
11. Becker D, Hansler JM, Strobel D, Hahn EG. Percutaneous ethanol injection and radio frequency ablation for the treatment of non resectable colorectal liver metastases – techniques and results. *Langenbecks Arch Surg* 1999; **384**: 339–343.
12. Rust C, Gores GJ. Locoregional management of hepatocellular carcinoma. Surgical and ablation therapies. *Clin Liver Dis* 2001; **5**: 161–173.
13. Ryder SD, Rizza PM, Metivier E, Karani J, Williams R. Chemoembolisation with lipiodol and doxorubicin: applicability in British patients with HCC. *Gut* 1996; **38**: 125–128.
14. Pelletier G, Roche A, Ink O *et al.* A randomised trial of hepatic arterial chemoembolisation in patients with unresectable HCC. *Hepatology* 1990; **77**: 181–184.
15. Groupe d'Etude et de Traitement du Carcinome Hepatocellulaire. Comparison of lipiodol chemoembolisation and conservative treatment for unresectable HCC. *N Engl J Med* 1995; **332**: 1256–1261.
16. Kouroumalis E, Skordilis P, Thermos K *et al.* Treatment of HCC with octreotide: a randomised controlled study. *Gut* 1998; **42**; 442–447.
17. Taylor-Robinson SD, Toledano MB, Arora S *et al.* Increase in mortality rates for intrahepatic cholangiocarcinoma in England and Wales 1968–1998: *Gut* 2001; **48**: 816–820.
18. De Groen PC, Gores GJ, LaRusso NF, Gunderson LL, Nagorney DM. Biliary tract cancers. *N Engl J Med* 1999; **341**: 1368–1379.
19. Bismuth H, Castaing D. *Hepatobiliary Malignancy*. London: Edward Arnold, 1994; 416–424.
20. Magnuson TH, Bender JS, Duncan MD, Ahrendt SA, Harmon JW, Regan F. Utility of magnetic resonance cholangiography in the evaluation of biliary obstruction. *J Am Coll Surg* 1999; **189**: 63–72.
21. Wiersema MJ, Vilmann P, Giovannini M, Chang KJ, Wiersema LM. Endosonography-guided fine-needle aspiration biopsy: diagnostic accuracy and complication assessment. *Gastroenterology* 1997; **112**: 1087–1095.
22. Patel AH, Harnois DM, Klee GG, LaRusso NF, Gores GJ. The utility of CA 19–9 in the diagnoses of cholangiocarcinoma in patients without primary sclerosing cholangitis. *Am J Gastroenterol* 2000; **95**: 204–207.
23. Nimura Y, Kamiya J, Nagino M *et al.* Aggressive surgical treatment of hilar cholangiocarcinoma. *J Hepatobiliary Pancreat Surg* 1998; **5**: 52–61.
24. Madariaga JR, Iwatsuki S, Todo S, Lee RG, Irish W, Starzl TE. Liver resection for hilar and peripheral cholangiocarcinomas: a study of 62 cases. *Ann Surg* 1998; **227**: 70–79.
25. Hochwald SN, Burke EC, Jarnagin WR, Fong Y, Blumgart LH. Association of preoperative biliary stenting with increased postoperative infectious complications in proximal cholangiocarcinoma. *Arch Surg* 1999; **134**: 261–266.
26. Kawarada Y, Isaji S, Taoka H, Tabata M, Das BC, Yokoi H. S4a + S5 with caudate lobe

(S1) resection using the Taj Mahal liver parenchymal resection for carcinoma of the biliary tract. *J Gastrointest Surg* 1999; **3**: 369–373.

27. Wakabayashi H, Ishimura K, Okano K *et al*. Is preoperative portal vein embolization effective in improving prognosis after major hepatic resection in patients with advanced-stage hepatocellular carcinoma? *Cancer* 2001; **92**: 2384–2390.

28 Lammer J, Hausegger KA, Fluckiger F *et al*. Common bile duct obstruction due to malignancy: treatment with plastic versus metal stents. *Radiology* 1996; **201**: 167–172.

29. Kubicka S, Rudolph KL, Tietze MK, Lorenz M, Manns M. Phase II study of systemic gemcitabine chemotherapy for advanced unresectable hepatobiliary carcinomas. *Hepatogastroenterology* 2001; **48**: 783–789.

30. Hejna M, Pruckmayer M, Raderer M. The role of chemotherapy and radiation in the management of biliary cancer: a review of the literature. *Eur J Cancer* 1998; **34**: 977–986.

31. Dhiel AK. Gallstone size and the risk of gallbladder cancer. *JAMA* 1983; **250**: 2323–2326.

32. Wise PE, Shi YY, Washington MK *et al*. Radical resection improves survival for patients with pT2 gallbladder carcinoma. *Am Surg* 2001; **67**: 1041–1047.

33. Lundberg O. Port site metastases after laparoscopic cholecystectomy. *Eur J Surg* 2000; **Suppl 585**: 27–30.

Meheshinder Singh John R.T. Monson

10

Large bowel obstruction

There are considerable differences between obstruction of the small and large bowel. The large bowel becomes obstructed 3–4 times less frequently than its small bowel counterpart. Nonetheless, large bowel obstruction remains a common surgical emergency. The main causes are cancer (primary or recurrent) and sigmoid volvulus, the prevalence being subject to a wide geographical variation. Colorectal cancer accounts for four of every five obstructions in Western Europe and North America. In Eastern Europe and many other parts of the world, sigmoid volvulus predominates as the primary cause. Pseudo-obstruction of the large bowel is an important differential diagnosis. Other causes are benign strictures usually the result of diverticular disease, ischaemia or anastomotic strictures (Table 1).

Key point 1

• The main causes of large bowel obstruction are cancer and volvulus.

CLINICAL PRESENTATION

The clinical manifestations of large bowel obstruction largely depend upon the site of obstruction and function of the ileocaecal valve. An obstructing lesion at the ileocaecal valve produces signs and symptoms of small bowel obstruction.

Dr Meheshinder Singh MBBS MMed(S'pore) FRCS(Edin) FRCSI, Colorectal Clinical Fellow, Academic Surgical Unit, Castle Hill Hospital, Cottingham HU16 5JQ, UK

Prof. John R.T. Monson MD FRCS FRCSI FACS FRCPSGlas(Hon), Professor of Surgery and Head of Department, Academic Surgical Unit, Castle Hill Hospital, Cottingham HU16 5JQ, UK (for correspondence)

Table 1 Causes of lower bowel obstruction

Cancer
Sigmoid volvulus
Diverticular disease
Strictures – ischaemic, diverticular, malignant, anastomotic
IBD
Hernia
Faecal impaction
Pseudo-obstruction
Miscellaneous

Patency of the ileocaecal valve implies that the valve functions correctly and allows only antegrade passage of gas and faeces. When there is distal obstruction, the valve often becomes incompetent and both the small and large bowel distend. However, if the valve remains competent, it results in a closed loop obstruction of the segment of colon between the valve and the obstructing lesion. The colon distends progressively as the ileum continues to empty gas and fluid into the obstructed segment. Failure to decompress this allows the intracolonic pressure to build up rapidly which may ultimately result in ischaemia and perforation which is a disastrous complication of obstruction.

According to Laplace's law, the caecum dilates more easily than other parts of the colon because of its greater original diameter and thinner wall; hence, it is at a greater risk of perforation (Fig. 1). According to the law, tension (in this case, in the wall of the colon) is proportional to the radius, and is, therefore, higher in the caecum than elsewhere:

$$2T = PR \qquad\qquad \text{Eq. 1}$$

where T is wall tension, P is transmural pressure, and R is radius of a sphere.

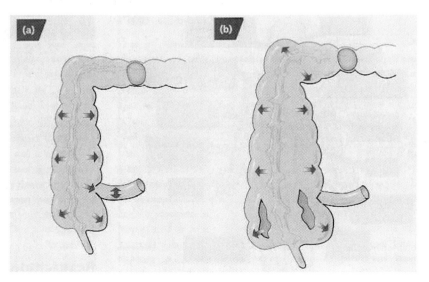

Fig. 1 Obstruction from a tumour in the transverse colon. In (a) ileocaecal valve remains open, but in (b) a competent valve results in a closed loop obstruction.

Key point 2

- A closed loop obstruction involves the segment of colon between a competent ileocaecal valve and the obstructing lesion. Failure to identify this may result in a caecal perforation.

DIAGNOSIS

The diagnosis of large bowel obstruction is made by means of a good history and clinical examination. A plain supine abdominal radiograph is mandatory. The use of an erect film does not yield any further significant information,[1] and has been abandoned in most centres.

Plain radiographs reveal gaseous distended colon down to the point of obstruction. There will be little or no gas in the colon or rectum distal to the obstruction. The level of obstruction is often estimated by the point of distal cut-off of the gas shadow. It is important to remember that this cut-off can be misleading as the gas shadows may terminate far short of the obstructing lesion, when the lumen immediately proximal to the obstruction is filled with fluid or semisolid faeces. In one series, the overall sensitivity of plain films in predicting the level of obstruction was 60%.[2]

In the case of a closed loop obstruction, the caecum may appear as a large, distended, gas-filled organ in the right lower quadrant (Fig. 2). The small bowel loops may be distended, although this would depend upon the competence of the ileocaecal valve.

Although plain abdominal films are helpful in diagnosing obstruction, they can be misleading in many instances (Table 2).

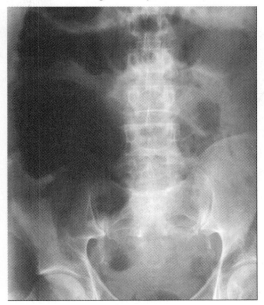

Fig. 2 Closed loop obstruction caused by a splenic flexure tumour. Note the dilated caecum.

Table 2 Drawbacks of plain radiographs

- Inaccurate localization of level of obstruction
- Misleading distribution of gas shadows (stopping short of the site of obstruction)
- Large bowel obstruction simulating appearance of small bowel obstruction
- Inability to differentiate a mechanical from a pseudo-obstruction

CONTRAST ENEMA

It is difficult differentiating between a mechanical obstruction and a pseudo-obstruction on a plain abdominal radiograph. Such a diagnostic error may result in an unnecessary laparotomy. For these reasons, we recommend the use of a water-soluble contrast enema in all patients with suspected large bowel obstruction (Fig. 3).

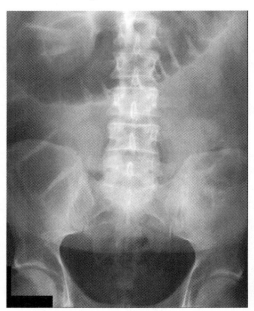

Fig. 3 Large bowel obstruction caused by an anastomotic stricture. Note the staple line.

Key point 3

- Contrast radiology is indicated in all cases of apparent large bowel obstruction except when the clinical condition dictates an emergency operation.

Pseudo-obstruction is confidently diagnosed only if the contrast flows freely around to the caecum. A positive finding on the enema may demonstrate a shouldered cut-off in the case of malignancy, the beak sign at the apex of a

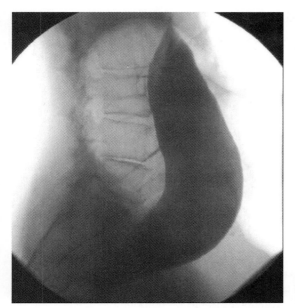

Fig. 4 Bird's beak sign diagnostic of sigmoid volvulus.

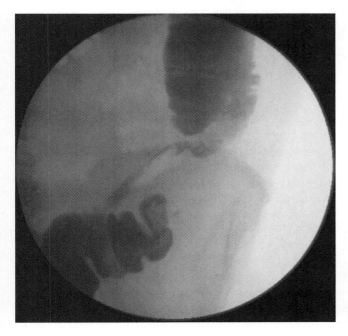

Fig. 5 Water-soluble contrast enema showing an anastomotic stricture

volvulus (Fig. 4), the coiled spring appearance in intussusception, or a long tapered stricture with mucosal oedema in the case of diverticular stricture.

The contrast media of choice is gastrograffin (Fig. 5), a water soluble hyperosmolar agent which draws fluid into the colon. This fact gives it significant therapeutic potential by softening the inspissated faeces and allowing it to pass through the obstruction. However, a single contrast study of this nature should never be considered a replacement for formal colonic evaluation should mechanical obstruction be excluded.

OTHER DIAGNOSTIC IMAGING

Ultrasonography has a limited role in the diagnosis of large bowel obstruction. Presence of dilated, gas-filled bowel hinders proper imaging. It offers a sensitivity of 23% in determining the aetiology of obstruction in comparison to plain films (7%).[2] Ultrasonography may provide useful information particularly if there is a large palpable mass or presence of liver metastases, especially when the decision to operate on an elderly patient is otherwise borderline

Computerized tomography (CT) is a very good modality in evaluating patients with suspected obstruction.[3,4] It is a highly accurate method in determining the level and cause of obstruction and should be the technique of choice when clinical or plain radiographic findings are equivocal. In one series, CT successfully diagnosed colonic obstruction in 45 of 47 patients (96% sensitivity) and correctly localized the point of obstruction in 44 of 47 patients (94%). CT is also superior (87%) to both ultrasonography (23%) and plain radiography (7%) in determining the aetiology of obstruction.[2]

CT can provide useful information particularly when there is a large palpable mass which might be fixed to the surrounding structures. This would be of assistance in anticipating an area of difficult dissection. CT might also demonstrate invasion of a ureter from an obstructing cancer or presence of liver metastases and may visualize small quantities of free intraperitoneal gas which may not be visible on plain radiographs.

Key point 4

- CT is highly accurate in determining the level and cause of obstruction.

CT colonography is an exciting and promising technique with an enormous potential for colorectal screening in the future.[5] However, its use in the acute setting is still in its infancy. It makes use of volumetric CT data combined with specialized computer software to produce three-dimensional endoluminal images of the colon and rectum.

The unique capabilities of CT colonography include the display of the proximal colon that is inaccessible at colonoscopy because of the obstructing lesion. At the same time, it can stage the cancer as well as identify any synchronous lesions.[5,6] In one series, a total of 97% (87/90) of all colonic segments were adequately visualized at CT colonography in patients with obstructing colorectal lesions compared with 60% (26/42) of segments at barium enema.[6]

Magnetic resonance imaging (MRI) has evolved with improvements in software design that allows faster imaging but current low levels of availability in the acute setting preclude its wider use.[7]

Key point 5

- MRI and CT colonography are advanced modalities of imaging and their role in large bowel obstruction is uncertain.

Chou *et al.*[8] demonstrated the use of MRI in bowel obstruction. By retrograde insufflation of 1 l of air through a Foley catheter placed in the rectum, they were able to delineate the level of obstruction in 7 of 9 patients.

An algorithm for the investigation of large bowel obstruction is shown in Figure 6.

PRINCIPLES OF MANAGEMENT

Although the majority of patients with large bowel obstruction present with incomplete obstruction, invariably they have lost a considerable volume of fluid and electrolytes and may, in addition, be chronically malnourished. Also, most of them are elderly individuals with frequent co-morbidity. These factors should be taken into consideration before planning surgery.

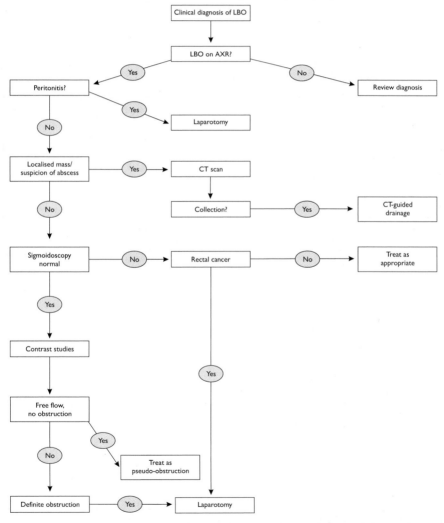

Fig. 6 Algorithm for diagnosis of large bowel obstruction (LBO). AXR, abdominal radiograph.

Key point 6

- Initial treatment should be aimed at: (i) restoring the circulating blood volume; (ii) replacing the fluid and electrolyte deficits; and (iii) optimizing and preparing for surgery (if there is a need).

On the other hand, patients with acute large bowel obstruction are usually unwell and require aggressive resuscitation ideally within a HDU/ITU setting. Therefore, delay in resuscitation, and in planning and starting operative treatment, is to be avoided. Most patients with acute on chronic obstruction due to a mechanical obstruction will require an operation at some stage. The degree of urgency will depend upon: (i) the severity of obstruction; (ii) the general state of the patient; and (iii) the judgement of the surgeon as to whether strangulation or impending perforation is likely.

The precise choice of techniques and approach (surgery, interventional radiology) depends on the cause of the obstruction, its site, and the general condition of the patient.

Key point 7

- Surgery should not be unduly delayed especially when there are signs suggesting underlying ischaemia or impending perforation.

MANAGEMENT OF OBSTRUCTION CAUSED BY MALIGNANCY

Despite increasing efforts in early detection of colorectal cancers, advanced disease presenting with acute obstruction accounts for 8–30% of all cancers.[9–11]

In the past, the safest mode of treatment of an obstructing carcinoma of the colon was to decompress the obstructed segment or bypass the growth and perform resection at a later stage irrespective of tumour location. Currently, it is widely accepted that obstructive right-sided colonic tumours can be treated by a primary resection and anastomosis. In contrast, the management of obstructive left-sided lesions is still a topic of controversy with various differing opinions.

Right-sided obstruction

Goligher and Smiddy[12] were the pioneers who described right hemicolectomy as the procedure of choice for obstructing tumours of the right colon. Even when a closed loop obstruction exists and the caecum is markedly distended, a right hemicolectomy is feasible provided extreme care is taken to avoid caecal perforation. Intestinal continuity may be restored by an end-to-end, end-to-side or side-to-side ileotransverse anastomosis (stapled or hand-sewn), depending on the relative discrepancy in the width of the bowel ends, and on the surgeon's preference. Our preferred technique is a side-to-side stapled ileotransverse anastomosis using a linear cutter stapler (Multifire GIA80, Autosuture). When the colon is obstructed by a carcinoma of the splenic flexure, an extended right hemicolectomy is the procedure of choice with anastomosis between the ileum and the descending colon.

If the lesion is inoperable because of fixity, a bypass procedure like an ileotransverse anastomosis is appropriate. In the presence of perforation and significant soiling, resection and formation of an ileostomy and a mucus fistula is a safe and effective option.

Left-sided obstructions

Traditionally, left-sided obstructions were treated by a three stage procedure consisting of a primary colostomy, subsequent definitive resection, and finally reversal of the colostomy. This three stage procedure was gradually replaced by a two stage (Hartmann's procedure) and, more recently, by single stage operations.

There are a number of factors which influence the choice of an operative procedure (Table 3). When the patient's general status is poor, a staged procedure with the creation of a colostomy is the safest option. Most surgeons would opt for a Hartmann's procedure, wherein the obstructing tumour is resected and the proximal colon is brought out as an end colostomy with the distal end (rectum) stapled or oversewn. The principal advantages of this procedure are that the lesion has been resected and that potential for an anastomotic leakage is avoided. The major disadvantage is the difficulty in reversal once the patient has fully recovered from the initial operation.

Single-stage procedure

Fear of septic complications especially anastomotic leakage has traditionally turned surgeons away from doing anastomosis in the face of an acute left-sided colonic obstruction. However, experience has accumulated to show that primary anastomosis is associated with minimum morbidity and mortality in the acute setting.[14,15] Therefore, it is not surprising that many centres currently propose a primary resection of the tumour followed by immediate restoration of intestinal continuity. This can be either in the form of a subtotal colectomy with primary ileosigmoid or ileorectal anastomoses,[16] or an intra-operative colonic lavage with immediate colocolonic or colorectal anastomosis.[17,18] Present data also support the notion that single staged resections with primary anastomosis in the emergency setting is generally safe[19] with results that are comparable to those of elective surgery.[20,21] There are, however, conflicting data with regard to the preferred type of single stage procedure.

The SCOTIA (subtotal colectomy *versus* on-table irrigation with anastomosis) study group[22] performed the first randomized trial comparing these techniques for

Table 3 Factors which influence the choice of an operative procedure (from Torralba *et al.*[13])

Patient's general status – poor	
Operative findings	Presence of a synchronous lesion Significant peritoneal dissemination Status of proximal bowel
Status of sphincter function or anal continence	
Most importantly – the Surgeon's experience	

the management of left-sided malignant colonic obstruction. Of the 91 eligible patients recruited by 12 centres, 47 were randomized to subtotal colectomy and 44 to on-table irrigation and segmental colectomy. Hospital mortality rates were similar in the two groups. However, postoperative morbidity was somewhat higher in the subtotal colectomy group; this was related to a significantly higher bowel frequency in this group. The SCOTIA study group concluded that segmental resection following intra-operative irrigation was the preferred option except in cases of perforation of the caecum, when subtotal colectomy was more appropriate.

By contrast, Torralba *et al.*[13] favour subtotal colectomy and they claim that intra-operative colonic lavage should only be performed when the anastomosis must be in the rectum or in patients with a history of incontinence. One major advantage of subtotal colectomy is the ease of follow-up and the ability to deal with both synchronous and metachronous tumours.

Key point 8

- In favourable circumstances, a single-stage procedure is a safe option in the management of malignant left-sided colonic obstruction.

In general, a single-stage procedure is suitable in patients with acute left-sided obstruction except in those who are haemodynamically unstable or who have peritonitis.

Currently, the use of self-expandable metallic stents (SEMS) in relieving left-sided colonic obstruction has become popular (Fig. 7). SEMS have proven effectiveness in relieving obstructions of the oesophagus and the biliary tree. The use of SEMS in colonic obstruction was first reported by Itabashi in 1993.[23]

SEMS are effective in relieving colonic obstruction temporarily in preparation for subsequent surgery, hence avoiding an operation in the emergency setting.[24–26] Patients could subsequently undergo a single staged operation and could avoid a stoma in favourable circumstances.[27] SEMS also provide a good means of palliating unresectable obstructing tumours.[26,28]

Tejero,[29] in 1997, introduced a three-staged procedure for the relief of malignant left-colonic obstruction: (i) resolution of the obstruction by means of a stent placed at the site of the tumour; (ii) recovery of the general state of the patient; and (iii) elective and final surgery (if not suitable, the stent may be used as a definitive palliative treatment).

In this series, the obstruction was resolved in 35 of 38 patients (92%). In 22 patients, the three phases were completed and in 13 patients the stent constituted definitive palliative treatment. One patient (2.6%) died after resection of the tumour.

VOLVULUS

In the Western world, volvulus accounts for 1–7% of all intestinal obstruction.[30] However, in other areas (e.g., Africa) it is a more common cause of obstruction. The commonest site of volvulus is the sigmoid colon which

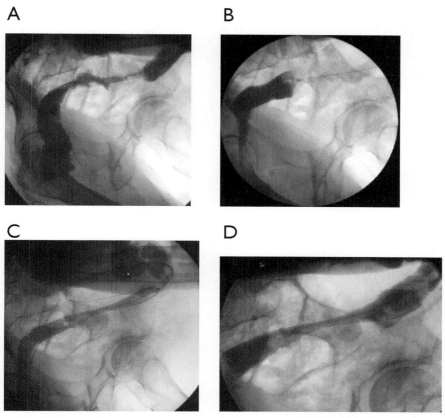

Fig. 7 An 87-year-old patient with an inoperable obstructing sigmoid cancer. (a) Malignant sigmoid stricture; (b) guide wire passed beyond the stricture; (c)Wall stent introduced over wire; (d)stent in place – note the spindle shape with the centre of the stent covering the obstruction site.

accounts for 70–80% of all large bowel volvulus. This is followed by volvulus of the caecum and, rarely, the transverse colon or splenic flexure.

Sigmoid volvulus

Plain abdominal radiographs are usually diagnostic showing a markedly distended sigmoid colon extending towards the right upper quadrant (Fig. 8). However, when in doubt, a water-soluble contrast enema may be useful provided the patient is fit enough to undergo the procedure. The contrast may reveal a complete obstruction to flow with a characteristic 'bird's beak' appearance at the base of the torsion (Fig. 4) If the contrast does get past the base, the distended sigmoid loop will be demonstrated. In some cases, this is therapeutic by itself.

The choice of treatment hinges upon whether or not there are signs of ischaemia or strangulation.

Endoscopic deflation

Since its introduction by Bruusgaard in 1947, non-operative decompression has become the treatment of choice for patients without any signs of peritonitis. This

127

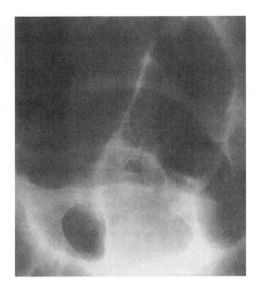

Fig. 8 Sigmoid volvulus

is achieved by introducing a rigid sigmoidoscope up to the point of the twist. Once this point is reached, the mucosa is inspected. If there are any signs of ischaemia or if blood stained fluid is seen through the lumen, then strangulation must be suspected and an immediate laparotomy should be performed. However, if the mucosa looks normal, a well lubricated rectal tube is introduced through the sigmoidoscope and secured in place. It is wise for the operator to be suitably clothed as there will be a massive discharge of flatus and liquid faeces once the tube negotiates the torsion. If the base of the volvulus cannot be reached with a rigid sigmoidoscope, flexible sigmoidoscopy may be used.[31] A further advantage of the water-soluble contrast enema is that it allows an opportunity to place a decompressing flatus tube under direct radiological guidance.

Key point 9

- Endoscopic decompression is the initial management of patients with sigmoid volvulus provided there are no signs of peritonitis.

Elective surgery

Following successful decompression, there is a well recognized propensity for recurrence which is reportedly as high as 90% with accompanying mortality rates as high as 40%.[32] This has prompted many surgeons to recommend an interval sigmoid colectomy.[33]

One problem frequently encountered at laparotomy, especially when the volvulus is chronic or recurrent, is the discrepancy between the proximal and distal bowel lumen. Moreover, the wall of the proximal bowel may be much thicker making it difficult for stapling. If a primary anastomosis has been decided upon, this can be undertaken by a hand sutured end-to-end anastomosis by taking wider bites of the proximal bowel. Alternatively, we prefer a stapled end-to-side anastomosis using a circular stapler. This is

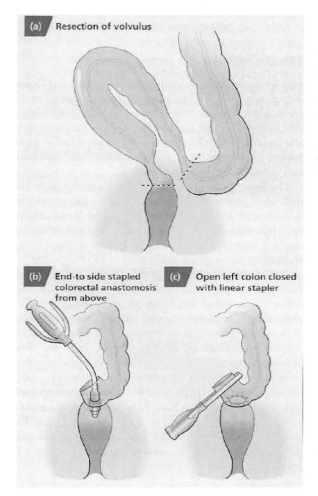

(a) Resection of volvulus

(b) End-to side stapled colorectal anastomosis from above

(c) Open left colon closed with linear stapler

Fig. 9 Stapled anastomosis after resection of sigmoid volvulus.

fashioned by placing the anvil into the rectal stump, using a purse string and passing the gun into the open end of the proximal bowel. The spike is advanced to pass through the antimesenteric aspect of the bowel leaving enough length beyond the staple line for subsequent closure once the gun is fired. The open end is then closed using a linear stapler (Fig. 9).

Emergency surgery

The indications for emergency laparotomy are: (i) the presence of peritonitis; (ii) the failure to decompress endoscopically; or (iii) when ischaemia or strangulation is suspected. The exact procedure will depend upon the viability of the colon. If the colon is gangrenous, there is no alternative to resection, taking care not to untwist the torsion. After excision, the arguments for an immediate anastomosis are similar to those in obstruction from a cancer. However, there are insufficient trials comparing patients treated with or without a primary anastomosis in this condition. Similarly, on-table lavage has not been widely employed for volvulus. We strongly believe that a Hartmann's procedure should be the treatment of choice when an infarcted colon complicates a volvulus.

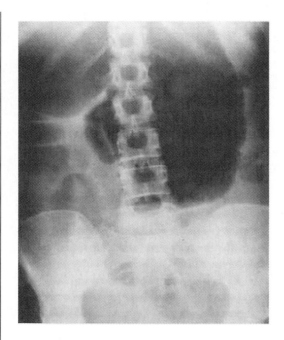

Fig. 10 Caecal volvulus. Plain abdominal radiograph.

If the colon remains viable following derotation, primary resection and anastomosis may be performed in favourable circumstances. However, if there is the slightest fear of a leak, exteriorizing both ends is the safest option. Mesosigmoidopexy, even though advocated by some, has a high recurrence rate (30–80%).[32,34] Bhatnagar et al.[35] introduced a technique of extraperitonealizing the whole segment of the sigmoid colon with favourable results. Other ingenious techniques which are not widely practised are procedures like a laparoscopic sigmoid fixation or laparoscopic resection.[36]

Caecal volvulus

Caecal volvulus is primarily a consequence of mobility of a non-fixed caecum. Diagnosis is apparent on a plain abdominal radiograph showing a distended caecum assuming a 'comma' shape with its concavity facing inferiorly and to the right (Fig. 10).

Treatment is principally surgical although occasional cases of successful colonoscopic decompression have been described. Generally, we reserve colonoscopic reduction for patients who are in poor general condition and in whom laparotomy is contra-indicated.

At laparotomy, as in sigmoid volvulus, if the bowel is gangrenous, resection in the form of a right hemicolectomy is necessary. If the bowel is viable, various options between resection and various fixation procedures are available. Methods of fixation include caecopexy (suturing the right colon to the right paracolic gutter) and caecostomy which has an added advantage of decompressing the bowel in addition to fixation.[37,38] Resection has the best long-term results and we generally perform a stapled side-to-side anastomosis following a right hemicolectomy as described for an obstructing right colonic cancer. Recurrence following this procedure is uncommon.

OGILVIE'S SYNDROME (ACUTE COLONIC PSEUDO-OBSTRUCTION)

This is a common and potentially dangerous condition. It presents with signs and symptoms and radiological appearances of large bowel obstruction but without any apparent mechanical cause. If left untreated, it can lead to ischaemic necrosis and colonic perforation. The pathogenesis of this syndrome is unknown, but current evidence points towards an autonomic imbalance caused by parasympathetic suppression.[39,40]

Key point 10

- Neostigmine appears to be effective in the early resolution of acute colonic pseudo-obstruction.

Diagnosis is based on history, clinical examination and plain radiographs which show the appearance of a large bowel obstruction. A water soluble contrast enema should be performed to confirm the diagnosis and rule out a mechanical cause. Besides, the osmotic effect of the water soluble contrast is often therapeutic in decompressing the colon.[41]

Once the diagnosis is confirmed, management is initially conservative and should be continued for 48–72 h provided there are no signs of peritonitis or increasing caecal diameter. During this period, decompression with a flatus tube or a colonoscope may be attempted. However, this has a high incidence of recurrence.

Indications for surgery are failure of conservative treatment or colonoscopic decompression, or clinical signs of impending or actual perforation. In the absence of ischaemia or perforation, a tube caecostomy is ideal for decompression.[42] Decompressing colostomies and ileostomies have higher mortality rates. In the presence of ischaemia or perforation, resection is indicated and it is safest to exteriorize both ends as an ileostomy and mucus fistula.

Currently, pharmacological treatment has proved to be of value. Motility enhancing drugs such as erythromycin have been effective in treating pseudo-obstruction. There are various reports of the success of neostigmine in achieving decompression.[40,43] Turegano-Fuentes *et al.*[39] reported a satisfactory clinical and radiological decompression in 12 of 18 patients after a single dose of neostigmine (2.5 mg in 100 ml of normal saline over 60 min).

Key points for clinical practice

- The main causes of large bowel obstruction are cancer and volvulus.

- A closed loop obstruction involves the segment of colon between a competent ileocaecal valve and the obstructing lesion. Failure to identify this may result in a caecal perforation.

(continued on next page)

Key points for clinical practice (continued)

- Contrast radiology is indicated in all cases of apparent large bowel obstruction except when the clinical condition dictates an emergency operation.

- CT is highly accurate in determining the level and cause of obstruction.

- MRI and CT colonography are advanced modalities of imaging and their role in large bowel obstruction is uncertain.

- Initial treatment should be aimed at: (i) restoring the circulating blood volume; (ii) replacing the fluid and electrolyte deficits; and (iii) optimizing and preparing for surgery (if there is a need).

- Surgery should not be unduly delayed especially when there are signs suggesting underlying ischaemia or impending perforation.

- In favourable circumstances, a single-stage procedure is a safe option in the management of malignant left-sided colonic obstruction.

- Endoscopic decompression is the initial management of patients with sigmoid volvulus provided there are no signs of peritonitis.

- Neostigmine appears to be effective in the early resolution of acute colonic pseudo-obstruction.

ACKNOWLEDGEMENT

We thank Dr James Cast, Consultant Radiologist, Castle Hill Hospital.

References

1. Field S, Guy PJ, Upsdell SM, Scourfield AE. The erect abdominal radiograph in the acute abdomen: should its use be abandoned? *BMJ* 1985; **290**: 1934–1936.
2. Suri S, Gupta S, Sudhakar PJ, Venkataramu NK, Sood B, Wig JD. Comparative evaluation of plain films, ultrasound and CT in the diagnosis of intestinal obstruction. *Acta Radiol* 1999; **40**: 422–428.
3. Frager D, Rovno HD, Baer JW, Bashist B, Friedman M. Prospective evaluation of colonic obstruction with computed tomography. *Abdom Imaging* 1998; **23**: 141–146.
4. ShaffMI, Tarr RW, Partain LL, James AE Jr. Computed tomography and magnetic resonance imaging of the acute abdomen. *Surg Clin N Am* 1988; **68**: 233–254.
5. Johnson CD, Dachman AH. CT colonography: the next colon screening examination? *Radiology* 2000; **216**: 331–341.
6. Marrin MM, Farrell RJ, Raptopoulos V, McGee JB, Bleday R, Kruskal JB. Role of virtual computed tomographic colonography in patients with colorectal cancers and obstructing colorectal lesions. *Dis Colon Rectum* 2000; **43**: 303–311.
7. Gupta H, Dupuy DE. Advances in imaging in acute abdomen. *Surg Clin North Am* 1997; **77**: 1245–1263.
8. Chou CK, Liu GC, Chen LT, Jaw TS. Use of MRI in bowel obstruction. *Abdom Imaging* 1993; **18**: 131–135.
9. Ohman U. Prognosis in patients with obstructing colorectal carcinoma. *Am J Surg* 1982; **143**: 742–747.
10. Phillips RK, Hittinger R, Fry JS, Fielding LP. Malignant large bowel obstruction. *Br J Surg* 1985; **72**: 290–302.

11. Serpell JW, McDermott FT, Katrivessis H, Hughes ES. Obstructing carcinomas of the colon. *Br J Surg* 1989; **76**: 965–969.
12. Goligher JC, Smiddy FG. The treatment of acute obstruction and perforation of the colon and rectum. *Br J Surg* 1957; **47**: 270–276.
13. Torralba JA, Robles PE, Parilla P, Lujon JA, Liren R, Pinero A, Fernandez JA. Subtotal colectomy vs intraoperative colonic irrigation in the management of obstructed left colonic carcinoma. *Dis Colon Rectum* 1998; 41: 18–22.
14. Hughes ES, McDermott FT, Polglase AL, Nottle P. Total and subtotal colectomy for colonic obstruction. *Dis Colon Rectum* 1985; **28**: 162–163.
15. Foster ME, Johnson CD, Billings PJ, Davies PW, Leaper DJ. Intraoperative antegrade lavage and anastomotic healing in acute colonic obstruction. *Dis Colon Rectum* 1986; **29**: 255–259.
16. Stephenson BM, Shandall AA, Farouk R, Griffith G. Malignant left sided large bowel obstruction managed by subtotal colectomy/total colectomy. *Br J Surg* 1990; **77**: 1098–1102.
17. Forloni B, Reduzzi R, Paludetti A, Colpani L, Cavallari G, Frosali D. Intraoperative colonic lavage in emergency surgical treatment of left sided colonic obstruction. *Dis Colon Rectum* 1998; **41**: 23–27.
18. Runkel S, Hinz U, Lehnert T, Buhr HJ, Herfarth C. Improved outcome after emergency surgery for cancer of the large intestine. *Br J Surg* 1998; **85**; 1260–1265.
19. Deans GT, Krukowski ZH, Irwin ST. Malignant obstruction of the left colon. *Br J Surg* 1994; **81**: 1270–1276.
20. Koruth NM, Krukowski ZH, Youngson GG. Intraoperative colonic irrigation in the management of left sided large bowel emergencies. *Br J Surg* 1985; **72**: 708–711.
21. Murray JJ, Schoetz Jr DJ, Coller JA, Roberts PL, Veidenheimer MC. Intraoperative colonic lavage and primary anastomoses in non-elective colon resection. *Dis Colon Rectum* 1991; **34**: 527–531.
22. SCOTIA Study Group. Single-stage treatment for malignant left-sided colonic obstruction: a prospective randomized clinical trial comparing subtotal colectomy with segmental resection following intraoperative irrigation. *Br J Surg* 1995; **82**; 1622–1627.
23. Itabashi M, Hamano K, Kameoka S, Asahina K. Self expanding stainless steel stent application in rectosigmoid strictures. *Dis Colon Rectum* 1993; **36**: 508–511.
24. Campbell KL, Hussey JK, Eremin O. Expandable metal stent application in obstructing carcinoma of the proximal colon: report of a case. *Dis Colon Rectum* 1997; **40**: 1391–1393.
25. Mainar S, De Gregorio AMA, Tejero E *et al*. Acute colorectal obstruction: treatment with self expanding metallic stents before scheduled surgery – results of a multicentre study. *Radiology* 1999; **210**: 65–69.
26. Law WL, Chu KW, Ho WC, Tung HM, Law YK, Chu KM. Self expanding metallic stent in the treatment of colonic obstruction caused by advanced malignancies. *Dis Colon Rectum* 2000; **43**: 1522–1527.
27. Boorman P, Soonawalla Z, Sathananthan N, MacFarlane P, Parker MC. Endoluminal stenting of obstructed colorectal tumours. *Ann R Coll Surg Engl* 199; **81**: 251–254.
28. Akle CA. Endoprosthesis for colonic strictures. *Br J Surg* 1998; **85**: 310–314.
29. Tejero E, Mainar A, Montes C *et al*. Initial results of a new procedure for treatment of malignant obstruction of the left colon. *Dis Colon Rectum* 1997; **40**: 432–436.
30. Ballantyne GH. Review of sigmoid volvulus: clinical patterns and pathogenesis. *Dis Colon Rectum* 1982; **25**: 823–830.
31. Arigbabu A, Badejo O, Akinola M. Colonoscopy in the emergency treatment of colonic volvulus in Nigeria. *Dis Colon Rectum* 1985; **28**: 795–798.
32. Wertkin MG, Aufses Jr AH. Management of volvulus of the colon. *Dis Colon Rectum* 1978; **21**: 40–45.
33. Grossman EM, Longo WE, Stratton MD, Virgo KS, Johnson FE. Sigmoid volvulus in department of veterans affairs medical center. *Dis Colon Rectum* 2000; **43**: 414–418.
34. Morissey TB, Deitch EA. Recurrence of sigmoid volvulus after surgical intervention. *Am Surg* 1994; **60**: 29–31.
35. Bhatnagar BNS, Sharma CLN. Non-resective alternative for the cure of non-gangrenous sigmoid volvulus. *Dis Colon Rectum* 1998; **41**: 381–388.
36. Chung RS. Colectomy for sigmoid volvulus. *Dis Colon Rectum* 1997; **40**: 363–365.

37. Benacci JC, Wolff BG. Caecostomy: therapeutic indications and results. *Dis Colon Rectum* 1995; **38**: 530–534.
38. Perrier G, Peillon C, Liberge N, Steinmetz L, Boyet L, Testart J. Caecostomy is a useful procedure. Study of 113 colonic obstructions caused by cancer. *Dis Colon Rectum* 2000; **43**: 50–54.
39. Turegano-Fuentes F, Munoz-Jimenez F, Valle-Hernandez E *et al*. Early resolution of Ogilvie's syndrome with intravenous neostigmine. A simple and effective treatment. *Dis Colon Rectum* 1997; **40**: 1353–1357.
40. Trevisani GT, Hyman NH, Church JM. Neostigmine. Safe and effective treatment for acute colonic pseudo-obstruction. *Dis Colon Rectum* 2000; **43**: 599–603.
41. Vanek VW, Al Salti M. Acute pseudo-obstruction of the colon (Ogilvie's syndrome): an analysis of 400 cases. *Dis Colon Rectum* 1986; **29**: 203–210.
42. JosephC, Benacci B, Wolff G. Caecostomy. Therapeutic indications and results. *Dis Colon Rectum* 1995; **38**: 530–534
43. Stephenson BM, Morgan AR, Salaman JR, Wheeler MH. Ogilvie syndrome: a new approach to an old problem. *Dis Colon Rectum* 1995; **38**: 424–427.

Ayo Oshowo Irving Taylor

11

Local recurrence of rectal cancer

Local recurrence remains a significant problem in rectal cancer treatment. Over the last few decades, the reported incidence of recurrence has not changed appreciably, ranging from 5–45%.[1–6] This causes disabling and profound complications, with resultant severe impairment in quality-of-life. The survival rate after recurrence is low, with only 5–10% living longer than 5 years.[7,8] Often, a diagnosis of recurrent cancer is more devastating to a patient than the initial rectal cancer diagnosis.

Significant advances have been made recently in achieving long-term cure based on improved surgical technique and a multidisciplinary approach. Although there are a number of controversies about the best method of management, a number of therapeutic options now exists. It is imperative to identify a proven standard of care and adopt this in order to prevent local recurrence. This review aims to discuss local recurrence of rectal cancer in the context of the recent data from on-going published trials.

DEFINITION, EPIDEMIOLOGY AND PREVENTION

Local recurrence is defined as any evidence of cancer re-growth in the operative field in the pelvis following a 'curative' resection. It is presumed that all visible tumour had been removed at the time of the primary surgery. This recurrence may be intramural, along the bowel anastomosis and surgical scar, or extramural in the original tumour bed, mesenteric lymph nodes, pericolic

Mr Ayo Oshowo MS FRCS(Gen), Specialist Registrar, Department of Surgery, Royal Free and University College London Medical School, University College London, Charles Bell House, 67–73 Riding House Street, London W1W 7EJ, UK (for correspondence)

Prof. Irving Taylor MD ChM FRCS, David Patey Professor of Surgery, Head of Department of Surgery, Royal Free and University College London Medical School, University College London, Charles Bell House, 67–73 Riding House Street, London W1W 7EJ, UK

fat or pelvic sidewall and adjacent pelvic structures. Most will argue that local recurrence is not a spread, but rather a failure of the primary treatment. Thus, malignant cells remain in the original site, and then grow as isolated deposits with no systemic dissemination.[9–11]

Key point 1

- Local recurrence is defined as any evidence of cancer re-growth in the operative field in the pelvis following a 'curative' resection. Recurrent cancer is often more devastating to a patient than the initial rectal cancer diagnosis.

PATTERNS OF RECURRENCE

The most common pattern of recurrence from rectal cancer is loco-regional although systemic recurrence to liver, lungs, peritoneum, bone and brain can also occur. Rectal cancer tends to recur as isolated deposits in 50% of cases, unaccompanied by systemic dissemination.[9,12] Synchronous systemic recurrences occur in approximately 30%, while systemic recurrence alone occurs in 6–20%.[11,13,14] In contrast, colonic cancer recurrences are often accompanied by disseminated disease.[15] The increased local recurrence rate in patients with rectal cancer is most likely attributable to the limited space in the pelvis. This is similarly reflected in the higher recurrence rate from mid and low rectal tumours.[9]

Length of time to recurrence is variable and generally underestimated. It depends on when the patient becomes symptomatic, the time at which recurrence was determined and the methods for determining the recurrence patterns. The exact sites, sequence and time of recurrence are often difficult to predict. Some 85% of recurrences occur in the first 2 postoperative years, with a peak incidence at 6–12 months. Nearly all (95%) occur within 5 years; recurrence is rare after this.[2,14] This implies that a concentrated follow-up programme in the first 2 years should identify most cases.

Key point 2

- Loco-regional is the commonest pattern of rectal cancer recurrence. Most cases occur in the first 2 postoperative years.

The median life expectancy in inoperable, recurrent pelvic disease is about 10 months.[13] Only half the patients will be suitable for further surgical treatment and 5-year survival is poor (20%).[16,17] In addition, these patients suffer from intractable pelvic pain, ulcerating perineal lesions, episodes of intestinal obstruction, enterocutaneous fistulas, continence problems, persistent rectal discharge, bleeding and sepsis. Occlusion of the pelvic lymphovascular system may be complicated by leg swelling and thrombo-embolism.

PREDICTORS OF LOCAL RECURRENCE

It may be possible to minimize the risk of local recurrence if reasons why it occurs can be identified. Factors that influence local recurrence are related to the tumour, the patient and the surgical technique.

Tumour-related factors

There is unanimity about the prognostic significance of the tumour characteristics. The frequency of local recurrence decreases when the cancer is more than 13 cm from the anal verge.[9,18,19] Tumours located in the upper, mid and low rectum have recurrence rates in the order of 3.6%, 9.5% and 31.7%, respectively.[20] This may be due to the increasingly limited space and, therefore, easier contiguous spread coupled with the technical difficulty of resection in the lower pelvis.[9] Larger tumour size (4 cm or greater) is also associated with a high recurrence rate. Large tumours are more likely to be pathologically advanced and obstructing.[21] When there is increased depth of invasion or serosal invasion, patients are at increased risk of local recurrence and, accordingly, poor survival.

Early recurrence rates are associated with the tumour type – gross or histological. Patients with exophytic, localized tumours have a lower recurrence rate than infiltrative or diffuse types.[22] Ulcero-infiltrating and ulcero-fungating types also show a higher incidence of recurrence than fungating lesions. Similarly, poorly differentiated tumours are associated with early recurrence.[23] Mucin production has been associated with high recurrence rates due to a tendency to fixation to contiguous tissue.[24,25] Lymphovascular invasion is a poor prognostic factor which may predict more aggressive, disseminated disease and hence poor overall survival. In general, local recurrence increases with advancing stage of the disease and correlates well with Dukes' stage. This is more pronounced when the advanced Dukes' stage is associated with more distal tumours.[26]

Patient factors

The female pelvis is broader and shallower and this facilitates easier dissection and resection. There is no relationship between the age of the patient and local recurrence, especially when disease-related survival is considered and other variables are controlled.[27] Patient-related risk factors, such as the presence of cardiovascular disease, correlate with postoperative complications. Recurrence rate is thought to be higher in patients who have sustained an anastomotic leak.[28,29]

Surgical technique

Advances have been made in the technique of radical resection and reconstruction, and in determining the place of adjuvant chemotherapy and radiation therapy. It is important to identify patients with a substantial risk of local recurrence based on both accurate staging and patient factors. Such patients may be offered adjuvant therapy, to reduce their risk of recurrence.

Surgery is the mainstay and most effective form of primary tumour control. Surgical technique determines the outcome of rectal cancer management. Excellent results have been achieved in many centres with total mesorectal excision (TME).[30–36]

Table Local recurrence after 'curative' resection. Differing rates of local recurrence with or without total mesorectal excision (TME) in large series of rectal resection

Authors	n	Surgery	Pre-operative radiotherapy	Local recurrence (%)
Kapiteijn et al. 2001[37]	937	TME	–	8.2 (at 2 yr)
Kapiteijn et al. 2001[37]	924	TME	Yes	2.4 (at 2 yr)
Martling et al. 2001[38]	272	–	Yes	12
Arbman et al. 1996[39]	128	TME	–	7
MacFarlane et al. 1993[40]	135	TME	–	5
Cawthorn et al. 1990[33]	122	TME	–	7
Enker et al. 1995[36]	204	TME	–	6
Bjerkset et al. 1996[41]	107	TME	–	9
Kusunoki et al. 1997[42]	91	–	–	16
Paty et al. 1994[43]	134	–	–	11
Stipa et al. 1991[44]	235	–	–	18.3

This procedure significantly decreases the risk of local recurrence for resectable rectal cancer to 7% or less (Table 1).

TME is applicable to both sphincter-sparing and abdominoperineal excisions. TME, as opposed to the conventional surgical approach, uses sharp dissection to obtain a more distal, circumferential margin. The potential tumour deposits in the distal mesentery are removed as an intact unit by precise, sharp dissection, along the visceral fascia, thus avoiding tumour spillage from the disrupted mesentery.

Key point 3

- Surgery is the best form of primary control. Excellent results have been achieved with total mesorectal excision (TME).

The use of circular staplers has been shown to lead to a reduction in local recurrence compared with sutured anastomosis in a study[45] of colonic and rectal resections. However, these findings require careful consideration because in that study recurrence rates were high and anastomotic site had no effect on the recurrence rate.

The margin of resection (lateral or circumferential)[30–33] correlates with local recurrence. The issue of what constitutes an 'acceptable' distal resection margin is still hotly debated, but should be regarded as the minimum margin required to achieve a low local recurrence rate and which allows a safe anastomosis to be performed. A minimal distal margin of 2 cm for potentially curable carcinomas should be adequate.[46,47] Some advocate abdominoperineal resection as a means of achieving a safe, adequate resection margin for low-lying tumours. This is probably inappropriate advice, because local recurrence rates following low anterior resection are the same as for abdominoperineal resection when comparing the degree of differentiation and stage of tumour.[9,11]

The experience of the surgeon and facilities available in a unit have a profound influence on local recurrence. Excellent results can be achieved by surgeons provided they are trained in standardized procedures. This is exemplified by the technique of total mesorectal excision when compared with conventional non-standardized surgery; recurrence rates are 7% and 15–45%, respectively. In the era before the wide-spread application of TME, local recurrence rates were related to surgical teams, rather than grade of surgeon, suggesting that technique is more important than experience.[60]

Other novel surgical techniques have been developed in recent years and have a significant bearing on the recurrence rate.[47] Laparoscopic colorectal cancer surgery is technically feasible and functionally advantageous. Early reports described difficulty with larger tumours and inadequate oncological radicality. Likewise, port site tumour implantation and local recurrence with the potential for under-staging due to inadequate nodal sampling have been described.[48–50] The effect of pneumoperitoneum on the spread of cancer cells is still being investigated. However, these problems may relate to operator factors during the learning curve. This is the subject of on-going prospective randomised trials such as the MRC CLASICC (Conventional versus Laparoscopic-Assisted Surgery In Colorectal Cancer) trial.

Endo-anal excision with sparing of the anal sphincter in low-lying early T-stage tumours has been attempted. This is performed in selected patients in whom pre-operative staging has confirmed an early tumour and the absence of obvious nodal or perirectal deposits.

Transanal endoscopic microsurgery (TEMS) is another minimally invasive technique which is suitable for early stages, especially in the elderly. However, when patients are operated with this technique for locally invasive tumours, or in the presence of nodal metastases, there is a high risk of local recurrence.[51]

The long-term effect of these techniques is still being assessed in several prospective randomised trials.

Adjuvant radiotherapy

There is good evidence that radiotherapy reduces local recurrence by about 50%.[37] The optimal dose and timing (pre-, intra-, postoperative or 'sandwich' technique) must be considered by the multidisciplinary team on an individual patient basis. The risk of local recurrence should be balanced against overtreatment, plus the risk of early and late complications of radiotherapy. The effect of radiotherapy may be most evident in large, high grade tumours with a minimal margin of clearance. It allows tumour shrinkage and thus permits better local control and hopefully long-term disease-free survival. Regardless of any impact on mortality rates, it can be argued that the improvement in morbidity rates due to a lower local recurrence warrants the adjunctive use of radiation, at least in Dukes' B or C cancer.

Key point 4

- The addition of radiotherapy to TME has shown most significant beneficial effect in stages 2 and 3 rectal cancers situated within 10 cm of the anal verge.

ADJUVANT CHEMOTHERAPY

Chemotherapy has been shown to be of most benefit in Dukes' stage C colorectal cancer. The standard therapy is offered as a prolonged 6-cycle course using 5-fluorouracil with folinic acid. The effect of chemotherapy after resection of Dukes' stage B tumours is still the subject of on-going randomised clinical trials and patients should be encouraged to participate in these. Chemotherapy is not recommended for patients with Dukes' A cancer. Absolute benefits are likely to be less for patients with earlier stage disease because of the lower risk of recurrence and mortality rate.

Neo-adjuvant chemotherapy (often combined with radiotherapy) is offered to suitable patients with low, locally advanced rectal cancer in whom local recurrence rate is predictably high. This can lead to tumour shrinkage sufficient enough to allow resection and sphincter-preserving procedures with long-term low recurrence rates and acceptable quality of life.[52]

MANAGEMENT OF LOCAL RECURRENCE

The most difficult problem following rectal cancer surgery is the management of locally recurrent disease. Survival after recurrence is low. Patients with inoperable, recurrent pelvic disease have a median life expectancy of less than 10 months. Improved survival may be achieved through early diagnosis, repeat resection for cure, palliative resection, chemotherapy and/or radiotherapy.

EARLY DIAGNOSIS

Early detection of local recurrence should be sought in order to identify those patients who will benefit from a 'curative re-resection'. The pattern of recurrence shows a peak incidence between 6–12 months. This suggests that concentrated, intensive follow-up, during the first 2 years should be beneficial.[2,13,14] Subsequent follow-up can be scheduled less frequently. Many patients may be symptom-free, in whom recurrent disease is identified on digital rectal and procto-sigmoidoscopic examination. A rising level of carcino-embryonic antigen (CEA) may indicate recurrent disease, although it is not uniformly sensitive or specific,[54] and 30% of colorectal cancers do not express this antigen. Colonoscopy is useful in identifying recurrent mucosal disease.[55] Barium enema has a sensitivity of about 88% for identifying mucosal lesions. Computed tomography (CT), magnetic resonance imaging, and endo-anal ultrasound are able to detect extraluminal recurrences. Fluoro-18-deoxyglucose (FDG) positron emission tomography (PET) has also been used to differentiate recurrent tumour from fibrosis and to exclude distant spread before proceeding to further major surgery.[56]

However, the value of such follow-up is debatable,[53] and the optimum frequency of clinical follow-up is still controversial. Intensive follow-up is expensive and would be valuable if early detection of recurrent tumours translated into improved long-term survival. This is because further curative resection is only possible in 5–20% of patients,[44] and appears to have little or no effect on overall survival rate.

The purpose of follow-up is to provide psychological support and to detect loco-regional recurrence and distant metastases. Follow-up also provides an opportunity for audit and participation in new trials. In our unit, patients are followed up at 6 weeks, 6-monthly for 2 years, then annually. Clinical examination and rigid sigmoidoscopy (for rectal cancer) is undertaken at each visit. This is supplemented by 3-monthly CEA and 6-monthly CT of liver and pelvis. After 2 years, CT is requested when clinically indicated.

RESECTION

A thorough pre-operative assessment is mandatory to determine resectability and to exclude metastatic disease. Surgery should be considered, as it may occasionally be curative in a small proportion of suitable patients who have no evidence of systemic spread. Anastomotic recurrences can be treated by local resection or an abdominoperineal (AP) excision with a 5-year survival rate of 30%. A more radical procedure, pelvic exenteration, may be indicated for locally extensive recurrence not amenable to AP resection.

Anterior pelvic exenteration is indicated if the recurrent disease involves only anterior structures such as the prostate, bladder or vagina. During dissection, anatomic planes are difficult to ascertain, but should include wide lateral margins, the mesorectum, iliac and perirectal nodes. An abdomino-sacral resection is required in patients with extensive, local recurrences in the presacral space to encompass the involved sacrum. Newer techniques of colo-anal anastomosis, urinary tract reconstruction or diversion and myocutaneous flaps for perineal reconstruction can greatly reduce the morbidity of these procedures. The presence of peritoneal serosal seedings, liver metastases, or aorto-iliac node involvement mitigates the likelihood of curative resection. With careful selection, 30% 5-year survival has been achieved,[16,17,57,58] but with an accompanying high morbidity rate.

RADIOTHERAPY AND CHEMOTHERAPY

Radiotherapy should be offered to patients with locally recurrent rectal cancer who have not previously undergone radiotherapy. In some patients, radiotherapy may allow tumour regression sufficient to permit further resection.

Unresectable recurrences carry a 5-year survival of only 5%. At this stage, palliative chemoradiotherapy may be offered, but the emphasis is on symptom control. Radiotherapy should be offered to patients with bone pain from metastases. External beam radiotherapy is palliative in patients with disabling symptoms with a few experiencing long-term relief of 6–8 months. Chemotherapy has been shown to improve symptom control and quality-of-life when given early, especially where there is accompanying systemic spread. Newer agents such as irinotecan (a topoisomerase 1 inhibitor) can be used as a second line treatment where initial standard treatment with 5-fluorouracil had failed to stop disease progression.[59] Patients whose symptoms are difficult to control should be referred to the palliative care team. The multidisciplinary team should balance the potential effectiveness of these agents in individual patients against the adverse effects.

Key point 5

- Aggressive surgical treatment of pelvic recurrence is possible in very few patients. Chemotherapy or radiotherapy may help palliate symptoms.

CONCLUSIONS

TME has resulted in a recurrence rate as low as 5% and should be regarded as the standard treatment of primary rectal cancer. The addition of radiotherapy to TME has shown most benefit in the prevention of local recurrence in stage 2 and 3 rectal cancers situated within 10 cm of the anal verge.[37]

Low recurrence rate should not be achieved at all cost. The issues of morbidity and quality-of-life need to be addressed when performing a supra-radical resection. The approach to recurrent rectal cancer requires a sophisticated multidisciplinary team to obtain optimum results.

Key points for clinical practice

- Local recurrence is defined as any evidence of cancer re-growth in the operative field in the pelvis following a 'curative' resection. Recurrent cancer is often more devastating to a patient than the initial rectal cancer diagnosis.

- Loco-regional is the commonest pattern of rectal cancer recurrence. Most cases occur in the first 2 postoperative years.

- Surgery is the best form of primary control. Excellent results have been achieved with total mesorectal excision (TME).

- The addition of radiotherapy to TME has shown most benefit in stages 2 and 3 rectal cancers situated within 10 cm of the anal verge.

- Aggressive surgical treatment of pelvic recurrence is possible in very few patients. Chemotherapy or radiotherapy may help palliate symptoms.

References

1. Kapiteijn E, Marijnen C, Colenbrander AC *et al* Local recurrence in patients with rectal cancer, diagnosed between 1988 and 1992: a population-based study in the west Netherlands. *Eur J Surg Oncol* 1998; **24**: 528–535.
2. Phillips RKS, Hittinger R, Blesovsky L, Fry JS, Fielding LP. Local recurrence following 'curative' surgery for large bowel cancer. *Br J Surg* 1984; **71**: 12–16.
3. Bruinvels DJ, Stiggelbout AM, Kievit J, Van Houwelingen HS, Habbema DF, van de Velde CJ. Follow-up of patients with colorectal cancer. A meta-analysis. *Ann Surg* 1994; **219**: 174–182..

4. Amato A, Pescatori M, Butti A. Local recurrence following abdominoperineal excision and anterior resection for rectal carcinoma. *Dis Colon Rectum* 1991; **34**: 317–322.

5. Dixon AR, Maxwell WA, Thornton Holmes J. Carcinoma of the rectum: a 10 year experience. *Br J Surg* 1991; **78**: 308–311.

6. Michelassi F, Vannucci L, Ayala JJ, Chappel R, Goldberg R, Block GE. Local recurrence after curative resection of colorectal adenocarcinoma. *Surgery* 1990; **108**: 787–793.

7. Gagliardi G, Hawley PR, Hershman MJ, Arnott SJ. Prognostic factors in surgery for local recurrence of rectal cancer. *Br J Surg* 1995; **82**: 1401–1405.

8. Sardi A, Minton JP, Nieroda C, Sickle-Santanello B, Young D, Martin Jr EW. Multiple reoperations in recurrent colorectal carcinoma. An analysis of morbidity, mortality and survival. *Cancer* 1988; **61**: 1913–1919.

9. Pilipshen SJ, Heilweil M, Quan SH, Sternberg SS, Enker WE. Patterns of pelvic recurrence following definitive resections of rectal cancer. *Cancer* 1984; **53**: 1354–1362.

10. Taylor FW. Cancer of the colon and rectum: a study of routes of metastases and death. *Surgery* 1962; **52**: 305–308.

11. McDermott FT, Hughes ESR, Pihl E *et al*. Local recurrence after potentially curative resection for rectal cancer in a series of 1008 patients. *Br J Surg* 1985; **72**: 34–37.

12. Rinnert-Gongora S, Tartter PI. Multivariate analysis of recurrence after anterior resection for colorectal carcinoma. *Am J Surg* 1989; **157**: 573–576.

13. Rao AR, Kagan AR, Chan PM *et al*. Patterns of recurrence following curative resection alone for adenocarcinoma of the rectum and sigmoid colon. *Cancer* 1981; **48**: 1492–1495.

14. Carlson U, Lasson A, Ekelund G. Recurrence rates after curative surgery for rectal cancer with special reference to their accuracy. *Dis Colon Rectum* 1987; **30**: 2861–2865.

15. Russell AH, Tong D, Dawson LE, Wisbeck W. Adenocarcinoma of the proximal colon. Sites of initial dissemination and patterns of recurrence following surgery alone. *Cancer* 1984; **53**: 360–367.

16. Hafner GH, Herrera L, Petrelli NJ. Morbidity and mortality after pelvic exenteration for colorectal adenocarcinoma. *Ann Surg* 1992; **215**: 63–67.

17. Williams Jr LF, Huddleston CB, Sawyers JL *et al*. Is total pelvic exenteration reasonable primary treatment for rectal carcinoma? *Ann Surg* 1988; **207**: 670–674.

18. Vandertoll DJ, Beahrs OH. Carcinoma of the rectum and low sigmoid. Evaluation of anterior resection in 1766 favourable lesions. *Arch Surg* 1965; **90**: 793–798.

19. Stearns Jr MW, Binkley GE. The influence of location on prognosis in operable rectal cancer. *Surg Gynaecol Obstet* 1983; **96**: 368–372.

20. Moosa AR, Ree PC, Marks JE, Levin B, Platz CE, Skinner DB. Factors influencing local recurrence after abdominoperineal resection for cancer of the rectum and rectosigmoid. *Br J Surg* 1975; **62**: 727–730.

21. Garcia-Valdecasas JC, Llovera JM, deLacy AM *et al*. Obstructing colorectal carcinomas. Prospective study. *Dis Colon Rectum* 1991; **34**: 759–762.

22. Michelassi F, Vannucci L, Montag A *et al*. Importance of tumour morphology for long term prognosis of rectal adenocarcinoma. *Am Surg* 1988; **54**: 376–379.

23. Steinberg SM, Barwick KW, Stablein DM. Importance of tumour pathology and morphology in patients with surgically resected colon cancer. Findings from the Gastro-Intestinal Tumour Study Group. *Cancer* 1986; **58**: 1340–1345.

24. Wang Q, Gao H, Wang Y, Chen Y. The clinical and biological significance of the transitional mucosa adjacent to colorectal cancer. *Surg Today* 1991; **21**: 253–261.

25. Dawson PM, Habib NA, Fane S, Rees HC, Wood CB, Allen-Mersh TG. Association between extent of colonic mucosal sialomucin change and subsequent local recurrence after curative excision of primary colorectal cancer. *Br J Surg* 1990; **77**: 1279–1283.

26. Bentzen SM, Balsev I, Pedersen M *et al*. Time to loco-regional recurrence after resection of Dukes' B and C colorectal cancer with and without adjuvant postoperative radiotherapy. A multivariate regression analysis. *Br J Cancer* 1992; **65**: 102–107.

27. Wiggers T, Arends JW, Volovics A. Regression analysis of prognostic factors in colorectal cancer after curative resections. *Dis Colon Rectum* 1988; **31**: 33–41.

28. Akyol AM, McGregor JR, Galloway DJ, Murray G, George WD. Anastomotic leaks in colorectal cancer surgery: a risk factor for recurrence? *Int J Colorectal Dis* 1991; **6**: 179–183.

29. Umpleby HC, Fermor B, Symes MO, Williamson RC. Viability of exfoliated colorectal carcinoma cells. *Br J Surg* 1984; **71**: 659–663.

30. Heald RJ, Husband EM, Ryall RD. The mesorectum in rectal cancer surgery – the clue to pelvic recurrence? *Br J Surg* 1982; **69**: 613–616.

31. Scott N, Jackson P, Al-Jaberi T *et al*. Total mesorectal excision and local recurrence: a study of tumour spread in the mesorectum distal to rectal cancer. *Br J Surg* 1995; **82**: 1031–1033.

32. Adam IJ, Mohamdee MO, Martin IG *et al*. Role of circumferential margin involvement in the local recurrence of rectal cancer. *Lancet* 1994; **344**: 707–711.

33. Cawthorn S, Parums D, Gibbs N *et al*. Extent of mesorectal spread and involvement of lateral resection margin as prognostic factors affecting surgery for rectal cancer. *Lancet* 1990; **335**: 1055.

34. Heald RJ. Total mesorectal excision is optimal surgery for rectal cancer: a Scandinavian consensus. *Br J Surg* 1995; **82**: 1297–1299.

35. Aitken RJ. Mesorectal excision for rectal cancer. *Br J Surg* 1996; **83**: 214–216.

36. Enker WE, Thaler HT, Cranor ML *et al*. Total mesorectal excision in the operative treatment of carcinoma of the rectum. *J Am Coll Surg* 1995; **181**: 335–346.

37. Kapiteijn E, Marijnen CAM, Nagtegaal ID *et al*. Preoperative radiotherapy combined with total mesorectal excision for resectable rectal cancer. *N Engl J Med* 2001; **345**: 638–646.

38. Martling A, Holm T, Johansson H, Rutqvist LE, Cedermark B. The Stockholm 11 trial on preoperative radiotherapy in rectal carcinoma: long-term follow-up of a population-based study. *Cancer* 2001; **92**: 896–902.

39. Arbman G, Nilson E, Hallbrook O *et al*. Local recurrence following total mesorectal excision for rectal cancer. *Br J Surg* 1996; **83**: 375–379.

40. MacFarlane JK, Ryall RDH, Heald RJ. Mesorectal excision for rectal cancer. *Lancet* 1993; **341**: 457–460.

41. Bjerkset T, Edna TH. Rectal cancer: the influence of type of operation on local recurrence and survival. *Eur J Surg* 1996; **162**: 643–648.

42. Kusunoki M, Yanagi H, Shoji Y *et al*. Anoabdominal rectal resection and colonic J pouch-anal anastomosis: 10 years' experience. *Br J Surg* 1997; **84**: 1277–1280.

43. Paty PB, Enker WE, McDermott K *et al*. Treatment of rectal cancer by low anterior resection with coloanal anastomosis. *Ann Surg* 1994; **219**: 365–373.

44. Stipa S, Nicolanti V, Botti C *et al*. Local recurrence after curative resection of colorectal cancer: frequency, risk factors and treatment. *J Surg Oncol Suppl* 1991; **2**: 155–160.

45. Akyol AM, McGregor JR, Galloway DJ, Murray G, George WD. Recurrence of colorectal cancer after sutured and stapled large bowel anastomosis. *Br J Surg* 1991; **78**: 1297–1300.

46. Madsen PM, Christiansen J. Distal intramural spread of rectal carcinomas. *Dis Colon Rectum* 1986; **29**: 279.

47. Guillem J, Cohen A. Current issues in colorectal cancer surgery. *Semin Oncol* 1999; **26**: 505–513.

48. Chew DK, Borromeo JR, Kimmelstiel FM. Peritoneal mucinous carcinomatosis after laparoscopic-assisted anterior resection for early rectal cancer: report of a case. *Dis Colon Rectum* 1999; **42**: 424–426.

49. Chen WS, Lin W, Kou YR, Kuo HS, Hsu H, Yang WK. Possible effect of pneumoperitoneum on the spreading of colon cancer tumour cells. *Dis Colon Rectum* 1997; **40**: 791–797.

50. Gutt CN, Riemer V, Kim ZG, Jacobi CA, Paolucci V, Lorenz M. Impact of laparoscopic colonic resection on tumour growth and spread in an experimental model. *Br J Surg* 1999; **86**: 1180-1184.

51. Banerjee AK, Shorthouse AJ. Local excision of rectal tumours. In: Taylor I, Johnson CD. (eds) *Recent Advances in Surgery*, vol 20. Edinburgh: Churchill Livingstone, 1997; 103–128.

52. Chaudhry V, Nittalla M, Prasad ML. Preoperative chemoradiation and coloanal reconstruction for low rectal cancer. *Am Surg* 2000; **66**: 387–393.

53. Ovsaka J, Jarvinen H, Kujari H, Perttila I, Mecklin JP. Follow-up of patients operated on for colorectal carcinoma. *Am J Surg* 1990; **159**: 593–596

54. Northover J. Carcinoembryonic antigen and recurrent colorectal cancer. *Gut* 1986; **27**: 117–122.

55. Juhl G, Larson GM, Mullins R, Bond S, Polk Jr HC. Six-year results of annual colonoscopy after resection of colorectal cancer. *World J Surg* 1990; **14**: 255–261.

56. Ruers TJM, Langenhoff BS, Neeleman N *et al*. Value of positron emission tomography with (F-18) fluorodeoxyglucose in patients with colorectal liver metastases: a prospective study. *J Clin Oncol* 2002; **2**: 388.
57. Boey J, Wong J, Ong GB. Pelvic exenteration for locally advanced colorectal carcinoma. *Ann Surg* 1982; **195**: 513–518.
58. Ledesma EJ, Bruno S, Mittelman A. Total pelvic exenteration in colorectal disease. *Ann Surg* 1981; **194**: 701–703.
59. Cunningham D, Pyrhonen S, James UD *et al*. Randomised trial of irinotecan plus supportive care versus supportive care alone after fluorouracil failure for patients with metastatic colorectal cancer. *Lancet* 1998; **352**: 1413–1418.
60. Phillips RK, Hittinger R, Blesovsky L, Fry JS, Fielding LP. Local recurrence following 'curative' surgery for large bowel cancer: I. The overall picture. *Br J Surg* 1984; **71**: 12–16.

K.P. Nugent

12

Benign anal disease

Anal disease accounts for a large number of general practitioner, general surgical and coloproctological referrals and consultations. Some of the commoner symptoms and benign diagnoses are discussed along with their recent advances in treatment. Many of the symptoms overlap between these diagnoses and with other more serious, potentially life threatening diagnoses; indeed the conditions may co-exist. Therefore, a full history and examination (including a sigmoidoscopy) should be undertaken in every patient.

FISTULA-IN-ANO (IDIOPATHIC)

Fistulas may be associated with some specific conditions but the majority seen in the UK are idiopathic or cryptoglandular in nature. The incidence is difficult to determine but in Scandinavia, where records are exemplary, the estimated incidence is around 1 in 10,000.[1] There is a male:female ratio of between 2:1 and 4:1 and the majority of fistulas occur in 30–60-year-olds.

AETIOLOGY AND SYMPTOMS

The most popular theory for the development of idiopathic fistula is that proposed by Sir Alan Parks – the cryptoglandular hypothesis.[2] An intersphincteric anal gland becomes infected and inflamed; once diseased, this becomes the seat of chronic infection. Sepsis spreads in any or all of three planes; vertically, horizontally or circumferentially resulting in fistula formation. Persistence of anal fistula may be due to partial epithelisation[3] or continuing sepsis.

Patients usually have had an episode of previous anal sepsis/abscess and later present with intermittent pain and purulent discharge. If the fistula is connected to the rectum, they may even pass faeces or wind through the external opening.

Miss Karen P. Nugent MA MS FRCS, Senior Lecturer/Honorary Consultant, University Surgical Unit, F Level, Centre Block (816), Southampton General Hospital, Tremona Road, Southampton SO16 6YD, UK

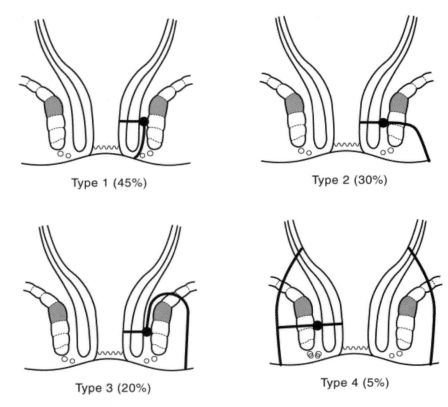

Type 1 (45%)

Type 2 (30%)

Type 3 (20%)

Type 4 (5%)

Fig. 1 Grades of fistulas.

CLASSIFICATION

Based on a series of 400 fistulas, the St Mark's Hospital classification divides fistula into 4 main categories (Fig. 1).[4] Intersphincteric fistulas are usually simple, although may co-exist with secondary tracks and occur in 45% of patients. Trans-sphincteric fistulas (29%) extend through the external sphincter, usually at the level of the anal glands. Suprasphincteric fistulas (20%) extend up to a level above puborectalis and then extend down through the levators to reach skin. Extrasphincteric fistulas (5%) are classified according to their pathogenesis.

ASSESSMENT

The majority of fistulas can be assessed by an 'educated finger'. It is important to delineate the internal and external opening, the pathway of the primary track and to trace any secondary tracks or extensions. More complicated fistulas plus those in the presence of scarring or which are failing to heal, may benefit from further imaging with magnetic resonance imaging (MRI); scans have been shown to correlate well with operative findings.[5] An alternative method of imaging more complex fistulas and their relationship to the anal sphincters is with peroxide-enhanced anal ultrasound. Peroxide (1 ml) is injected down the track and this allows increased resolution, especially of horseshoe and secondary extensions.[6] It is, however, operator-dependent.

> ## Key point 1
> - Complex fistulas should be assessed clinically and with MRI or ultrasound if they fail to heal or in the presence of scar tissue.

TREATMENT

Treatment of fistulas is aimed at draining sepsis, defining and eradicating fistulous tracts whilst preserving sphincter integrity and function.

Fistulotomy (with or without marsupulisation of the track) is the only sure way to get rid of a fistula and is the treatment of choice in first-time low simple fistulas. However, with more complex fistulas, this may result in excessive sphincter damage and, consequently, incontinence. Other methods have been employed to aid healing and to minimise trauma to the sphincter.

> ## Key point 2
> - The majority of fistulas are simple and can be treated with fistulotomy.

Setons

For more complex fistulas, insertion of a seton[7] (loose, tight or chemical) is often employed. A variety of different materials have been used from horse hair to silastic catheters. Each has a different mode of action.

Loose seton

A loose seton is used to mark a fistulous tract, stimulate fibrosis and facilitate drainage of sepsis. They may be left long-term in patients with on-going sepsis especially Crohn's disease or HIV infection. Short-term results of seton drainage alone are variable with reports of up to 78% of patients healing completely. In those in whom this method fails, there are other management options.[8] A fistulotomy may be performed (with or without defunctioning stoma) and the functional results assessed and dealt with after full healing; an advancement flap may be used after sepsis has been eradicated or the patient may elect to live with the seton in place.

Tight/cutting seton

The principle behind a cutting seton is the slow, controlled division of the enclosed sphincter mechanism with minimal separation of the transected ends. The majority of fistulas heal after the use of a cutting seton, but with considerable problems with incontinence in up to 66% especially incontinence to wind.

Chemical seton

These are used mostly in India where linen threads are covered in alkaline herbs (pH 8–9.2). The chemicals are caustic and cut through the tissues at a very slow rate. The chemicals have antifungal, antibacterial and anti-inflammatory properties. The setons are changed weekly and left snug. They cut through leaving very little in the way of deformity. The results are comparable with conventional surgical treatment but have economic advantages in a non-industrialised country.

Advancement flaps

Advancement flaps may be anocutaneous or mucosal in origin; success with either type is variable. The principle behind these advancement flaps is the same. The internal opening is exposed and the crypt bearing tissue is excised – some authors perform a full fistulectomy. An inverted U-shaped flap, including peri-anal skin and fat for anocutaneous flaps and mucosa or submucosa and a few muscle fibres for mucosal flaps, is raised with the base being twice the width of the apex. This is sutured to the mucosa and underlying internal anal sphincter covering the closed internal opening.[9,10] In a recent series of 26 patients undergoing anocutaneous flaps, successful healing occurred in approximately half but continence deteriorated in 30%. Greater success has been reported with mucosal advancement flaps. In a recent series of 103 patients with high and suprasphincteric fistulas treated with core fistulectomy and advancement flap, successful healing occurred in 93% and only 8% showed deterioration in continence.[11] Other series show initial healing rates of between 71%[12] and 81%[10] with poor outcome seen in patients who have had numerous previous procedures. The majority of recurrences occur within the first 15 months.

Fibrin glue

Fibrin adhesive has been used successfully to heal both primary and recurrent fistula-in-ano. After curettage of the tract, fibrin glue is injected into the tract until adhesive is seen coming out of the other opening. Successful healing has been seen in up to 85% when used on all fistulas[13] and in 60% of recurrent fistulas.[14] Most treatment failures occur within the first 3 months.[15]

Martius graft

Complex peri-anal fistulas may be very difficult to treat and may only heal with grafting of new vascularised tissue. Some have tried utilising omentum or leg muscles, but success has also been seen using the labial fat tissue (modified Martius graft) in combination with advancement flaps or sphincter repairs. In one series of 8 such grafts,[16] all of which were covered with a defunctioning stoma, the fistula healed in 6 (75%).

Key point 3

- Higher cure rates with complex procedures may be obtained at the expense of continence – a permanent loose seton may be the most acceptable option to the patient.

PERI-ANAL FISTULAS IN CROHN'S DISEASE

Peri-anal fistula may occur in up to 43% of patients with Crohn's disease. In view of the chronic and relapsing nature of Crohn's disease, fistulas in this condition should be treated as conservatively as possible.[17] The location and type of fistula should be determined along with an examination of the rectum (looking for inflammation). Abscesses should be drained and superficial, low intersphincteric and low trans-sphincteric fistulas may be treated by fistulotomy. More complex fistulas are best treated with non-cutting setons, antibiotics and azathioprine. Early results with infliximab have been promising, but may be associated with a high recurrence rate with time.

HAEMORRHOIDS

Symptoms from haemorrhoids have probably been treated for thousands of years and yet their aetiology is not completely understood and their treatment is still evolving. They are an extremely common problem, as seen by the high number of over-the-counter medicines available for the treatment of symptomatic piles, although precise data on incidence and prevalence are lacking.

AETIOLOGY AND SYMPTOMS

The cause of haemorrhoidal disease is not known. It has been proposed that haemorrhoids are caused by slippage of the normal lining of the anal canal.[18] This leads to a loss in organisation, muscular hypertrophy and fragmentation of the muscle and elastin components. Once the sliding process has started, then shearing forces at the time of defecation exacerbate the problem. This results in certain abnormalities including raised resting anal pressures, which return to normal after haemorrhoidectomy.[19]

Common symptoms include bleeding (usually bright red), pain, itching and the presence of anal lumps or prolapsing tissue. Other pathology should be excluded where appropriate and all patients should undergo sigmoidoscopic examination.

CLASSIFICATION

Haemorrhoids can be classified into external and internal. The internal group can be further subclassified into first degree (symptomatic enlarged masses of haemorrhoidal tissue which do not prolapse out of the anal canal), second degree (masses that prolapse and reduce spontaneously), third degree (masses which prolapse and need to be manually reduced) and fourth degree (permanently prolapsed) as summarised in Figure 2.

TREATMENT

Most treatment modalities work by causing fixation of the sliding tissue back onto the muscle wall by fibrosis or tissue destruction. A meta-analysis in 1995 suggested that banding is more efficacious than injection and that surgical excision is the definitive treatment.[20]

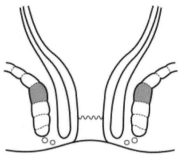

Type 1 No displacement

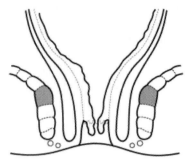

Type 2 Some prolapse spontaneous reduction

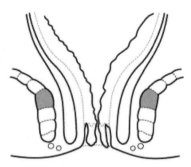

Type 3 Prolapse manual reduction

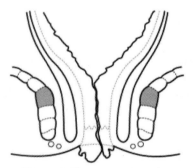

Type 4 Permanent prolapse

Fig. 2 Grades of haemorrhoids.

Creams and ointments

Bland soothing agents containing mild astringents sometimes give relief in haemorrhoids especially when presenting symptoms include itching. Many of these are combined with local anaesthetic agents to relieve pain. If combined with low dose corticosteroids (*e.g.* proctosedyl), they should only be used short-term.

Diet and bulking agents

These may act by softening motions and reducing shearing forces and seem to give some symptom relief especially in first- and second-degree haemorrhoids.

Injection sclerotherapy

The key to treatment in an out-patient setting is understanding that there are no sensory fibres above the dentate line so that haemorrhoids above this line can be treated without an anaesthetic.

Phenol in oil is the most commonly used solution for injection of haemorrhoids. It is quick to do, but may need repeated treatments and is best used for grade 1 and 2 haemorrhoids. A recent survey of surgeons in the South East Thames area showed that three–quarters of first-degree haemorrhoids were treated with injection sclerotherapy alone. However, 31% of surgeons reported complications with injection sclerotherapy, the majority of which were urological including impotence and prostatitis. These complications are likely to be secondary to sclerotherapy of anterior haemorrhoids.[21] More serious complications include retroperitoneal sepsis, necrotising fasciitis and multiple hepatic abscesses.[22]

Rubber banding

Barron's banding was developed in the 1960s and causes fixation and fibrosis by removing excess tissue followed by healing by secondary intention. A disadvantage has been that two people are needed, one to hold the proctoscope and one to apply the bands; a recent advance is the use of suction rubber banding which allows the technique to be performed by a single operator. It has higher rates of cure than sclerotherapy, but is associated with more pain.[20] Severe pain can be caused if the bands are placed too low and there is a small risk of perineal sepsis.

Other out-patient treatments

The infrared coagulator uses high intensity infrared light to coagulate vessels and tether mucosa to subcutaneous tissues. It is quick to do, but needs to be repeated on several occasions. Radio frequency probes are said to be able to treat all haemorrhoids in a single session by using the probe for two seconds in three or four areas. None of these is used routinely yet in the UK.

Out-patient treatment of internal haemorrhoids is quick and relatively painless; patients loose little time from work and cure rates are high. Patients should be warned that they may have some bleeding initially and again at 10–14 days. Failures can be re-treated with minimal side-effects.

Key point 4

- First- and second-degree haemorrhoids can be treated in the out-patient setting by simple, non-painful means with minimal side-effects.

Surgical/in-patient treatment

This usually reserved for symptomatic third- or fourth-degree haemorrhoids. The focus in recent years has been on minimising the complications of surgery and better pain relief.

Closed/open haemorrhoidectomy

Classical Milligan-Morgan or open haemorrhoidectomy has been practised for years in the UK; the Ferguson or closed technique is used more widely in the US. A recent randomised study comparing the two techniques suggests that the main advantage of the closed technique is not in pain control but in wound healing rates.[24] At 3 weeks, 86% of 'Ferguson' patients had healed wounds in contrast to 18% of 'Milligan-Morgan' patients and these latter patients had symptoms due to the delayed wound healing. A further study in day-case patients showed a high wound dehiscence in closed haemorrhoidectomy patients (10 of 18) and no difference between the two groups for final wound healing rates, pain, patient satisfaction or return to normal activity.[25] The choice of type of haemorrhoidectomy remains with the individual surgeon according to preference and training.

Stapled haemorrhoidectomy

Stapled or circumferential haemorrhoidectomy was initially advocated by Longo and colleagues. It aims to perform a mucosectomy 2 cm proximal to the dentate line in order to 'hitch up' the prolapsing anal lining and disrupt the proximal blood flow; it is said to reduce dramatically postoperative pain and hasten speed of healing.[27] Several randomised trials have shown a marked decrease in pain after stapled haemorrhoidectomy;[28] the pain after stapled haemorrhoidectomy is different, being dull and tenesmoid in nature. There has been one report of 5 patients of 22 treated with persistent pain; 4 of these had muscle within their stapled doughnuts,[29] but this level of pain has not been confirmed in any of the larger studies.

There have been few complications associated with the stapling technique; these include a case of pelvic sepsis,[30] and a patient with a rectovaginal fistula.[31] A potential problem is that the conventional stapled haemorrhoidectomy involves the use of a large circular anal dilator; there have been concerns that this may cause damage to the internal sphincter. One study from Singapore has shown significant, but asymptomatic, damage to the internal anal sphincter in 4 of 29 patients.[32] This has not been confirmed in a further study of 20 patients.[33]

Although the stapling device is expensive (the same cost as an intestinal circular stapler), this increased instrument cost appears to be off-set by the shorter convalescence period and less pain. It can be used in third- and fourth-degree haemorrhoids as well as thrombosed prolapsed circumferential haemorrhoids and the residual skin tags tend to shrivel by the third month after operation. The concerns with this procedure appear to rest around leaving a residual staple line and any muscular damage caused at the time of surgery.

Key point 5

- Promising results with the stapled haemorrhoidectomy technique and better peri-operative pain management mean that third- and fourth-degree haemorrhoids can be treated by day-case surgery with a swift return to work.

Secondary procedures/pain relief

With the move to day-case surgery and the emphasis on postoperative pain relief, it is important to design a careful peri-operative pain package. Pain sometimes increases a few days after haemorrhoidectomy possibly due to infection. One study randomised patients to receive metronidazole or a placebo for 7 days.[26] Patients had no anal pack and were also given diclofenac, 0.2% glyceryl-trinitrate (GTN) ointment and lactulose. Patients in the metronidazole group had significantly less pain.

Manual anal dilatation was introduced in the 1960s by Lord to reduce resting anal pressures. It is effective as is internal sphincterotomy; however, both procedures are associated with high levels of incontinence and the raised pressures are probably a result, rather than the cause, of haemorrhoids. Since spasm of the internal sphincter may be a source of anal pain after haemorrhoid surgery, other non-permanent alternatives have been tried. In a randomised trial of GTN ointment postoperatively for 7 days, the use of narcotic analgesics on the second day was reduced in the GTN group; however, the side-effect of headaches and a subsequent need for non-narcotic medications may limit its benefits.[23]

It appears that laxatives, non-steroidal analgesics and metronidazole are the combination of choice for post-operative pain relief post-haemorrhoidectomy. The role of GTN or diltiazem ointment has yet to be determined.

Key point 6

- Postoperative patients should receive laxatives, non-steroidal analgesics and a 7-day course of metronidazole. The role of sphincter relaxation with GTN or other agents has yet to be determined.

FISSURE

Fissure-in-ano is a linear tear in the lining of the distal anal canal below the level of the dentate line. It is a common condition affecting all age groups but usually young adults.

SYMPTOMS

Classic symptoms are anal pain during or after defecation accompanied by bright red rectal bleeding. The pain is often severe and described as a 'tearing pain' – it may last for minutes or for hours. Itching may accompany fissure in up to half the cases. Examination may reveal a split in the lining of the anal canal, but often pain and spasm prevent any examination. Secondary changes, such as a sentinel skin tag or a degree of anal stenosis, frequently accompany chronic anal fissures.

Most anal fissures are acute and settle spontaneously or with stool softening laxatives. Chronic fissures are those failing to heal within 6 weeks and usually need further intervention or treatment to heal. The majority of fissures occur posteriorly in the midline of the anal canal, although after childbirth women tend to have anterior fissures. Abnormally lying or multiple fissures should raise the suspicion of an underlying pathology (*e.g.* Crohn's disease, HIV infection or syphilis).

AETIOLOGY

The true aetiology of anal fissures is unknown. A popular theory is based around the severe internal sphincter spasm, which predates fissure formation, and the paucity of blood supply in the posterior midline.[34] This combination may lead to ischaemia and failure to heal is due to continuing ischaemia. This theory may also explain the relapses seen after non-permanent sphincterotomies in comparison to surgical sphincterotomies, due to a return to high resting pressures after cessation of treatment.

TREATMENT

Acute fissures usually heal spontaneously. A high-fibre diet and/or stool softening laxatives with a high water consumption are usually all that is needed. A small proportion (<10%) of chronic fissures heal without intervention.[35] However, because most of these patients have a raised resting anal pressure, treatment is usually directed at reducing spasm in the anal canal.

Chemical sphincterotomy

Nitric oxide is the neurotransmitter involved in mediating relaxation of the internal sphincter. The first chemicals successfully used to treat chronic anal fissures were nitric oxide donors – GTN ointment and isosorbide dinitrate. A pea-sized amount of 0.2% GTN ointment applied twice or three times a day to the anal canal for 8 weeks heals up to two-thirds of chronic anal fissures.[36] More than half the patients experience headaches, although these diminish in intensity with continuing application; however, this side-effect reduces compliance. Patients with a long history or who have a sentinel pile are less likely to heal with GTN ointment.[37]

A recurrence of symptoms occurs in about one-quarter of patients within a median of 2 years, associated with a rise in resting anal pressures, but most of these fissures heal with further GTN treatment.[38] Those patients whose symptoms recur, however, may benefit from a more permanent reduction in their resting pressure (surgical intervention) which is associated with a higher cure rate (97% *versus* 61%).[39]

Alternatives to GTN ointment are nifedipine and diltiazem, which are calcium channel blockers; they cause relaxation of smooth muscle. A recent randomised trial showed similar efficacy to GTN ointment, 65% healing with topical diltiazem 2% for 8 weeks, with no reported side-effects.[40]

Key point 7

• Chronic fissure should initially be treated by chemical sphincterotomy. Only non-healers or patients who recur should then be treated surgically.

Botulinum toxin

Botulinum toxin A is a lethal biological neurotoxin. It binds to presynaptic cholinergic terminals and inhibits the release of acetylcholine at the neuromuscular junction. Paralysis occurs within hours of injection and the effect lasts for 3–4 months (until axonal regeneration). The result of injecting botulinum toxin into the anal sphincter is to produce a prolonged, but reversible, sphincter relaxation, any incontinence is therefore transient. Healing rates of up to 96% have been recorded with a dose of 20 U[41] with no adverse effects; the rate of healing is related to the dose,[42] but it is still not clear where the injection should be placed.

Surgery

Although pharmacological agents may be employed as first-line treatment for chronic anal fissures, failure of treatment or recurrence of symptoms may warrant surgical intervention. A recent Cochrane Review[43] succinctly details the commonest techniques used for fissures: anal stretch, open lateral sphincterotomy, closed lateral sphincterotomy and anal advancement flap. Using the two commonest end points – those of persistence of the fissure and postoperative incontinence of flatus – all reports of direct comparisons between techniques were reviewed. The conclusion was that anal stretch is associated with a significantly higher risk of minor incontinence and should be abandoned in favour of open or closed partial lateral internal sphincterotomy.

There is probably little difference in the outcomes between open or closed internal sphincterotomy.[35] Healing occurs in 98% and the length of incision should be limited to the length of fissure.[44] Varying degrees of incontinence are reported to occur in 30% of patients (more frequently in women).[45] To avoid this complication, especially in patients who have had previous anal surgery or women who have had children, it is recommended that these patients undergo anal ultrasound and anorectal physiological assessment of their sphincters. If the sphincter is already compromised an anal advancement flap may be the preferred treatment.

Key point 8

- For patients requiring surgery for anal fissure, open and closed partial lateral internal sphincterotomy are equally efficacious. Anal stretch has a high risk of incontinence and should not be used for the treatment of fissure.

Key point 9

- There is a significant risk of incontinence after sphincterotomy and patients at risk should be carefully counselled.

CONCLUSIONS

Benign anal disease causes considerable morbidity and is a frequent finding in patients within primary and secondary care settings. Treatment of fissures, fistulas and haemorrhoids should be aimed at pain-free symptomatic control with as little disruption to the sphincter mechanism as possible.

Key points for clinical practice

- Complex fistulas should be assessed clinically and with MRI or ultrasound if they fail to heal or in the presence of scar tissue.

- The majority of fistulas are simple and can be treated with fistulotomy.

- Higher cure rates with complex procedures may be obtained at the expense of continence – a permanent loose seton may be the most acceptable option to the patient.

- First- and second-degree haemorrhoids can be treated in the out-patient setting by simple, non-painful means with minimal side-effects.

- Promising results with the stapled haemorrhoidectomy technique and better peri-operative pain management mean that third- and fourth-degree haemorrhoids can be treated by day-case surgery with a swift return to work.

- Postoperative patients should receive laxatives, non-steroidal analgesics and a 7-day course of metronidazole. The role of sphincter relaxation with GTN or other agents has yet to be determined.

- Chronic fissure should initially be treated by chemical sphincterotomy. Only non-healers or patients who recur should then be treated surgically.

- For patients requiring surgery for anal fissure, open and closed partial lateral internal sphincterotomy are equally efficacious. Anal stretch has a high risk of incontinence and should not be used for the treatment of fissure.

- There is a significant risk of incontinence after sphincterotomy and patients at risk should be carefully counselled.

References

1. Ewerth S, Ahlberg J, Collste G, Holmstrom B. Fistula-in-ano. A six year follow up study of 143 operated patients. *Acta Chir Scand* 1978; **482 (Suppl)**: 53–55.
2. Parks AG. The pathogenesis and treatment of fistula-in ano. *BMJ* 1961; **i**: 463–469.
3. Lunniss PJ, Sheffield JP, Talbot IC, Thomson JPS, Phillips RKS. Persistence of anal fistula may be related to epithelialisation. *Br J Surg* 1995; **82**: 32–33.
4. Parks AG, Gordon PH, Hardcastle JD. A classification of fistula-in-ano. *Br J Surg* 1976; **63**: 1–12.
5. Lunniss PJ, Barker PG, Sultan AH *et al*. Magnetic resonance imaging of fistula-in-ano. *Dis Colon Rectum* 1994; **37**: 708–718.
6. Ratto C, Gentile E, Merico M *et al*. How can the assessment of fistula-in-ano be improved? *Dis Colon Rectum* 2000; **43**: 1375–1382.
7. McCourtney JS, Finlay IG. Setons in the surgical management of fistula-in-ano. *Br J Surg* 1995; **82**: 448–452.
8. Phillips RKS, Lunniss PJ. *Anal Fistula. Surgical Evaluation and Management*. London: Chapman and Hall, 1996.
9. Zimmerman DD, Briel JW, Gosselink MP, Schouten WR. Anocutaneous advancement flap repair of transsphincteric fistulas. *Dis Colon Rectum* 2001; **44**: 1474–1480.

10. Hyman N. Endoanal advancement flap repair for complex anorectal fistulas. *Am J Surg* 1999; **178**: 337–340.

11. Ortiz H, Marzo J. Endorectal flap advancement repair and fistulectomy for high trans-sphincteric and suprasphincteric fistulas. *Br J Surg* 2000; **87**: 1680–1683.

12. Ozuner G, Hull TL, Cartmill J, Fazio VW. Long-term analysis of the use of transanal rectal advancement flaps for complicated anorectal/vaginal fistulas. *Dis Colon Rectum* 1996; **39**: 10–14.

13. Sentovich SM. Fibrin glue for all anal fistulas. *J Gastrointest Surg* 2001; **5**: 158–161.

14. Venkatesh KS, Ramanujam P. Fibrin glue application in the treatment of recurrent anorectal fistulas. *Dis Colon Rectum* 1999; **42**: 1136–1139.

15. Cinron JR, Park JJ, Orsay CP *et al*. Repair of fistulas-in-ano using fibrin adhesive: long-term follow-up. *Dis Colon Rectum* 2000; **43**: 944–949.

16. Pinedo G, Phillips R. Labial fat pad grafts (modified Martius graft) in complex perianal fistulas. *Ann R Coll Surg Engl* 1998; **80**: 410–412.

17. Schwartz DA, Pemberton JH, Sandborn WJ. Diagnosis and treatment of perianal fistulas in Crohn's disease. *Ann Intern Med* 2001; **135**: 906–918.

18. Gass OC, Adams J. Haemorrhoids: etiology and pathology. *Am J Surg* 1950: **79**: 40–43.

19. Hulme-Moir M, Bartolo DC. Hemorrhoids *Gastroenterol Clin North Am* 2001; **30**: 183–197.

20. MacRae HM, McLeod RS. Comparison of hemorrhoid treatment modalities: a meta-analysis. *Dis Colon Rectum* 1995; **38**: 687–694.

21. Al-Ghnaniem R, Leather AJ, Rennie JA. Survey of methods of treatment of haemorrhoids and complications of injection sclerotherapy. *Ann R Coll Surg Engl* 2001; **83**: 325–328.

22. Murray-Lyon IM, Kirkham JS. Hepatic abscesses complicating injection sclerotherapy of haemorrhoids. *Eur J Gastroenterol Hepatol* 2001; **13**: 971–972.

23. Wasvary HJ, Hain J, Mosed-Vogel M, Bendick P, Barkel DC, Klein SN. Randomized, prospective, double-blind, placebo-controlled trial of effect of nitroglycerin ointment on pain after hemorrhoidectomy. *Dis Colon Rectum* 2001; **44**: 1069–1073.

24. Arbman G, Krook H, Haapaniemi S. Closed vs. open hemorrhoidectomy – is there any difference? *Dis Colon Rectum* 2000; **43**: 1174–1175.

25. Carapeti E, Kamm M, McDonald P, Chadwick S, Phillips RKS. Randomised trial of open versus closed day-case haemorrhoidectomy. *Br J Surg* 1999; **86**: 612.

26. Carapeti EA, Kamm MA, McDonald PJ, Phillips RKS. Double-blind randomised controlled trial of effect of metronidazole on pain after day-case haemorrhoidectomy. *Lancet* 1998; **351**: 169–172.

27. Longo A. Treatment of haemorrhoids disease by reduction of mucosa and haemorrhoidal prolapse with a circular-suturing device: a new procedure. *Proc Sixth World Congress of Endoscopic Surgery, Rome, Italy* 1998; **777**: 84.

28. Seow-Choen F. Stapled haemorrhoidectomy: pain or gain? *Br J Surg* 2001; **88**: 1–3.

29. Cheetham MJ, Mortensen NJM, Nystrom P-O, Kamm MA, Phillips RKS. Persistent pain and faecal urgency after stapled haemorrhoidectomy. *Lancet* 2000; **356**: 730–733.

30. Molloy RG, Kingsmore D. Life threatening pelvic sepsis after stapled haemorrhoidectomy. *Lancet* 2000; **355**: 810.

31. Pescatori M. Stapled rectal prolapsectomy. *Dis Colon Rectum* 2000; **43**: 876–877.

32. Ho YH, Seow-Choen F, Tsang C, Eu KW. Randomized trial assessing anal sphincter injuries after stapled haemorrhoidectomy. *Br J Surg* 2001; **88**: 1449–155

33. Altomare DF, Rinaldi M, Sallustio PL, Martino P, De Fazio M, Memeo V. Long-term effects of stapled haemorrhoidectomy on internal anal function and sensitivity. *Br J Surg* 2001; **88**: 1487.

34. Klosterhalfen B, Vogel P, Rixen H *et al*. Topography of the inferior rectal artery: a possible cause of chronic, primary anal fissure. *Dis Colon Rectum* 1989; **32**: 43–52.

35. Jonas M, Scholefield JH. Anal fissure. *Gastroenterol Clin North Am* 2001; **30**: 167–181.

36. Lund JN, Scholefield JH. A randomised, prospective, double-blind, placebo-controlled trial of glyceryl trinitrate ointment in the treatment of anal fissure. *Lancet* 1997; **349**: 11–14.

37. Pitt J, Williams S, Dawson PM. Reasons for failure of glyceryl trinitrate treatment of chronic fissure-in-ano: a multivariate analysis. *Dis Colon Rectum* 2001; **44**: 964–967.

38. Lund JN, Scholefield JH. Follow-up of patients with chronic anal fissure treated with topical glyceryl trinitrate. *Lancet* 1988; **352**: 1681.

39. Evans J, Luck A, Hewett P. Glyceryl trinitrate vs. lateral sphincterotomy for chronic anal fissure: prospective, randomized trial. *Dis Colon Rectum* 2001; **44**: 93–97.
40. Jonas M, Neal KR, Abercrombie JF, Scholefield JH. A randomised trial of oral vs topical diltiazem for chronic anal fissures. *Dis Colon Rectum* 2001; **44**: 1074–1078.
41. Brisinda G, Maria G, Bentivoglio AR, Cassetta E, Gui D, Albanese A. A comparison of injections of botulinum toxin and topical nitroglycerin ointment for the treatment of chronic anal fissure. *N Engl J Med* 1999; **341**: 65–69.
42. Minguez M, Melo F, Espi A *et al*. Therapeutic effects of different doses of botulinum toxin in chronic anal fissure. *Dis Colon Rectum* 1999; **42**: 1016-1021.
43. Nelson R. Operative procedures for fissure in ano (Cochrane Review). *Cochrane Database Systematic Rev* 2001; **3**: CD 002199.
44. Garcia-Aguilar J, Belmonte Montes C, Perez JJ, Jensen L, Madoff RD, Wong WD. Incontinence after lateral internal sphincterotomy: anatomic and functional evaluation. *Dis Colon Rectum* 1998; **41**: 423–427.
45. Nyam DC, Pemberton JH. Long-term results of lateral internal sphincterotomy for chronic anal fissure with particular reference to incidence of fecal incontinence *Dis Colon Rectum* 1999; **42**: 1306–1310.

Jonathan D. Beard Peter A. Gaines

13

Angioplasty for critical limb ischaemia

DEFINITION, EPIDEMIOLOGY AND PROGNOSIS

The term chronic critical lower limb ischaemia (CLI) includes patients with chronic ischaemic rest pain, ulcers or gangrene due to peripheral arterial disease.[1] Without revascularisation, most will require a major amputation. The prevalence of CLI in the UK has recently been estimated at 20,000 patients per year, *i.e.* 40 per 100,000 population.[2]

The workload generated by CLI continues to increase due to the expanding elderly population and the increasing availability of therapeutic techniques. The majority of patients with CLI can now be offered revascularisation, mainly due to an increase in endovascular procedures.[3] The published results seem good in specialist centres, but intervention is often technically demanding and utilises significant hospital resources.[4] Furthermore, the prognosis for patients with CLI seems poor, as about 25% will die within a year and 50% within 5 years, mainly from coronary and cerebral vascular disease. Many studies have shown that the presence of diabetes and renal failure result in worse outcomes in terms of limb salvage and mortality rates.[5,6] Therefore, treatment of CLI requires relatively short-term objectives, especially in patients with significant co-morbidity. There is some evidence that increased rates of vascular reconstruction are associated with a lower incidence of amputation.[7] A national survey by the Vascular Surgical Society of Great Britain and Ireland showed that 70% of patients with CLI underwent revascularisation, with a 75% chance of successful limb salvage.[2]

Mr Jonathan D. Beard, BSc ChM FRCS(Lond), Consultant Vascular Surgeon, Sheffield Vascular Institute, Northern General Hospital, Sheffield S5 7AU, UK

Mr Peter A. Gaines MRCP FRCR, Consultant Vascular Radiologist, Sheffield Vascular Institute, Northern General Hospital, Sheffield S5 7AU, UK

RISK FACTOR IDENTIFICATION AND MODIFICATION

Identification and modification of risk factors normally forms the first line of treatment for patients with peripheral arterial disease. Although immediate attention is focused on limb salvage for patients with CLI, risk factor modification must always be remembered. This includes cessation of smoking, and good control of hypertension, hypercholesterolaemia and diabetes.[8] Antiplatelet therapy with aspirin or clopidogrel also reduces the risk of vascular death, myocardial infarction and stroke by 25%.[9] Failure to address these factors may also result in failure of the revascularisation procedure.[10]

Renal impairment is often associated with peripheral arterial disease and requires detection and treatment, if possible, before proceeding to diagnostic arteriography or endovascular intervention.

Key point 1

- Assessment and treatment of co-morbidity and risk factors for atherosclerosis must not be forgotten in patients with CLI.

PATIENT SELECTION AND ANALGESIA

Most patients with CLI require intervention. There are some situations when this would be inappropriate and these patients should not undergo unnecessary investigation. If their general condition appears poor, and the chances of survival are limited due to co-existent pathology, it seems reasonable to treat such patients with analgesia alone. However, if their quality-of-life seems reasonable and they are likely to survive for more than few months, it seems better to attempt revascularisation whenever possible. Some patients present with such advanced ischaemia that there is little viable tissue left on the weight-bearing area of the foot. A below-knee amputation is the best option in these cases. A through-knee (Gritti-Stokes) amputation is more appropriate for chair-or bed-bound patients. An algorithm outlining the management of patients with CLI is shown in Figure 1.

Prompt and adequate pain control is essential for patients with CLI. This usually requires oral opioids. Attention must also be paid to treatment of concomitant co-morbidity as well as to achieving adequate hydration, oxygenation and nutrition.

ENDOVASCULAR TREATMENT VERSUS OPEN SURGERY

The evidence for endovascular intervention compared to open surgery in CLI remains weak. There have been few randomised trials in patients with peripheral arterial disease, and none in those with CLI alone. Holm et al.[11] randomised 102 patients (66% with CLI), and Wolf et al.[12] randomised 263

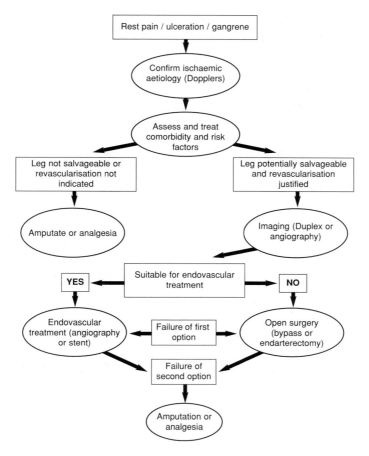

Fig. 1 Management pathway for patients with chronic critical lower limb ischaemia (CLI).

patients (73% with claudication), to either angioplasty or surgery. In each case the lesion had to be suitable for both techniques. At follow-up, they found significant improvement in quality-of-life with no significant difference in outcome between the two techniques. As for open surgery, the results for endovascular intervention depend upon the level of the disease (proximal better than distal), the severity of the lesion (stenosis better than occlusion), and the quality of the in-flow and run-off.

The primary success and subsequent patency rates of open surgery and endovascular intervention are at least 10–15% lower in patients with CLI compared to claudicants. However, even a short-term improvement may result in

Key point 2

- Few randomised studies comparing endovascular intervention against open surgery for peripheral arterial disease exist, and none for those with CLI alone.

healing, and re-occlusion does not necessarily result in clinical deterioration.[13] In
addition, these patients are likely to die from other causes before requiring re-
intervention. For these reasons, many institutions have now turned to a strategy
of endovascular intervention in the first instance, and this seems applicable for
approximately 50–75% of cases.[14]

CLI is usually due to vascular disease at 2 or 3 levels. Aorto-iliac disease
should be treated first, as it may convert rest pain to claudication and, if left alone,
would jeopardise any infra-inguinal intervention. When there is tissue loss, then
treatment of the in-flow to the limb alone appears less likely to result in healing,
as in-line flow to the foot is often required. The infra-inguinal disease can be
managed by surgery or angioplasty as a combined procedure, or may be delayed
according to the clinical situation. A variety of combinations may be appropriate.
When an occlusion of the ipsilateral iliac segment seems too long for
endovascular treatment, then the contralateral side can be treated by angioplasty
or stenting to facilitate a femoro-femoral cross-over.[15] Endovascular intervention
proximal to such a cross-over graft does not appear to interfere with the
durability of the graft.[16] Pre- or peri-operative angioplasty or stenting can
improve graft in-flow or run-off resulting in better patency and a reduction in the
length of the bypass. Pre-operative angioplasty of a superficial femoral artery
stenosis may permit a short popliteal-pedal bypass rather than a full-length
bypass from the femoral artery. Angioplasty of a tibial artery stenosis at the time
of femoro-popliteal bypass may avoid the need for a jump graft.

SUPRA-INGUINAL DISEASE

Aortobifemoral bypass is considered the 'gold' standard for the treatment of
extensive aorto-iliac disease, with 5-year patency rates of about 90%.[17]
However, it carries a mortality rate of 5% as well as the risk of graft infection
and postoperative impotence. Femorofemoral and iliofemoral bypass provide
satisfactory ways of dealing with unilateral iliac disease, albeit with lower
patencies of 80% at 3 years.[18] Extra-anatomic axillobifemoral bypass has a poor

patency of only 60% at 5 years, due to the long graft and lower flow rate.[19] Therefore, fit patients with extensive aorto-iliac disease are best treated with an aortobifemoral graft. Unfit patients and those with localised disease should undergo femorofemoral or iliofemoral bypass or angioplasty/stenting depending upon the pattern of disease.

> **Key point 5**
>
> • Endovascular intervention for supra-inguinal disease has become the treatment of choice for most patients. Aortobifemoral grafting remains the gold standard for extensive bilateral disease.

Axillofemoral bypass should be reserved for those in whom endovascular intervention is unsuitable or fails. With the advent of percutaneous angioplasty and stenting, endarterectomy for localised aorto-iliac disease seems rarely justified. Localised stenosis or occlusion of the common femoral artery seems best treated by endarterectomy. Angioplasty of the femoral bifurcation does not work well, because of difficulties with access from the opposite groin and the bulky calcified disease. Stents cannot be used at this level because the artery flexes with movements of the hip.

Infrarenal aortic stenoses usually occur in women, often in association with hyperlipidaemia. Simple lesions seem best treated by balloon dilatation, with primary success in greater than 90% of cases, and long-term patencies of 70–90% at 4 years.[20] There are no randomised data to suggest that aortic stents are better than angioplasty alone and neither is there likely to be, since this disease pattern is uncommon. If stents restrict distal embolisation, they may well have a role in bulky or eccentric stenoses. The initial technical success with stents is in the region of 90–100% with patencies at 4 years of around 90%.[21]

Iliac stenosis

Simple iliac stenoses appear relatively easy to treat by balloon dilatation. The primary success rate exceeds 90% for all reported series, with long-term patencies of 75–95% at 1 year, 60–90% at 3 years and 60–80% at 5 years.[22–25] The primary success rate and long-term patency rate seem better for common iliac compared to external iliac lesions and when the superficial femoral artery is patent. The use of stents for iliac stenoses has continued despite the lack of supporting data. In general, stents are used when the lesion is thought to be at high risk from primary failure and embolisation (*e.g.* eccentric stenosis) or when angioplasty fails (usually defined as residual stenosis of greater than 50%, a residual pressure gradient or an extensive dissection). Large series of stents, used mainly for iliac stenoses, have shown a primary technical success 95–100% and long-term patencies of 78–95% at 1 year, 53–81% at 3 years and 54–72% at 5 years.[26–28] These results appear to be similar to angioplasty alone, but the studies are all non-randomised. Recently, a meta-analysis of the results of angioplasty and stent placement for aorta iliac occlusive disease[29] concluded that compared to angioplasty, stents have: (i) an improved technical success rate; (b) a similar complication rate; and (c) a 39% reduction in the risk of long-term failure.

The long-awaited randomised trial by Richter has yet to be published although abstracts have appeared.[30] In this study, stenoses were randomised between angioplasty and stent placement with a significantly improved primary success rate in the stent group and a better 5-year angiographic patency (64.6% *versus* 93.6%). Similarly, the 5-year clinical success rates rose from 69.7% to 92.7% in the stent group. The Dutch Iliac Stent Trial Group has published a randomised trial of primary stent placement *versus* selective stent placement in patients with iliac artery occlusive disease.[31] In this study, 279 patients with intermittent claudication (including only 12 iliac occlusions) were randomised to either primary stent placement or stent placement after angioplasty if there was a residual mean gradient of greater than 10 mmHg. No difference was found in the two strategies at short- and long-term follow-up, but the policy of selective stent placement was cheaper. However, the trial was based on the premise that a residual gradient following angioplasty predicts poor outcome, something for which there is no good scientific base. In summary, angioplasty for iliac stenoses is effective and relatively safe; stents are only required for the management of complications.

Iliac occlusion

Iliac occlusions can also be treated by balloon angioplasty. Two recent series of chronic iliac occlusions treated by simple balloon dilatation report a primary success of 78% and 89%.[32,33] Leu *et al.* reported a clinical success (including primary failures) at 1, 4 and 10 years of 64%, 57% and 57%, respectively.[32] If primary failures were excluded, then the primary clinical success at each interval rises to 75%, 68% and 68%, respectively. The secondary clinical success in those patients who had subsequent placement of a stent rose to 94% at 1 year, and 92% at 4 years and 10 years. In this study, there was a high risk of embolisation (24%), but in the majority of cases this was either not clinically significant or was treated by aspiration thrombo-embolectomy at the time of the primary procedure. Gupta *et al.* reported a clinical success (including primary failures) of around 58% at 1 year and 55% at 3 and 5 years.[33] Embolisation occurred in only 8% of cases.

Stents seem an ideal way of treating iliac occlusions because of their ability to scaffold the large bulk of disease and reduce embolisation (Fig. 2). The available data on the subject appear limited,[34,35] but indicate primary patency rates of 85%, 80% and 55% at 1-, 3-, and 5-year follow-up. These results seem little different from angioplasty alone and we await the result of an on-going UK randomised trial (STAG). However, stents may reduce the embolisation rate to less than 5%.

Key point 6

- Little evidence exists for the use of stents for iliac disease, except for the treatment of complications following angioplasty. The results of randomised trials are awaited.

INFRA-INGUINAL DISEASE

The conventional treatment for the majority of patients with CLI due to infra-inguinal disease is bypass grafting to the infrageniculate vessels. A meta-analysis

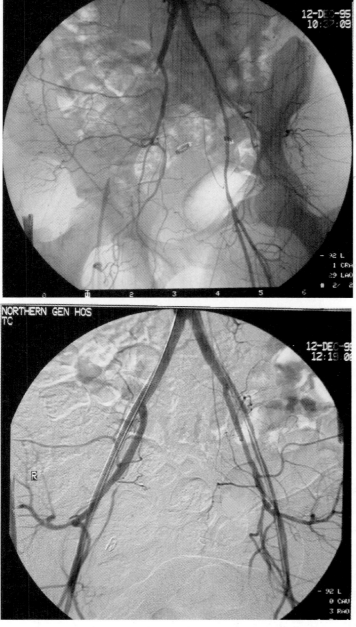

Fig. 2 Long right iliac occlusion (a), successfully treated with a self-expanding Wallstent (b).

by Hunink *et al.*[36] re-analysed the data from 1572 patients with CLI treated with a femoropopliteal bypass graft. The primary patency rate for below-knee vein grafts was 66% at 5 years compared to only 33% for prosthetic grafts (PTFE). Vein graft patency depends upon many factors including the quality of

167

the vein and the run-off.[37] It seems unlikely that endovascular intervention for extensive infra-inguinal disease will match the patency rates of a good quality vein graft. However, infra-inguinal bypass surgery for CLI has a mortality of 5% and a wound complication rate of 20%.[38] A recent study found that only 20% of patients achieved an ideal outcome without complications.[39] Graft infection seems particularly disastrous and often results in amputation. Angioplasty seems appropriate for those with localised disease (uncommon in CLI), and those unfit for surgery or who lack of a good long saphenous vein.

The overall primary success of angioplasty in patients with localised infra-inguinal disease (mostly claudicants) is 84% with 1- and 5-year patencies of 64% and 52%.[40] The extent of disease and severity of ischaemia affect the outcome and durability of the intervention. A recent meta-analysis of 923 angioplasties for femoropopliteal disease in patients with claudication or CLI was performed by Muradin et al.[41] Combined 3-year patencies were 61% for stenoses and claudication, 48% for occlusions and claudication, 43% for stenoses and CLI, and 30% for occlusions and CLI. Taking these factors into consideration along with the complications of intervention, the Standards of Practise Committee of the Society of Cardiovascular and Interventional Radiology indicated that suitable lesions to treat would be stenoses or occlusions up to 10 cm in length, limited to the superficial femoral artery.[42] Many devices have been used in the femoropopliteal segment in an attempt to improve the outcome of simple angioplasty. Stents have been studied in at least 2 randomised trials[43,44] and have shown no benefit over angioplasty. They cannot be deployed in the popliteal artery because of knee flexion and should only be used to rescue a flow-limiting dissection or thrombosis, or as part of a randomised trial. Similarly, lasers and atherectomy devices have no role to play in native arterial disease.

Key point 7

- Angioplasty is the treatment of choice for localised disease (stenosis or occlusion < 10 cm) of the superficial femoral artery. A randomised trial of surgery *versus* angioplasty for intermediate disease has commenced in the UK.

More extensive infra-inguinal disease can be considered for endovascular intervention in patients with CLI compared to claudicants, because a higher complication rate seems acceptable in the threatened limb. Lesions suitable for angioplasty, therefore, include occlusions up to 15 cm in length affecting the superficial femoral, popliteal and the tibial arteries. Intentional subintimal angioplasty is currently becoming popular. This permits any length of lesion to be treated, including flush occlusions of the superficial femoral artery. Bolia and colleagues have reported a series of 200 subintimal angioplasties for long femoropopliteal occlusions with an initial success rate of 80%.[45] In this technique, the guide wire is deliberately directed into the subintimal plane at the level of the occlusion which is then crossed in the same plane before balloon angioplasty (Fig. 3). For the technique to be successful, the distal

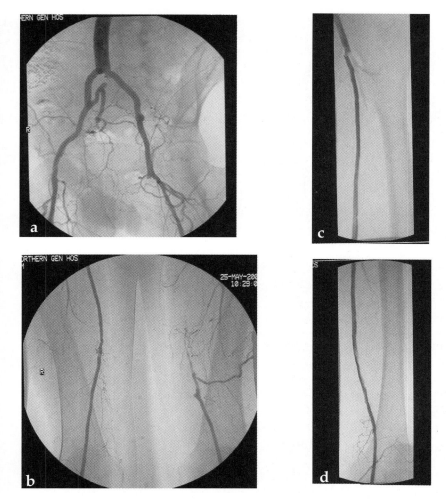

Fig. 3 Occlusion of the entire superficial artery from its origin (a, b), treated successfully by subintimal angioplasty (c, d).

Key point 8

- Subintimal angioplasty permits the endovascular treatment of extensive infra-inguinal disease but randomised trials against vein bypass are required.

segment of artery, into which the dissection extends, must be relatively free of disease to allow re-entry back into the true lumen.

CURRENT RECOMMENDATIONS FOR TREATMENT

Because the severity of disease and quality of run-off affects the success of angioplasty, patency rates in critical limb ischaemia seem likely to be at least

169

10% lower than the figures quoted for claudication. Nevertheless, limb salvage rates of between 50–89% at 1 and 2 years have been reported for femoropopliteal angioplasty.[46,47] Infrapopliteal angioplasty has also achieved limb salvage rates of 44–96% at 1 year.[48,49] Based on the current evidence, the Transatlantic Intersociety Consensus (TASC) recommends the following:[37]

- Endovascular procedure is the treatment of choice for type A lesions (single stenosis or occlusion of the superficial femoral or popliteal artery < 3 cm).

- Surgery is the procedure of choice for type D lesions (complete occlusion of the superficial femoral or popliteal artery).

- More evidence is required regarding the treatment of intermediate type B and C lesions (multiple stenoses and longer occlusions). (A randomised controlled trial of angioplasty versus surgery [BASIL trial] for this intermediate disease has commenced in the UK.)

PREVENTION OF COMPLICATIONS

The complication rate from angioplasty in CLI seems higher than that for claudication[50] presumably because of the severity of co-morbid disease and the tendency to treat more extensive lesions. Acute deterioration in the severity of ischaemia is usually due to distal embolisation, or dissection which removes collaterals or occludes flow. Embolisation should be managed by thrombo-aspiration in the first instance. If this fails, then surgical embolectomy or thrombolysis may be required. The administration of heparin during the procedure helps to limit thrombus formation. Spasm should be treated by the liberal use of antispasmodics, such as Tolazoline 12.5 mg, particularly in the tibial vessels. Clearly these high-risk interventions should only be performed when surgical cover is available.

Key points for clinical practice

- Assessment and treatment of co-morbidity and risk factors for atherosclerosis must not be forgotten in patients with CLI.

- Few randomised studies comparing endovascular intervention against open surgery for peripheral arterial disease exist, and none for those with CLI alone.

- The primary success and subsequent patency of endovascular intervention depends upon the level of the disease (supra-inguinal better than infra-inguinal), severity of disease (stenosis better than occlusion), and quality of in-flow/run-off.

- Like surgery, endovascular intervention for CLI has a 10–15% lower success rate than that for claudication, due to the presence of more extensive disease.

- Endovascular intervention for supra-inguinal disease has become the treatment of choice for most patients. Aortobifemoral grafting remains the gold standard for extensive bilateral disease.

(continued on next page)

Key points for clinical practice (continued)

- Little evidence exists for the use of stents for iliac disease, except for the treatment of complications following angioplasty. The results of randomised trials are awaited.

- Angioplasty is the treatment of choice for localised disease (stenosis or occlusion < 10 cm) of the superficial femoral artery. A randomised trial of surgery *versus* angioplasty for intermediate disease has commenced in the UK.

- Subintimal angioplasty permits the endovascular treatment of extensive infra-inguinal disease but randomised trials against vein bypass are required.

References

1. Transatlantic Inter-Society Consensus (TASC). Management of peripheral arterial disease (PAD). *Eur J Vasc Endovasc Surg* 2000; **19 (Suppl)**: S144–S150.
2. The Vascular Surgical Society of Great Britain and Ireland. Critical limb ischaemia: managuelet and outcome. Report of a National Survey. *Eur J Vasc Endovasc Surg* 1995; **10**: 108—113.
3. Pell JP, Wyman MR, Fowkes FG, Gillespie I, Ruckley CV. Trends in vascular surgery since the introduction of percutaneous transluminal angioplasty. *Br J Surg* 1994; **81**: 932—935.
4. Holdsworth RJ, McCollum PT. Results and implications of treating end-stage limb ischaemia. *Eur J Vasc Endovasc Surg* 1997; **13**: 164–173.
5. Fratezi, AC, Albers M, De Luccia N, Pereira CAB. Outcome and quality of life of patients with severe chronic limb ischaemia: a cohort study on the influence of diabetes. *Eur J Vasc Surg* 1995; **10**: 459–465.
6. Leers SA, Reifsnyder T, Delmonte R, Caron M. Realistic expectations for pedal bypass grafts in patients with end-stage renal disease. *J Vasc Surg* 1998; **28**: 976–983.
7. Karlstrom L, Bergqvist D. Effects of vascular surgery on amputation rates and mortality. *Eur J Vasc Endovasc Surg* 1997; **14**: 273–283.
8. Anon. Joint British recommendations on prevention of coronary heart disease in clinical practice. *Heart* 1998; **80 (Suppl 2)**: S1–S29.
9. Antiplatelet trialists collaboration. Collaboration overview of randomised trials on antiplatelet therapy. 1. Prevention of death, myocardial infarction and stroke by prolonged antiplatelet therapy in various categories of patients. *BMJ* 1994; **308**: 81—106.
10. Cavender JB, Rogers WJ, Fisher LD, Bush BJ, Coggin CJ, Meyers WO. Effects of smoking on survival and morbidity in patients randomised to medical or surgical therapy in the Coronary Artery Surgery Study (CASS): 10-year follow-up. *J Am Coll Cardiol* 1992; **20**: 287–294.
11. Holm J, Arfvidsson B, Jivegard L. Chronic lower limb ischaemia. A prospective randomised controlled study comparing the 1-year results of vascular surgery and percutaneous transluminal angioplasty (PTA). *Eur J Vasc Endovasc Surg* 1991; **5**: 517–522.
12. Wolf GL, Wilson SE, Cross AP. Surgery or balloon angioplasty for peripheral vascular disease: a randomised clinical trial. *J Vasc Interv Radiol* 1993; **4**: 639–648.
13. Ray SA, Minty I, Buckenham TM *et al*. Clinical outcome and restenosis following percutaneous transluminal angioplasty for ischaemic rest pain or ulceration. *Br J Surg* 1995; **82**: 1217–1221.
14. London NJM, Varty K, Sayers RD *et al*. Percutaneous transluminal angioplasty for lower-limb critical ischaemia. *Br J Surg* 1995; **82**: 1232–1235.
15. Whitbread T, Cleveland TJ, Beard JD, Gaines PA. The treatment of aortoiliac occlusions by endovascular stenting with or without adjuvant femorofemoral crossover grafting. *Eur J Vasc Endovasc Surg* 1998; **15**: 169–174.

16. Perler BA, Williams GM. Does donor iliac artery percutaneous transluminal angioplasty or stent placement influence the results of femorofemoral bypass? Analysis of 70 consecutive cases with long-term follow up. *J Vasc Surg* 1996; **24**: 363–370.

17. de Vries SO, Hunink MG. Results of aortic bifurcation grafts for aortoiliac occlusive disease: a meta analysis. *J Vasc Surg* 1997; **26**: 558–569.

18. Ricco JB. Unilateral iliac occlusive disease: a randomised multicenter trial examining direct revascularisation versus crossover bypass. *Ann Vasc Surg* 1992; **6**: 209–219.

19. Naylor AR, Ah-See AK, Engeset J. Axillofemoral bypass as a limb salvage procedure in high risk patients with aortoiliac disease. *Br J Surg* 1990; **77**: 659.

20. Joosten AH, Ho GH, Breuking FA *et al.* Percutaneous transluminal angioplasty of the infrarenal aorta: initial outcome and long term clinical and angiographic results. *Eur J Vasc Endovasc Surg* 1996: **12**: 201-206.

21. Sheeran SR, Hallisey MJ, Ferguson D. Percutaneous stent placement in the abdominal aorta. *J Vasc Interv Radiol* 1997; **8**: 55–60.

22. Johnston KW. Iliac arteries: re-analysis of results of balloon angioplasty. *Radiology* 1993; **186**: 382–386.

23. Jorgensen B, Skovgaard N, Norgard J, Karle A, Holstein P. Percutaneous transluminal angioplasty in 226 iliac artery stenoses: role of the superficial femoral artery for clinical success. *Vasa* 1992; **21**: 382–386.

24. Tegtmeyer CJ, Hartwell CD, Selby JB, Robertson R, Kron IL, Tribbloe CG. Results and complications of angioplasty in aortoiliac disease. *Circulation* 1991; **81**: 207–218.

25. Jeans WD, Armstrong S, Cole SEA *et al.* Fate of patients undergoing transluminal angioplasty for lower limb ischaemia. *Radiology* 1990; **177**: 559–564.

26. Murphy KD, Encarnacion CE, Le VA, Palmaz JC. Iliac artery stent placement with the Palmaz stent: follow up study. *J Vasc Surg* 1995; **6**: 321–329.

27. Martin EC, Katzen BT, Benenati JF *et al.* Multicenter trial of the Wallstent in the iliac and femoral arteries. *J Vasc Interv Radiol* 1995; **6**: 843–849.

28. Murphy TP, Webb MS, Lambiase RE *et al.* Percutaneous revascularisation of complex iliac artery stenoses and occlusions with use of Wallstents. Three year experience. *J Vasc Interv Radiol* 1996; **7**: 21–27.

29. Bosch JL, Hunink MG. Meta-analysis of the results of percutaneous transluminal angioplasty and stent placement for aortoiliac occlusive disease. *Radiology* 1997; **204**: 87–96.

30. Richter GM, Roeren T, Brado M *et al.* Further update of the randomised trial. Iliac stent placement versus PTA – morphology, clinical success rates, and failure analysis [abstract]. *J Vasc Interv Radiol* 1993; **4**: 30–31.

31. Tetteroo E, van der Graaf Y, Bosch JL *et al.* Randomised comparison of primary stent placement versus primary angioplasty followed by selective stent placement in patients with iliac artery occlusive disease. *Lancet* 1998; **351**: 1153–1159.

32. Leu AJ, Schneider E, Canova CR, Hoffman U. Long term results after recanalisation of chronic iliac artery occlusions by combined catheter therapy without stent placement. *Eur J Vasc Endovasc Surg* 1999; **18**: 499–505.

33. Gupta AK, Ravimandalam K, Rao KRV *et al.* Total occlusion of iliac arteries: results of balloon angioplasty. *Cardiovasc Interv Radiol* 1993; **16**: 165–177.

34. Dyet JF, Gaines PA, Nicholson AA *et al.* Treatment of chronic iliac artery occlusions by means of percutaneous endovascular stent placement. *J Vasc Interv Radiol* 1997; **8**: 349–353.

35. Vorwerk D, Guenther RW, Schürmann K *et al.* Primary stent placement for chronic iliac artery occlusions; follow up results in 103 patients. *Radiology* 1995; **194**: 745–749.

36. Hunink WG, Wong JB, Donaldson MC, Meyerovitz MF, Harrington DP. Patency rates of percutaneous and surgical revascularisation for femoropopliteal arterial disease. *Med Decis Making* 1994; **14**: 71–81.

37. Transatlantic Inter-Society Consensus (TASC). Management of peripheral arterial disease (PAD). *Eur J Vasc Endovasc Surg* 2000; **19 (Suppl)**: S182–S197.

38. Taylor LM, Edwards JM, Porter JM. Present status of reversed vein bypass grafting: five year results of a modern series. *J Vasc Surg* 1990; **11**: 193–206.

39. Nicoloff AD, Taylor LM, McLafferty RB, Moneta GL, Porter JM. Patient recovery after infrainguinal bypass grafting for limb salvage. *J Vasc Surg* 1998; **27**: 256–266.

40. Adar R, Critchfield GC, Eddy DM. A confidence profile analysis of the results of femoropopliteal percutaneous transluminal angioplasty in the treatment of lower extremity ischaemia. *J Vasc Surg* 1999; **10**: 57–59.

41. Muradin GSR, Basch JL, Hunink MGM. Balloon dilatation and stent implantation for treatment of femoropopliteal arterial disease: a meta-analysis. *Radiology* 2001; **221**: 137–145.

42. Standards of Practise Committee of the Society of Cardiovascular and Interventional Radiology. Guidelines for percutaneous transluminal angioplasty. *Radiology* 1990; **177**: 619.

43. Cejina M, Schoder M, Lammer J. PTA versus stent in femoro-popliteal obstruction. *Radiology* 1999; **39**: 144–150.

44. Vroegindeweij D, Vos LD, Tielbeeck AV *et al*. Balloon angioplasty combined with primary stenting versus balloon angioplasty alone in femoropopliteal obstructions: a comparative randomised study. *Cardiovasc Interv Radiol* 1997; **20**: 420–425.

45. London NJM, Srinivasan R, Sayers RD, Bell PRF, Bolia A. Subintimal angioplasty of femoropopliteal artery occlusion: the long-term results. *Eur J Vasc Surg* 1994; **8**: 148–155.

46. Ray SA, Minty I, Buckenham TM *et al*. Clinical outcome and restenosis following percutaneous transluminal angioplasty for ischaemic rest pain or ulceration. *Br J Surg* 1995; **82**: 1217–1221.

47. London NJM, Varty K, Sayers RD *et al*. Percutaneous transluminal angioplasty for lower-limb critical ischaemia. *Br J Surg* 1995; **82**: 1232–1235.

48. Schwarten DE. Clinical and anatomical considerations for non-operative therapy in tibial disease and the results of angioplasty. *Circulation* 1991; **83 (Suppl I)**: 86–93.

49. Brown KT, Schoenbert NY, Moore ED *et al*. Percutaneous transluminal angioplasty of infrapopliteal vessels: preliminary results and technical considerations. *Radiology* 1998; **169**: 75–79.

50. Belli AM, Cumberland DC, Knox AM. The complication rate of percutaneous peripheral balloon angioplasty. *Clin Radiol* 1990; **41**: 380–383.

Tan Arulampalam Irving Taylor

14

The clinical application of PET in surgical oncology

Since the discovery of X-rays by Roentgen in 1895, medical imaging has developed into a complex speciality. Imaging modalities can be broadly subdivided into two distinct categories. In the first, there are the techniques which give detailed morphological information relating to the physical properties of the tissue under investigation. These include planar X-ray, computed tomography (CT), ultrasound (USS) and magnetic resonance imaging (MRI). In the second category, the techniques are those that produce functional images using dynamic scintigraphy. These radioisotope imaging techniques include single photon emission computed tomography (SPECT) and positron emission tomography (PET). In addition to these, magnetic resonance spectroscopy and functional MRI are becoming available. Traditionally, the surgical oncologist has relied heavily on morphological imaging not only when planning a surgical procedure, but also in selecting patients not suitable for major intervention. This chapter examines the role of PET in oncological imaging based on current evidence.

Abbreviations: Computed tomography (CT), ultrasound (USS), magnetic resonance imaging (MR), single photon emission computed tomography (SPECT), positron emission tomography (PET), carbon 11 (^{11}C), oxygen 15 (^{15}O), fluorine 18 (^{18}F), nitrogen 13 (^{13}N), thallium doped sodium iodide (NaI (TI)), bismuth germanate oxide (BGO), standardised uptake values (SUV), 2-[^{18}F] fluoro-2-deoxy-D-glucose (FDG), [^{18}F]-fluorouracil ([^{18}F]-FU), glucose transporter molecule (GLUT), non-small cell lung cancer (NSCLC), European Organisation for Research and Treatment of Cancer (EORTC), fluorothymidine (FLT).

Mr Tan Arulampalam FRCS, Department of Surgery and Institute of Nuclear Medicine, Royal Free and University College Medical School, Middlesex Hospital, Mortimer Street, London W1N 8AA, UK

Prof. Irving Taylor MD ChM FRCS, David Patey Professor of Surgery, Head of Department of Surgery, Royal Free and University College London Medical School, University College London, Charles Bell House, 67–73 Riding House Street, London W1W 7EJ, UK

THE BIOLOGICAL BASIS OF PET

POSITRON DECAY

PET is a minimally-invasive, metabolic imaging modality that uses radiolabelled ligands to deliver high-resolution images of pathological disease processes, such as cancer. Cancer leads to alterations in cellular biochemical reactions and it is possible to synthesise positron-emitting analogues of naturally occurring compounds that target these aberrant biochemical processes and organ functions. Positron emitting nuclei (^{11}C, ^{15}O, ^{18}F and ^{13}N) do not occur in nature and, therefore, have to be synthesised in a cyclotron or linear accelerator.

Positron decay ultimately results in the emission of two 511 keV photons that can be detected by external detector assemblies (Fig. 1). This form of radioactive decay can be quantitated and an image of the biodistribution of the tracer can be tomographically reconstructed in the transaxial, sagittal and coronal planes. Furthermore, dynamic modelling of tracer kinetics allows tomographic images of other functional parameters such as tissue perfusion, metabolic rate and the density of targeted receptors to be reconstructed. Conceptually, this is far removed from conventional anatomical imaging of disease. The deranged biochemical processes resulting from malignant change detected by PET tend to precede morphological changes detected by conventional imaging. These factors confer advantages when imaging malignant disease.

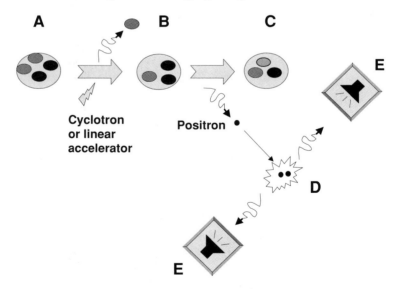

Fig. 1 Schematic diagram of positron decay. An atomic nucleus is usually found in an electrostatic stable state (A). After processing in a cyclotron or linear accelerator a neutron deficient state is induced (B). In order to return to a stable state (C), a proton transmutates and causes the release of a positron from the nucleus. Within 0.2–2 mm, this positron collides with an electron forming a quasi-stable 'positronium', which then annihilates (D) resulting in the discharge of two 511 keV photons that travel at 180 degrees to each other. These co-incident gamma rays are detected by the opposing PET co-incidence detection cameras (E). Using computer software, the point of origin of the annihilation event can be calculated. This very closely approximates to the point of actual positron decay.

> **Key point 1**
>
> • PET is a functional imaging technique that is well suited for cancer imaging.

PET INSTRUMENTATION

There are a variety of detectors capable of imaging positron-emitting tracers and these can be broadly divided into four classes: (i) the thallium-doped sodium iodide (NaI (Tl)) gamma camera with lead collimators; (ii) the dual-head rotating NaI (Tl) camera with modified electronics for coincidence detection; (iii) the dedicated NaI (Tl) PET camera with a ring detection system; and (iv) the dedicated bismuth germanate oxide (BGO) PET camera with a ring detection system (Fig. 2). The performance of these camera types varies and with the wide range comes a wide difference in price. A multicrystal BGO PET camera has a sensitivity for cancer lesions of 4–6 mm, but in clinical practice the detection of such lesions is dependent on the differential uptake of FDG between normal and malignant tissue. The actual resolution may, therefore, be 6–10 mm. Most nuclear medicine departments can afford to operate an adapted Anger gamma camera, which is PET capable, but inferior in terms of data quality. A state-of-the-art full ring, multicrystal dedicated BGO PET camera costs £1–1.5 million. Debate continues as to which system can meet clinical demand effectively and at a sustainable cost.

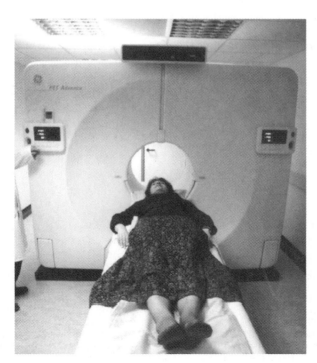

Fig. 2 A full ring dedicated BGO-PET scanner. Courtesy of the Institute of Nuclear Medicine, Royal Free and University College Medical School, London, UK.

IMAGE ACQUISITION, RECONSTRUCTION AND QUANTITATION

The key advantage of functional imaging with PET is the ability to relate detected radioactivity to specific metabolic parameters. This allows comparison between lesions in one patient over time, for example to monitor treatment, or between different patients in order to compare disease.

Patients are scanned after a period of fasting in order to ensure basal serum glucose levels. Patients are weighed and measured prior to intravenous administration of the tracer. Usually, the average tracer activity is approximately 370 MBq. A period of 45 min or so is allowed for uptake in the tissues. Images can be acquired after tracer injection in a static or dynamic mode. In the former, the body is imaged in sections of 15 cm for emitted activity and then transmitted activity from a germanium source. Dynamic imaging is the acquisition of multiple images over a set time period over a region or regions of the body. Both these techniques allow functional metabolic parameters to be calculated. This means that an area of high FDG uptake could be quantified with respect to glucose metabolism and tissue perfusion, for example.

Image reconstruction is the process of producing a 2- or 3-dimensional image from the acquired data sets using either iterative or Fourier techniques. Iterative reconstruction techniques lead to a more accurate reconstructed image by allowing for the effects of noise. This technique is computationally demanding and, therefore, Fourier techniques are more often used.

Having reconstructed the image, it is possible to derive indices that relate detected activity to metabolic parameters. It is impractical to obtain quantitative tracer calculations in routine clinical practice. This is because continuous invasive blood sampling would be required and the procedure would be extremely labour-intensive. Instead, FDG uptake is expressed in terms of a semiquantitative standardised uptake value (SUV). The number obtained is a measure of the activity concentration in a volume of tissue corrected for the injected activity and the patients body weight.

SUV corrected for weight =

$$\frac{[\text{Average tumour activity concentration (MBq/l)} \times \text{Body weight (kg)}]}{[\text{Injected activity (MBq)}]}$$

PET TRACERS

The tracer most frequently used for oncological applications of PET is the fluorinated glucose analogue 2-[^{18}F]-fluoro-2-deoxy-D-glucose (FDG). Many studies demonstrate its high sensitivity and specificity,[1] although the latter can be a problem due to false positive FDG uptake in highly metabolic benign lesions, most notably inflammatory tissue. Other tracers such as [^{18}F]-fluorouracil ([^{18}F]-FU) are available to predict and monitor treatment response. [^{15}O]-water has also been used for assessing metastatic adenocarcinoma and is a marker of tissue perfusion and vascularity.

[^{11}C]-Methionine is a marker of amino acid metabolism, but is not widely used in clinical practice. Likewise, [^{11}C]-thymidine is a marker of cellular proliferation as this compound is a substrate for DNA synthesis. Unfortunately,

[^{11}C]-thymidine is erratically metabolised in the body and, therefore, is not as helpful as other tracers. The field of tracer development in oncological imaging continues to expand and we speculate that one of the fluorinated thymidine analogues may prove to be of great value in this respect.

THE BIOLOGICAL BASIS FOR THE USE OF FDG

FDG is commonly used in oncological applications of PET because it is able to target malignant tissue on the basis of increased glucose metabolism in this tissue. Glucose is preferentially concentrated in malignant cells due to an increase in membrane glucose transporters[2] as well as an increase in the principal enzymes such as hexokinase, phosphofructokinase and pyruvate dehydrogenase.[3] The activation of the gene coding for the synthesis of the glucose transporter, GLUT1, is a major early marker of cellular malignant transformation. Once transported into the cell, FDG is phosphorylated by hexokinase, but takes no further part in glycolysis. FDG-6-phosphate becomes metabolically trapped as accessory metabolic pathways are too slow for the half-life of FDG and it proceeds to decay by positron emission. The detected activity of [^{18}F]-fluorine closely approximates to the accumulated FDG-6-phosphate (Fig. 3).

Although this model is widely accepted, there are certain important physiological factors that influence FDG uptake. These include tissue oxygenation and glucose utilisation, regional blood flow and the inflammatory reaction surrounding the tumour,[4,5] all of which may interfere with the specificity of FDG-PET for malignant tissue.

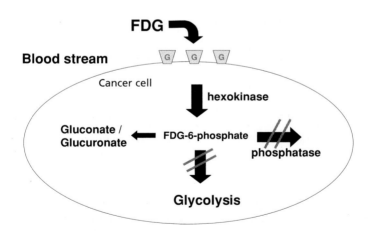

Fig. 3 Intravenously injected FDG preferentially accumulates in cancer cells due to an up-regulation of glucose transporter molecules (G). Once within the cell, FDG is phosphorylated to FDG-6-phosphate by hexokinase, an enzyme that is also up-regulated by malignant transformation. Unlike glucose-6-phosphate, FDG-6-phosphate does not take any further part in glycolysis. Phosphatase activity is low in these cells so dephosphorylation is not an option. Alternative metabolic pathways to gluconate or glucuronate are too slow for the half-life of FDG and, since it cannot diffuse out of the cell, it becomes metabolically trapped. The FDG proceeds to decay by positron emission.

CLINICAL APPLICATION OF PET IN ONCOLOGY

In order to analyse the areas where FDG-PET may be of clinical efficacy, it is necessary to assess this modality in terms of screening, detection and staging of primary disease, detecting and evaluating the extent of recurrent disease and finally the assessment of subclinical response to therapy.

Key point 2

- There is good evidence for the accuracy of PET over conventional anatomical imaging methods (CT and MRI) for a variety of cancers. The main indications for PET in oncology are detection and staging of primary disease, detection and staging of recurrence/metastasis and the evaluation of subclinical therapy response.

SCREENING FOR PRIMARY CANCER

Screening for cancer with FDG-PET may seem a logical application, but when one examines this in the context of FDG uptake in normal tissues it is understandable why FDG-PET has not played a major role. Since interpretation of FDG-PET scans relies on the differential uptake between normal and malignant tissues, screening for cancer in asymptomatic individuals is hazardous as there can be an unacceptable number of false positives. Yasuda *et al.*[6] examined PET for screening 3165 asymptomatic patients for a variety of cancers and found an unacceptably high rate of both false negative and false positive PET studies. It is generally accepted that the high cost, both financial and in time, precludes PET from being a cost-effective screening tool at present. Investigation into targeted screening programmes may, however, be useful.

DETECTING PRIMARY CANCER

The impact of FDG-PET for detecting primary disease has probably been greatest in the realm of diagnosing the nature of solitary pulmonary nodules. The incidence of these in the US is approximately 130,000 per year of which 50–60% are benign.[7] Non-small cell lung cancer (NSCLC) comprises 75% of all lung cancers and diagnosis is inaccurate, primarily due to a lack of sensitivity of diagnostic investigations (sputum cytology, bronchoscopy, transthoracic needle aspiration and CT). Although bronchoscopy is widely available, the procedure fails to reach a diagnosis in 60% of patients with small (less than 2 cm) lesions. A significant number of patients, therefore, undergo diagnostic thoracotomy and resection, of whom 20–40% are found to have benign lesions.[8] FDG-PET (Fig. 4), however, shows clear superiority in diagnosis with an average sensitivity and specificity of 95% and 81%, respectively (555 patients),[9] and this is superior even to invasive transthoracic fine-needle aspiration.[10] There can be problems of false positive (granulomatous diseases, such as tuberculosis) and false negative (small lesions less than 6 mm) studies, but the evidence suggests that FDG-PET is more

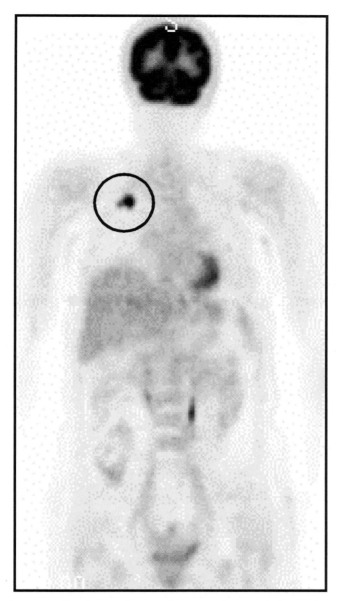

Fig. 4 Coronal FDG-PET showing a solitary malignant pulmonary lesion in the apex of the right upper lobe (circled). Courtesy of the Institute of Nuclear Medicine, Royal Free and University College Medical School, London, UK.

accurate than other diagnostic techniques. The high cost of PET may be off-set by a significant reduction in thoracotomies.[11] Costs are further reduced when one considers that the complications of surgery and invasive investigation are avoided.

Pancreatic cancer is another malignant disease for which FDG-PET holds many advantages. One of the main diagnostic challenges remains the differentiation between benign mass-forming pancreatitis and adenocarcinoma. Several studies in the mid 1990s demonstrated a sensitivity for adenocarcinoma of approximately

95% and a specificity range of 78–90%.[12] This is significantly better than that which can be achieved with CT or endoluminal USS. However, for colorectal cancer the data are equivocal. Colorectal cancer is a common disease, but it is evident that although FDG-PET can accurately diagnose the primary lesion, currently available techniques such as colonoscopy, CT colonography and barium enema are equally accurate, cheaper and more widely available.[13] A future role in detecting primary colorectal cancer and other malignant diseases may rest on the ability of PET to provide metabolic data on tumour biology, for example correlation of tracer uptake with histopathological characteristics. FDG-PET has been used to detect a variety of other primary tumours, but the examples above represent a significant proportion of the clinical workload for this application.

STAGING PRIMARY CANCER

The cost savings from PET tend to accrue due to accurate staging of malignant disease. This is because appropriate treatments can be instituted which might give the greatest chance of cure as well as avoiding unnecessary surgery due to the presence of disseminated disease. Morphological imaging has been shown to be poor for detecting additional disease and there are several malignant tumours where incorporation of FDG-PET into the clinical imaging algorithm has led to a significant reduction in morbidity along with cost savings.

A recent meta-analysis of 2226 patients with NSCLC demonstrated the superiority of FDG-PET over CT (sensitivity 79%, specificity 91% compared to 60% and 77%, respectively, for CT).[14] Therefore, resection of tumour may be avoided due to the discovery of malignant mediastinal lymphadenopathy on FDG-PET. The incorporation of FDG-PET into the staging of lung cancer is now included in the guidelines of the British Thoracic Society.

The importance and superiority of FDG-PET over other morphological techniques has been similarly demonstrated in malignancies, such as lymphoma[15] and melanoma.[16] Studies of patients with lymphoma have shown that up to 8% of patients were upstaged[17] and management altered in approximately 14% (44 patients).[18] The application of FDG-PET is not, however, a universally accepted staging technique in oncology and this is demonstrated by the equivocal data for staging head and neck cancers, breast cancer and colorectal cancer. Although, overall, FDG-PET is more accurate for staging primary colorectal cancer, both FDG-PET and CT have a reported sensitivity of around 29% for detecting malignant lymph nodes. The superiority of PET for demonstrating liver metastases is much greater. There is a need for multicentre trials of FDG-PET against conventional imaging, to document clinical benefit and to justify cost.

Key point 3

- The benefits of PET are through altered clinical management, mainly the ability to detect disease early as well as preventing unnecessary or inappropriate surgical procedures.

Coronal FDG-PET

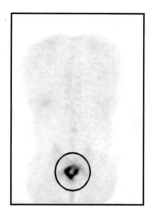

CT Pelvis

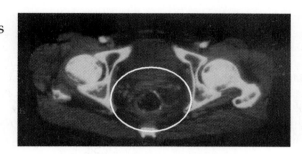

Fig. 5 Coronal FDG-PET showing a loco-regional recurrence (circled) in the pelvis of a patient who previously underwent anterior resection of an adenocarcinoma of the rectum. The concurrent transaxial CT through the pelvis does not show any diagnostic features of recurrence. Courtesy of the Institute of Nuclear Medicine, Royal Free and University College Medical School, London, UK.

DETECTING RECURRENT CANCER

The area where FDG-PET has a definite place is in the detection of recurrent disease. This is because the advantages of imaging a metabolic signal over conventional morphological imaging of tissues are clearly seen for differentiating postoperative or post-radiotherapy fibrosis from recurrence, as well as in the evaluation of patients with rising tumour markers and normal/equivocal morphological imaging.

Several authors have demonstrated the benefits of FDG-PET over CT for assessing metastatic disease,[19] post-therapy 'scar' tissue (Fig. 5),[20] and rising tumour markers.[21,22] Huebner *et al.*[1] have published a meta-analysis of FDG-PET for detecting recurrent colorectal cancer. In 11 studies the sensitivity and specificity were 97% and 76%, respectively. The clinical impact of FDG-PET is through altered patient management, that is the commencement of chemotherapy, resection of recurrent disease and the avoidance of surgical intervention. Experience suggests that FDG-PET changes management in a third of cases if incorporated into the imaging algorithm for recurrent colorectal cancer.[1]

These principles hold for the imaging of recurrent lung cancer, lymphoma and melanoma. In fact, for lymphoma, studies have shown not only high sensitivity and specificity (96% and 94%, respectively), but also positive and negative predictive values of 90% or above.[23] Similarly, in the detection of recurrent melanoma, new disease can be detected in 20% of cases and management altered in 15%.[24]

EVALUATING THE EXTENT OF RECURRENT CANCER

Ultimately, when recurrent or metastatic disease is confirmed, appropriate treatment can only be decided once the true extent of disease has been accurately delineated. This allows the selection of patients for surgical resection, which at this stage is usually a demanding procedure with a higher rate of complications, increased cost and poorer outcome when compared to the treatment of primary disease. FDG-PET appears to be well suited to the task of evaluating these patients.

The management of colorectal liver metastases serves as a good example for the utility of FDG-PET. It is estimated that with careful selection the 5-year survival after liver resection may be 25–38%, but CT remains a disappointing imaging technique for this task. Newer contrast enhanced MRI techniques are emerging as the gold standard, but they remain as expensive as PET and are not routinely used. It has been demonstrated in patients with colorectal liver metastases that the sensitivity and specificity of FDG-PET are significantly better than CT for detecting multifocal liver metastasis (Fig. 6) and the presence of additional extrahepatic disease.[25]

So, FDG-PET may not only detect recurrence at an earlier stage, but may also aid the decision-making process as to how best to treat the detected disease. The assessment of the extent of recurrence with FDG-PET is valuable in lymphoma, melanoma and lung cancer.

Key point 4

- PET is expensive, but cost savings accrue due to earlier diagnosis (decreased number of investigations) and prevention of inappropriate surgery.

EVALUATING SUBCLINICAL RESPONSE TO THERAPY

Accurate information regarding the response to radiotherapy and/or chemotherapy in patients being treated for colorectal cancer provides useful guidance in predicting, planning and revising on-going adjuvant therapy. This is particularly important when considered in the context of the unwanted side-effects of some of these treatments. Studies assessing the uptake of FDG measured by PET and correlation with the antitumour effects of chemotherapy have been reported for various tumour types including pancreatic adenocarcinoma, lymphoma and colorectal cancer.

Response to chemotherapy

The available data with respect to colorectal cancer suggest highest concentration of $[^{18}F]$-FU in responsive tumours.[26] Strauss and Conti[27]

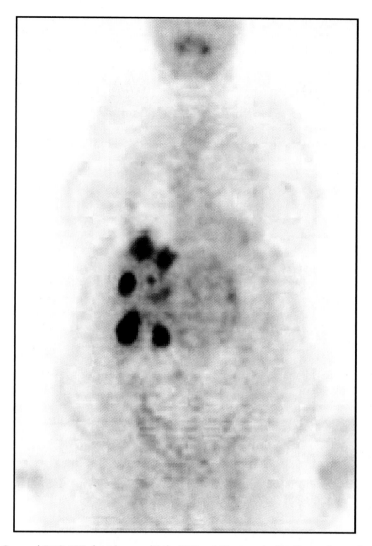

Fig. 6 Coronal FDG-PET showing multiple FDG avid lesions in the liver of a patient previously treated for carcinoma of the colon. Courtesy of the Institute of Nuclear Medicine, Royal Free and University College Medical School, London, UK.

demonstrated that lesions with low [^{18}F]-FU uptake had a significant increase in volume and no response to treatment. An important study was conducted by Findlay *et al.*[28] which evaluated the metabolism of colorectal liver metastases using FDG-PET before and at intervals after treatment. The findings were compared with tumour outcome conventionally assessed using change in size on CT in 18 patients with assessable liver metastases. The results were expressed as a ratio of FDG uptake in tumour and normal liver (T:L) and these showed that the T:L ratio 4–5 weeks after treatment was able to discriminate response from non-response both lesion-by-lesion and for overall patient response (sensitivity 100%, specificity 90% and 75%, respectively). Debate continues as to whether [^{18}F]-FU is superior to FDG in predicting the response to treatment on an individual patient basis. There are also encouraging data emerging from those that have looked at PET evaluation of treatment response in upper gastrointestinal malignancies.[29]

The potential role of PET in this aspect of oncology and particularly in the management of colorectal cancer is, therefore, set to change. The EORTC and EC PET Oncology Concerted Action Group reviewed the data of 31 European PET centres and found a satisfactory methodology for functionally assessing tumour response.[30] We now have guidelines from the EORTC regarding the optimal approach to assessing tumour response with FDG-PET in terms of which particular tumours to study and standard methodology.[31]

Response to radiotherapy

Similar promise was thought to be present for PET in the evaluation of radiotherapy response. There are some problems, most notably demonstrated by Haberkorn et al.[32] who evaluated FDG-PET in 21 patients (41 examinations) with recurrent colorectal cancer undergoing pelvic radiotherapy. A correlation was made between the palliative benefit and reduction in FDG uptake in 50% of patients (this was also more accurate than the tumour marker, CEA). This was an underestimation of true response and it is more likely than not that in patients with good response, the inflammatory reaction to radiotherapy caused FDG uptake resulting in some patients being incorrectly labelled as 'non-responders'.

More recently, Guillem et al.[33] have demonstrated that FDG-PET augments conventional morphological imaging modalities when used pre-operatively to assess response to chemoradiation for rectal carcinoma. This is primarily because information is available pre-operatively that allows sphincter-saving surgery to be accurately planned. The additional information gathered on FDG-PET complements CT and MRI.

A further application of FDG-PET is the potential ability to reduce radiotherapy treatment fields by restricting the target volume to the metabolically active tumour. This is usually smaller than the target volume designated by conventional CT, in lung and other cancers.[34,35] Such an approach could possibly reduce unwanted side-effects of radiotherapy. This is a contentious area and still the subject of on-going clinical evaluation.

CURRENT STATUS

The benefits of metabolic imaging for cancer are clearly demonstrated in several key areas: (i) the diagnosis and staging of primary disease; (ii) the detection and staging of recurrent disease; and (iii) the evaluation of treatment response at a subclinical stage. The range of malignancies in which these benefits have been demonstrated include lung cancer, colorectal cancer, lymphoma, melanoma, head and neck cancer and oesophageal cancer. Although this list appears limited, it is noteworthy that 60% of all 'cancer decisions' are covered and there is continued research into all other fields of oncology. One must consider very carefully the issues surrounding the evaluation of a new medical technology, because the theoretical benefits of PET may be lost in the translation of research work into clinical practice. Brennan[36] makes reference to this in an important editorial that comments on the use of FDG-PET in three important areas: (i) the assessment of FDG-PET in recurrent colorectal cancer, (ii) the evaluation of therapy response in oesophageal cancer; and (iii) the influence on decision-making models.

FDG-PET has a clear clinical impact through altering management in patients with cancer. These changes may lead to cost savings through operations that are avoided.[37] In colorectal cancer, it is estimated that an approximate saving of US$3000 can be made when FDG-PET is incorporated into the management algorithm for recurrent disease. These costs have to be set against the capital costs for a PET scanner, radiochemistry laboratory, cyclotron and staff (medical, physicists, radiographers and laboratory scientists) all of which is estimated to be around US$5 million.[38] Currently, a whole-body FDG-PET study costs approximately US$1000–1500, which is about 30% more than the cost of a 2 part CT. The issues of costs are made more complicated by the fact that PET is a technology capable of allowing oncological intervention at a stage where previously this would not have been possible. Apart from confirming PET to be both sensitive and specific for various oncological applications, data are now required on the outcome of the resultant interventions. In this respect, Brennan suggests that the surgical oncologist needs to take a lead in the development of PET for the various applications put forward. This includes long-term follow-up studies in the common cancers, such as lung cancer and colorectal cancer.

There are several developments on the horizon, which will serve to expand the utility and availability of PET. Multimodality PET/CT and PET/MRI scanners are now available. There are many advantages other than the accurate co-registration of both anatomical and metabolic data. These include reduced scan times allowing 2–3 patients to be scanned per hour rather than the conventional one per hour. The increased through-put results in reduced unit costs and increased availability. New detector materials that are more suitable for high energy photons produced by positron decay and are based on lutetium have been developed. Manufacturers have also made available PET cameras with a partial multicrystal BGO ring, which reduces costs substantially without an equivalent loss in specification.

Key point 5

- New multimodality PET/CT and PET/MRI scanners are becoming available. These offer the benefits of both morphological and functional imaging.

In terms of making PET more available, there are initiatives to develop mobile PET, but the optimal solution remains the investment into PET facilities and a cyclotron network capable of producing and distributing [^{18}F]-labelled ligands to these peripheral sites. Development of new tracers will enable specific metabolic pathways to be studied and may help improve both sensitivity and specificity for particular cancers. Currently, fluoro-thymidine, a marker a DNA proliferation, holds the greatest promise for oncological imaging. Other tracers that have been developed recently are listed in Table 1.

Table 1 New tracers for PET

Tracer	Reaction
Fluoroethyl tyrosine	An amino acid analogue
Fluoro misonidazole	Hypoxia ligand
Fluoro oestradiol	Oestrogen analogue
Fluoro thymidine	DNA proliferation

Possibly the area of greatest interest other than tracer development is the study of metabolic response to chemotherapy. There are concerns as to how to measure anatomical parameters which have been adopted by WHO[39] and it is expected that metabolic parameters will become accepted in due course.

CONCLUSIONS

PET has significant advantages over current anatomical imaging modalities in defined applications for a variety of solid tumours. These applications may vary between different tumours, but their impact on clinical decision making is now beyond question.[40] Despite these data, one must accept that continued study on a multicentre basis is still needed in order to compare changing conventional imaging techniques with PET. Long-term outcome measures as a result of altered management instigated by PET need to be examined closely. Currently, FDG-PET is a valuable imaging modality in many solid tumours and is a powerful adjunct to CT and MRI. With the expected changes in its availability and the expansion of indications for PET, this technique stands on the brink of being incorporated into gold standard oncological imaging algorithms.

Key points for clinical practice

- PET is a functional imaging technique that is well suited for cancer imaging.

- There is good evidence for the accuracy of PET over conventional anatomical imaging methods (CT and MRI) for a variety of cancers. The main indications for PET in oncology are detection and staging of primary disease, detection and staging of recurrence/metastasis and the evaluation of subclinical therapy response.

- The benefits of PET are through altered clinical management, mainly the ability to detect disease early as well as preventing unnecessary or inappropriate surgical procedures.

- PET is expensive, but cost savings accrue due to earlier diagnosis (decreased number of investigations) and prevention of inappropriate surgery.

- New multimodality PET/CT and PET/MRI scanners are becoming available. These offer the benefits of both morphological and functional imaging.

ACKNOWLEDGEMENT

The authors wish to thank The Trustees of University College Hospitals NHS Trust for funding FDG-PET scans and Professor Peter Ell and Dr Durval Costa for the opportunity to use data and select appropriate cases to present. In addition we thank Dr Dimitris Visvilis and Mrs Caroline Townsend for expert physics and radiographic support.

References

1. Huebner RH, Park KC, Shepherd JE *et al*. A meta-analysis of the literature for whole-body FDG PET detection of recurrent colorectal cancer. *J Nucl Med* 2000; **41**: 1177–1189.
2. Hartung T, Buchler M, Grimmel S *et al*. Correlation of increased FDG-uptake and elevated expression of glucose transporter 1 gene in human pancreatic carcinoma. *Eur J Nucl Med* 1994; **21**: S17.
3. Monakhov NK, Neistadt EL, Shavlovskil MM, Shvartsman AL, Neifakh SA. Physicochemical properties and isoenzyme composition of hexokinase from normal and malignant human tissues. *J Natl Cancer Inst* 1978; **61**: 27–34.
4. Clavo AC, Wahl RL. Effects of hypoxia on the uptake of tritiated thymidine, L-leucine, L-methionine and FDG in cultured cancer cells. *J Nucl Med* 1996; **37**: 502–506.
5. Yao WJ, Hoh CK, Hawkins RA *et al*. Quantitative PET imaging of bone marrow glucose metabolic response to hematopoietic cytokines. *J Nucl Med* 1995; **36**: 794–799.
6. Yasuda S, Ide M, Fujii H *et al*. Application of positron emission tomography imaging to cancer screening. *Br J Cancer* 2000; **83**: 1607–1611.
7. Khouri NF, Meziane MA, Zerhouni EA, Fishman EK, Siegelman SS. The solitary pulmonary nodule. Assessment, diagnosis, and management. *Chest* 1987; **91**: 128–133.
8. Midthun DE, Swensen SJ, Jett JR. Clinical strategies for solitary pulmonary nodule. *Annu Rev Med* 1992; **43**: 195–208.
9. Lowe VJ, Naunheim KS. Positron emission tomography in lung cancer. *Ann Thorac Surg* 1998; **65**: 1821–1829.
10. Dewan NA, Reeb SD, Gupta NC, Gobar LS, Scott WJ. PET-FDG imaging and transthoracic needle lung aspiration biopsy in evaluation of pulmonary lesions. A comparative risk-benefit analysis. *Chest* 1995; **108**: 441–446.
11. Gambhir SS, Hoh CK, Phelps ME, Madar I, Maddahi J. Decision tree sensitivity analysis for cost-effectiveness of FDG-PET in the staging and management of non-small-cell lung carcinoma. *J Nucl Med* 1996; **37**: 1428–1436.
12. Stollfuss JC, Glatting G, Friess H, Kocher F, Berger HG, Reske SN. 2-(Fluorine-18)-fluoro-2-deoxy-D-glucose PET in detection of pancreatic cancer: value of quantitative image interpretation. *Radiology* 1995; **195**: 339–344.
13. Arulampalam TH, Costa DC, Loizidou M, Visvikis D, Ell PJ, Taylor I. Positron emission tomography and colorectal cancer. *Br J Surg* 2001; **88**: 176–189.
14. Dwamena BA, Sonnad SS, Angobaldo JO, Wahl RL. Metastases from non-small cell lung cancer: mediastinal staging in the 1990s – meta-analytic comparison of PET and CT. *Radiology* 1999; **213**: 530–536.
15. Klose T, Leidl R, Buchmann I, Brambs HJ, Reske SN. Primary staging of lymphomas: cost-effectiveness of FDG-PET versus computed tomography. *Eur J Nucl Med* 2000; **27**: 1457–1464.
16. Eigtved A, Andersson AP, Dahlstrom K *et al*. Use of fluorine-18 fluorodeoxyglucose positron emission tomography in the detection of silent metastases from malignant melanoma. *Eur J Nucl Med* 2000; **27**: 70–75.
17. Moog F, Bangerter M, Diederichs CG *et al*. Lymphoma: role of whole-body 2-deoxy-2-[F-18]fluoro-D-glucose (FDG) PET in nodal staging. *Radiology* 1997; **203**: 795–800.
18. Bangerter M, Moog F, Buchmann I *et al*. Whole-body 2-[^{18}F]-fluoro-2-deoxy-D-glucose positron emission tomography (FDG-PET) for accurate staging of Hodgkin's disease. *Ann Oncol* 1998; **9**: 1117–1122.
19. Arulampalam THA, Costa DC, Visvikis D, Boulos PB, Taylor I, Ell PJ. The impact of

FDG-PET on the management algorithm for recurrent colorectal cancer. *Eur J Nucl Med* 2001; **28**; 1758–1765.

20. Ogunbiyi OA, Flanagan FL, Dehdashti F *et al*. Detection of recurrent and metastatic colorectal cancer: comparison of positron emission tomography and computed tomography. *Ann Surg Oncol* 1997; **4**: 613–620.

21. Flanagan FL, Dehdashti F, Ogunbiyi OA, Kodner IJ, Siegel BA. Utility of FDG-PET for investigating unexplained plasma CEA elevation in patients with colorectal cancer [see comments]. *Ann Surg* 1998; **227**: 319–323.

22. Arulampalam THA, Ledermann J, Costa DC. Asymptomatic patient with an increasing CEA concentration. *Lancet Oncol* 2001; **2**: 172.

23. Bangerter M, Kotzerke J, Griesshammer M, Elsner K, Reske SN, Bergmann L. Positron emission tomography with 18-fluorodeoxyglucose in the staging and follow-up of lymphoma in the chest. *Acta Oncol* 1999; **38**: 799–804.

24. Tyler DS, Onaitis M, Kherani A *et al*. Positron emission tomography scanning in malignant melanoma. *Cancer* 2000; **89**: 1019–1025.

25. Arulampalam THA, Costa DC, Loizidou M, Ell PJ, Taylor I. Positron emission tomography for the evaluation of colorectal liver metastases. *Eur J Surg Oncol* 2001; **27**: 779–780.

26. Shani J, Young D, Schlesinger T *et al*. Dosimetry and preliminary human studies of ^{18}F-5-fluorouracil. *Int J Nucl Med Biol* 1982; **9**: 25–35.

27. Strauss LG, Conti PS. The applications of PET in clinical oncology. *J Nucl Med* 1991; **32**: 623–648.

28. Findlay M, Young H, Cunningham D *et al*. Non-invasive monitoring of tumor metabolism using fluorodeoxyglucose and positron emission tomography in colorectal cancer liver metastases: correlation with tumor response to fluorouracil. *J Clin Oncol* 1996; **14**: 700–708.

29. Couper GW, McAteer D, Wallis F *et al*. Detection of response to chemotherapy using positron emission tomography in patients with oesophageal and gastric cancer. *Br J Surg* 1998; **85**: 1403–1406.

30. Price P, Jones T. Can positron emission tomography (PET) be used to detect subclinical response to cancer therapy? The EC PET Oncology Concerted Action and the EORTC PET Study Group. *Eur J Cancer* 1995; **31A**: 1924–1927.

31. Young H, Baum R, Cremerius U *et al*. Measurement of clinical and subclinical tumour response using [^{18}F]-fluorodeoxyglucose and positron emission tomography: review and 1999 EORTC recommendations. European Organization for Research and Treatment of Cancer (EORTC) PET Study Group. *Eur J Cancer* 1999; **35**: 1773–1782.

32. Haberkorn U, Strauss LG, Dimitrakopoulou A *et al*. PET studies of fluorodeoxyglucose metabolism in patients with recurrent colorectal tumors receiving radiotherapy. *J Nucl Med* 1991; **32**: 1485–1490.

33. Guillem JG, Puig-La Calle Jr J, Akhurst T *et al*. Prospective assessment of primary rectal cancer response to preoperative radiation and chemotherapy using 18-fluorodeoxyglucose positron emission tomography. *Dis Colon Rectum* 2000; **43**: 18–24.

34. Kiffer JD, Berlangieri SU, Scott AM *et al*. The contribution of ^{18}F-fluoro-2-deoxy-glucose positron emission tomographic imaging to radiotherapy planning in lung cancer. *Lung Cancer* 1998; **19**: 167–177.

35. Rosenman J. Incorporating functional imaging information into radiation treatment. *Semin Radiat Oncol* 2001; **11**: 83–92.

36. Brennan MF. PET scanning in malignancy: infant, adolescent or mature citizen? *Ann Surg* 2001; **233**: 320–321.

37. Valk PE, Pounds TR, Tesar RD, Hopkins DM, Haseman MK. Cost-effectiveness of PET imaging in clinical oncology. *Nucl Med Biol* 1996; **23**: 737–743.

38. Wieler HJ, Coleman RE. *PET in Clinical Oncology*. Darmstadt: Springer, 2000.

39. Therasse P, Arbuck SG, Eisenhauer EA *et al*. New guidelines to evaluate the response to treatment in solid tumors. European Organization for Research and Treatment of Cancer, National Cancer Institute of the United States, National Cancer Institute of Canada. *J Natl Cancer Inst* 2000; **92**: 205–216.

40. Bomanji JB, Costa DC, Ell PJ. Clinical role of positron emission tomography in oncology. *Lancet Oncol* 2001; **2**: 157–164.

J. Michael Dixon

15

Adjuvant treatment in breast cancer

Breast cancer can either be non-invasive (carcinoma *in situ*) or invasive. The adjuvant treatments used in breast cancer include radiotherapy and systemic therapy; their role in non-invasive and invasive cancer will be considered separately.

CARCINOMA *IN SITU*

Carcinoma *in situ* can be separated histologically into two separate types: (i) ductal carcinoma *in situ* (DCIS), which accounts for 98% of non-invasive disease; and (ii) lobular carcinoma *in situ* (LCIS).[1]

DUCTAL CARCINOMA *IN SITU*

Role of radiotherapy
Widespread (≥ 4 cm) DCIS is best treated by mastectomy. Radiotherapy is not required after mastectomy providing complete histological assessment shows DCIS only.

Localised DCIS (< 4 cm) can be treated surgically by wide local excision. Randomised trials have evaluated the role of radiotherapy following wide excision. The two randomised controlled trials published to date have both shown that radiotherapy is associated with a reduced risk of DCIS recurrence and invasive breast cancer development.[2,3] The first trial from the National Surgical Adjuvant Breast Project in the US randomised 814 patients.[2] At 8 years, radiotherapy resulted in a significantly lower local recurrence rate; (26.8%) in those who did not receive radiotherapy *versus* 12.1% in those who did. Radiotherapy reduced the risk of recurrent DCIS from 13.4% to 8.2%, and reduced the risk of invasive cancer from 13.4% to 3.9%. At 8 years, there was no

Mr J.M. Dixon MD FRCS FRCSEd, Consultant Surgeon and Senior Lecturer, Academic Office, Edinburgh Breast Unit, Western General Hospital, Edinburgh EH4 2XU, UK

effect of radiotherapy on survival (94% in those who received no radiotherapy *versus* 95% in those who did). A second randomised trial of 1002 patients also showed that, after a median of 4.2 years, radiotherapy reduced local recurrence rates.[3] Local relapse-free survival was significantly better for patients receiving radiotherapy than surgery alone (84% *versus* 91%, a hazard ratio of 0.62. More women were free of DCIS recurrence at 4 years with radiotherapy but this difference was not significant (92% *versus* 95%; hazard ratio = 0.65; 95% CI = 0.43–1.03). There was a significant reduction in invasive cancer development with the addition of radiotherapy (92% *versus* 96%; hazard ratio = 0.60; 95% CI = 0.37–0.97). This EORTC study reported an increase in contralateral breast cancer in women who received radiotherapy (3% *versus* 1%; hazard ratio = 2.57; 95% CI = 1.24–5.33). Preliminary data from the UK trial have been presented but not yet published. There was a highly significant reduction in both recurrence of DCIS and development of invasive disease in patients who received postoperative radiotherapy.[4]

Data from the NSABP study could not identify any group who did not benefit from the addition of radiotherapy.[5,6] Within the EORTC trial, the best local control rates were in women who had both free margins and received radiotherapy.[6,7] The addition of radiotherapy in patients with involved margins produced local control rates similar to those in patients who had a complete excision but no radiotherapy.[6] There did not appear to be a significant benefit in the EORTC trial of giving radiotherapy to patients with well differentiated DCIS.

Silverstein suggested that patients treated by wide excision with a 10 mm margin did not benefit significantly from radiotherapy.[8]. However, not only were these patients not randomised, but women with a greater than 10 mm margin treated by wide excision alone had significantly smaller areas of DCIS than women who received radiotherapy. Women in these studies were treated sequentially over a decade during which time the type of DCIS being treated changed significantly. No firm conclusions on the role of radiotherapy can be drawn from these non-randomised data.

The current consensus view is that following wide excision the majority of patients should be treated with postoperative radiotherapy to the breast.[9,10] Only women considered at low risk of recurrence based on small size of DCIS with good pathology (low grade with minimal or absent comedo necrosis) and adequate excision can safely avoid radiotherapy.

Key point 1

- Following wide excision of localised DCIS, most women benefit from postoperative radiotherapy to the breast.

Role of tamoxifen in DCIS

One randomised controlled trial treated patients with DCIS by wide excision and radiotherapy and then randomised patients to tamoxifen 20 mg/day for 5 years (902 women) or placebo (902 women). At a median follow-up of 74 months, there were fewer breast cancer events in women treated with tamoxifen than placebo (hazard ratio = 0.63; 95% CI = 0.48–0.83) and fewer ipsilateral or contralateral breast cancers (hazard ratio = 0.58; 95% CI = 0.83-0.85).[11] The benefit from tamoxifen appeared greater in younger women although the only group not to benefit significantly from tamoxifen were those women who presented with clinically evident rather than radiologically diagnosed DCIS. No study has yet evaluated the interaction between the oestrogen receptor (ER) status and the benefit from tamoxifen in DCIS. Data presented but not yet published from the UK DCIS trial show that only in the absence of radiotherapy did tamoxifen produce any significant effects.[4] Tamoxifen significantly reduced ipsilateral DCIS recurrence (hazard ratio = 0.68; 95% CI = 0.47–0.99) and reduced all contralateral events (hazard ratio = 0.48; 095% CI = 0.16–0.94). There were no other significant effects.

Data from these two randomised studies do not show a consistent effect of tamoxifen in DCIS. A further evaluation of its role, particularly in ER-positive DCIS is required. As in invasive cancer, tamoxifen reduces contralateral breast cancer events. Studies comparing tamoxifen and aromatase inhibitors in oestrogen receptor positive DCIS are underway. There is no current consensus that tamoxifen should be prescribed for all patients with DCIS.[10]

LOBULAR CARCINOMA *in situ*

No studies have been performed on the value of radiotherapy in LCIS because it is considered a marker of increased risk rather than a lesion which itself eventually evolves into invasive cancer. The NSABP prevention study enrolled patients with LCIS.[12] When the trial was unblinded, there was a significant 56% reduction in the number of invasive breast cancers that developed in patients with LCIS randomised to receive tamoxifen.

RADIOTHERAPY FOR INVASIVE BREAST CANCER

One review[13] identified 9 randomised controlled trials involving 4891 patients comparing breast conserving surgery followed by radiotherapy with simple or modified radical mastectomy in women with invasive breast cancer. This review found no difference in survival rates at 10 years (22.9% *versus* 22.9%) or in local recurrence (6.2% *versus* 5.9%, using pooled data from 6 trials including 3107 women).[13] These trials form the basis for giving patients with operable breast cancer the choice of breast conserving therapy or mastectomy.

RADIOTHERAPY AFTER BREAST CONSERVING SURGERY

Follow-up data at 10 years from a systematic review of randomised trials comparing patients having breast conservation surgery with or without radiotherapy demonstrated that there was a significantly lower rate of local relapse with radiotherapy – 8.5% for radiotherapy compared with 24% without radiotherapy.[14,15] Data recently released following the 5th Early Breast Cancer Trialists' Group meeting showed that, in a group of 6100 women randomised for radiotherapy, there was a significant 3.9% (SE = 1.2) increase in survival in women receiving radiotherapy when mortality from breast cancer was considered in the absence of other causes of death.[15] All patients should thus have breast radiotherapy following breast conserving surgery unless there are specific contra-indications. No study has identified any group of patients who do not derive a benefit from radiotherapy. Trials in specific subgroups have been completed but have short follow-up or are currently recruiting.

Key point 3

- After breast conserving surgery for invasive cancer, all patients should receive radiotherapy to the breast.

RADIATION AFTER MASTECTOMY

A systematic review comparing mastectomy alone with mastectomy followed by radiotherapy to the chest wall found that radiotherapy reduced local recurrence by two-thirds and slightly reduced breast cancer mortality (odds ratio = 0.94; 95% CI = 0.88–1.0).[13] Three subsequent trials in high risk pre- and postmenopausal women receiving adjuvant chemotherapy after mastectomy found radiotherapy not only reduced locoregional relapse but also significantly improved survival.[14,15] There are concerns about these studies because of the extent of axillary surgery and the appropriateness of the adjuvant chemotherapy given. Further studies are on-going to identify women who benefit most from postoperative radiotherapy after mastectomy.

RADIOTHERAPY TO LYMPH NODES

Axilla

There is no evidence that radiotherapy following axillary clearance can improve local recurrence rates or survival, but this combination is associated with an extremely high rate of arm swelling and lymphoedema; the combination of treatments cannot be recommended.[14] Following a positive axillary node sampling, radiotherapy produces similar local control rates to axillary clearance.[15]

Key point 4

- Radiotherapy to the axilla after limited axillary surgery produces local control rates similar to that of axillary clearance alone.

Internal mammary chain

There is no direct evidence that radiotherapy to the internal mammary chain improves survival or breast cancer specific survival. There are concerns that treatment may increase radiation induced cardiac morbidity.[15]

Ipsilateral supraclavicular fossa

There is insufficient evidence to assess the impact on survival of irradiation of the ipsilateral supraclavicular fossa. Randomised controlled trials have identified that postoperative radiotherapy is associated with a reduced risk of supraclavicular fossa nodal recurrence.[14] Morbidity associated with this treatment is rare and tends to be mild and temporary.

Key point 5

- Radiotherapy to the chest wall after mastectomy given to women at high risk of local recurrence improves local control and may improve survival.

ADJUVANT SYSTEMIC THERAPY FOR INVASIVE BREAST CANCER

Up to 50% of patients with operable breast cancer and over 80% of those with locally advanced disease ultimately die of metastases even though many of these patients never develop local recurrence.[15] These observations indicate that, even in patients with apparently localised breast cancer, the majority have systemic metastases present at the time of diagnosis. One potential method of improving survival of these patients is to treat them with systemic therapy following the locoregional treatments of surgery and/or radiotherapy to try and eradicate or slow down the growth of metastases.[15] There are two major forms of systemic therapy in common usage – hormonal therapy and chemotherapy.

HORMONAL THERAPY

Oestrogens appear to play an important role in the progression of breast cancer. The level of ER and to a lesser extent progesterone receptor (PgR) in a cancer cell nucleus determines the responsiveness to endocrine therapy. There appears to be a direct correlation between the quantity of ER present and the probability and extent of response to both primary and adjuvant hormonal therapy. The major source of oestrogen in premenopausal women is the ovary. Circulating oestrogen levels in postmenopausal women are about 10% of the level in premenopausal women and they are synthesised peripherally, principally in fat (including breast fat), skin, muscle, liver and by breast cancers from androstenedione which is produced by the adrenal glands. The production of oestrogens requires the presence of the aromatase enzyme. Hormonal therapy or to be more exact anti-hormonal therapy dates back to 1896 when Beatson documented regression in premenopausal women with metastatic breast cancer after oophorectomy. Surgical oophorectomy is still an option, but a reduction in circulating oestrogens can also be produced by radiation to the ovaries or by giving GnRH agonists.[15]

Adjuvant tamoxifen

Tamoxifen is a synthetic partial oestrogen agonist widely used in breast cancer. It acts primarily by binding to ER and is given in a standard dose of 20 mg/day. It has a half-life of 7 days and it takes 4 weeks for the drug to reach a steady state in plasma.

Results from the Early Breast Cancer Trialists' Overview demonstrated that tamoxifen produced an overall 47% reduction in the annual odds of recurrence and a 26% reduction in annual odds of death after exclusion of patients with ER-poor disease.[16] This effect is consistent across all age groups (Table 1) There was a significantly greater reduction in recurrence with increasing duration of adjuvant tamoxifen up to 5 years (26% for 5 years of tamoxifen *versus* 12% for 1 year).[16] There is no evidence that prolonging treatment beyond 5 years produced benefit and some evidence that prolonged treatment may be of harm.[17,18] In one study of 11,053 women who completed 5 years of tamoxifen and were subsequently randomised to either placebo or 5 years of tamoxifen, disease-free survival after 4 years of further follow-up was greater for those who had switched to placebo rather than for those who had continued tamoxifen (92% *versus* 86%) although there was no significant difference in overall survival.[17] Other studies have shown either a detrimental effect or an improvement in survival in continuing tamoxifen after 5 years.[16,18]

Data presented from the 2000 overview but not yet published indicate that there is no benefit in either local recurrence or survival to giving patients with ER-negative disease tamoxifen.[15]

Table 1 Proportional risk reduction subdivided into age groups after exclusion of patients with oestrogen receptor (ER) poor disease

Tamoxifen for 5 years		% Proportional reduction in:	
Age (years)	% ER +ve	Annual odds of recurrence (SD)	Annual odds of death (SD)
< 50	92%	45 (8)	32 (10)
50–59	93%	37 (6)	11 (8)
60–69	95%	54 (5)	33 (6)
> 70	94%	54 (13)	34 (13)
Overall	94%	47 (3)	26 (4)

Side-effects of tamoxifen

The use of tamoxifen is associated with an increased risk of endometrial cancer – average hazard rate 2.58 for 5 years of tamoxifen; this is associated with a cumulative risk at 10 years of 2 deaths (95% CI = 0–4) per thousand women treated.[15] This risk is almost exclusively limited to postmenopausal women. Tamoxifen is also associated with an increased death rate from pulmonary embolism and stroke in postmenopausal women. Although tamoxifen produces bone loss in premenopausal women (1.4% bone loss per annum), it

> **Key point 6**
>
> • Tamoxifen should be considered for adjuvant therapy in both pre- and postmenopausal patients with oestrogen receptor positive breast cancer and should be given for 5 years (treatment for longer periods produces no further benefit). Tamoxifen is well tolerated and few women develop serious side-effects.

does not have this effect in postmenopausal women because of its partial oestrogen agonist effects.[19]

Although only 3% of patients given tamoxifen stop the drug because of toxic effects, side-effects are common. Hot flushes are the most common complaint. Premenopausal women experience decreased vaginal secretions and atrophy; postmenopausal women may complain of vaginal discharge.[20]

Aromatase inhibitors

New specific aromatase inhibitors include the non-steroidal triazole agents, anastrozole and letrozole and a steroidal inactivator, exemestane. These block oestrogen production in postmenopausal women. The first results of the use of adjuvant anastrozole were presented in December 2001.[21] Over 9000 postmenopausal women were randomised following locoregional therapy for early breast cancer to tamoxifen alone, anastrozole alone, or tamoxifen and anastrozole combined. At a median follow-up of 33.3 months (median duration of therapy 30.7 months), there was a significantly better event-free survival for patients treated with anastrozole alone compared with tamoxifen alone (hazard ratio = 0.83). There was no apparent difference between tamoxifen and the combination. In women with ER-positive breast cancer, the benefit of anastrozole over tamoxifen was greater (hazard ratio = 0.78). Trials are underway of letrozole and exemestane comparing 5 years of either drug with 5 years of tamoxifen. There are other trials using a sequence of an aromatase inhibitor with tamoxifen over 5 years. Other trials are assessing the value of giving an aromatase inhibitor after 5 years of tamoxifen.

Combined hormonal treatments

It has been hypothesised that complete hormonal blockade (achieved by LHRH agonists plus tamoxifen) might be an effective alternative to chemotherapy in young women with ER-positive, early stage disease. Several large studies have

> **Key point 7**
>
> • Preliminary data suggest that aromatase inhibitors could be superior to tamoxifen as adjuvant therapy for postmenopausal women with oestrogen receptor positive breast cancers. Further data are awaited. On-going studies are evaluating combined hormonal treatments in premenopausal women.

compared complete hormonal blockade to chemotherapy in premenopausal women and have revealed equivalence or superiority for complete hormonal blockade compared to CMF chemotherapy.[21–24] An unpublished combined analysis suggests that the combination of tamoxifen and ovarian suppression may be superior to standard chemotherapy in terms of disease-free and overall survival in premenopausal women with ER-positive breast cancer.

Ovarian ablation

One systematic review of 12 randomised controlled trials with at least 15-year follow-up of over 2000 premenopausal women demonstrated that more women with ovarian ablation survived (52% *versus* 46%) and more survived free of recurrence (45% *versus* 39%).[25] This benefit was independent of nodal status. Five randomised trials have compared ovarian ablation plus chemotherapy with chemotherapy alone and found the absolute benefit of ablation was smaller than in the trials of ovarian ablation alone.

CHEMOTHERAPY

The most commonly used regimens for adjuvant treatment have been cyclophosphamide, methotrexate and 5-fluorouracil (CMF) or an anthracycline containing regimen, either adriamycin (A) or epirubicin (E) combined with cyclophosphamide (C) alone (AC or EC) or these two drugs combined with 5-fluorouracil (FAC or FEC).

The Early Breast Cancer Trialists' review of 47 randomised controlled trials including 18,000 women demonstrated that chemotherapy significantly reduced any kind of recurrence and death from all causes.[27] These effects were most marked in young women (Table 2) The proportional benefits were similar in women with node negative or positive disease.

Table 2 Proportional risk reduction with polychemotherapy subdivided by age at randomisation

Age at randomisation (years)	% Proportional risk reductions	
	Recurrence (SD)	Mortality (SD)
< 40	37 (7)	27 (8)
40–49	34 (5)	27 (5)
50–59	22 (4)	14 (4)
60–69	18 (4)	8 (4)

Duration of treatment

The overview identified 11 randomised trials including 6104 women comparing shorter regimens of treatment of 4–6 months with longer durations varying from 8–12 months.[27] There appeared to be no additional benefit from a longer treatment duration.

A recently updated systematic review of 11 randomised controlled trials involving 5942 women compared regimens containing anthracyclines (either A or E) with standard CMF regimens.[27] It found a significant reduction in recurrence rates with anthracycline regimens and a modest, but significant, improvement in 5-year survival (69% *versus* 72%).

> **Key point 8**
>
> - Chemotherapy improves survival when given as adjuvant therapy. Regimens selected for individual patients are based on balancing the risks of recurrence and effectiveness against side-effects.

The role of taxanes (paclitaxel and docetaxel) in the adjuvant setting remains to be defined. Paclitaxel is approved in the US for the adjuvant treatment of early stage node positive breast cancer. Initial studies reported additional benefit for paclitaxel when added to an AC regimen,[28] but a subsequent large randomised clinical trial performed by the NSABP failed to confirm any longer term survival benefit of paclitaxel following the AC regimen. Further clinical trials of both paclitaxel and docetaxel are on-going.

A randomised controlled trial from Milan of patients with 4 or more positive nodes compared the sequence of doxorubicin plus adriamycin for 4 cycles followed by intravenous CMF for 8 courses, or CMF for 2 cycles followed by doxorubicin for one cycle repeated to a total of 12 courses. There was a highly significant improvement in disease-free and overall survival in patients treated with the sequence of adriamycin followed by CMF.[29] This sequence of 4 cycles of adriamycin or epirubicin followed by 4 to 8 cycles of CMF has become a commonly used regimen in the UK for high risk women, although there are only limited survival data available with this schedule.

Dosage and side-effects

There is clear evidence that suboptimal doses of chemotherapy do not produce any significant benefit compared to untreated controls.[30,31] High-dose chemotherapy with bone marrow or peripheral stem cell rescue in breast cancer has been tested in several randomised trials which have failed to show any benefit from these high-dose treatments.[32,33]

Side-effects of chemotherapy include nausea and vomiting, bone marrow suppression, fatigue and GI disturbance.[20] Fertility and ovarian function are often affected by chemotherapy particularly in women aged over 40 years.[34] Long-term potential risks of chemotherapy include a small risk of development of second cancers.[25] Current data suggest that, providing the cumulative dose of doxorubicin does not exceed 35 mg/m^2, the risk of cardiac failure is low at less than 1%.[14]

Choosing appropriate adjuvant therapy

Prolongation of life needs to be balanced against treatment side-effects and long-term toxicities when selecting adjuvant therapy for individual patients. The greatest absolute improvements in survival are seen in patients at high risk of recurrence and death. Patients in these categories may be prepared, therefore, to accept higher degrees of toxicity and more side-effects for the greater potential gain. The current philosophy in adjuvant therapy is to stratify patients in relation to their risk of recurrence and tailor adjuvant treatment to that risk. There are a variety of ways of assessing risk including the use of the Nottingham Prognostic Index which stratifies patients on the basis of the

Table 3 Definitions of risk groups and associated risk of relapse

Risk group	Age	% Survival without relapse at 5 years
Node-negative patients		
Low risk	> 35 years, tumour ≤ 1 cm in diameter	> 90
Intermediate risk	≤ 35 years, tumour ≤ 1 cm in diameter	75–80
	> 35 years, tumour > 1 cm grade 1 or 2	
High risk	≤ 35 years, tumour > 1 cm grade 1 or 2	50–60
	Any tumour > 1 cm grade 3	
Node-positive patients		
Low or intermediate risk	> 35 years, 1–3 positive nodes	40–50
High risk	≤ 35 years, 1–3 positive nodes	20–30
	> 35 years, 4–9 positive nodes	
Very high risk	≤ 35 years, ≥4 nodes involved	10–15
	> 35 years, ≥ 10 nodes involved	

Data from Goldhirsch et al.[36] with permission

number of involved nodes, tumour size, and grade.[20,35] Age is also a prognostic factor and was suggested by the St Gallen group as a factor that should be considered when prescribing adjuvant chemotherapy (Table 3).[36] Having identified risk groups, adjuvant therapy is then tailored to risk (Table 4).

Chemotherapy regimens vary between units. Some centres use 6 cycles of CMF for low risk women, 6 cycles of an anthracycline containing regimen for women at intermediate risk and use between 8 and 12 cycles of an anthracycline-

Table 4 Suggested adjuvant treatment for patients with early invasive breast cancer

	ER status	Premenopausal patients	Postmenopausal patients
Node negative patients			
Low risk	Positive	Tamoxifen or nil	Tamoxifen* or nil
	Negative	Nil	Nil
Intermediate risk	Positive	Tamoxifen ± GnRH	Tamoxifen*
	Negative	Chemotherapy	Chemotherapy
High risk	Positive	Chemotherapy + tamoxifen ± GnRh	Tamoxifen* + chemotherapy
	Negative	Chemotherapy	Chemotherapy
Node positive patients			
Low + intermediate risk	Positive	Chemotherapy + tamoxifen + GnRH	Chemotherapy + tamoxifen*
	Negative	Chemotherapy	Chemotherapy
High + very high risk	Positive	More intensive Chemotherapy + tamoxifen + GnRH	More intensive chemotherapy + tamoxifen* if fit
	Negative	More intensive chemotherapy	More intensive chemotherapy

Data from Dixon and Leonard[46] with permission.
ER, oestrogen receptor; GnRH, gonadotrophin releasing hormone.
*Aromatase inhibitors likely to replace tamoxifen if early results of superiority in the adjuvant setting are confirmed.

based regimen for high risk women. Alterations in duration of chemotherapy may need adjustment depending on individual patient tolerance. Over-expression of c-erbB-2 by breast cancer is associated with a poor prognosis and some have suggested that this can help predict response to anthracyclines in the adjuvant setting.[37]

COMBINATION OF HORMONAL THERAPY AND CHEMOTHERAPY

One randomised controlled trial of 2306 women with lymph node negative, ER-positive, early breast cancer compared tamoxifen alone with tamoxifen plus CMF chemotherapy[41] and it found that adding chemotherapy to tamoxifen resulted in an improvement in disease-free survival at 5 years (90% *versus* 85%) and an improvement in overall survival (97% *versus* 94%). The addition of LHRH agonists and tamoxifen to chemotherapy appears to be superior to the use of LHRH agonists alone.[42,43] The ABC Trial in the UK specifically addresses the question of whether combinations of treatment are better than single agents alone and the results of this study are eagerly awaited.

ADJUVANT IMMUNOTHERAPY

More than 20 randomised trials of adjuvant immunotherapy have been completed, but these show no benefit for this treatment.[14] Up to 20% of breast cancers overexpress the c-erbB-2 or HER-2/neu oncoprotein. In studies of patients with advanced disease, trastuzumab (herceptin), a humanised IgG3 anti-c-erbB-2 antibody, has been shown to have good activity both as a single agent and in combination with other cytotoxic agents.[26] It is uncertain whether these benefits of trastuzumab in patients with advanced disease will translate to the adjuvant setting, but trials investigating this agent are underway.

ADJUVANT BISPHOSPHONATES

In one study of patients with primary breast cancer, who had microscopic bone marrow involvement detected by sensitive assays, patients received standard adjuvant therapy and were randomised to receive clodronate for 2 years or placebo. After 3 years of follow-up, patients who received clodronate had a reduction in the incidence of bone metastases and also had a reduction in the incidence of soft tissue and visceral metastases.[44,45]

Key point 9

- Novel adjuvant therapies including immunotherapy and bisphosphonates are showing promise, but require further evaluation in the adjuvant setting before they are introduced into clinical practice.

Key points for clinical practice

- Following wide excision of localised DCIS, most women benefit from postoperative radiotherapy to the breast.

- There is no consistent evidence to support the use of tamoxifen for all patients with DCIS.

- After breast conserving surgery for invasive cancer, all patients should receive radiotherapy to the breast.

- Radiotherapy to the axilla after limited axillary surgery produces local control rates similar to that of axillary clearance alone.

- Radiotherapy to the chest wall after mastectomy given to women at high risk of local recurrence improves local control and may improve survival.

- Tamoxifen should be considered for adjuvant therapy in both pre- and postmenopausal patients with oestrogen receptor positive breast cancer and should be given for 5 years (treatment for longer periods produces no further benefit). Tamoxifen is well tolerated and few women develop serious side-effects.

- Preliminary data suggest that aromatase inhibitors could be superior to tamoxifen as adjuvant therapy for postmenopausal women with oestrogen receptor positive breast cancers. Further data are awaited. On-going studies are evaluating combined hormonal treatments.

- Chemotherapy improves survival when given as adjuvant therapy. Regimens selected for individual patients are based on balancing the risks of recurrence and effectiveness against side-effects.

- Novel adjuvant therapies including immunotherapy and bisphosphonates are showing promise, but require further evaluation in the adjuvant setting before they are introduced into clinical practice.

References

1. Page DL, Steel CM, Dixon JM. Carcinoma *in situ* and patients at high risk of breast cancer. In: Dixon JM. (ed) *ABC of Breast Diseases*, 2nd edn. London: BMJ Books, 2000; 90–96.
2. Fisher B, Dignam J, Wolmark N *et al*. Lumpectomy and radiation for the treatment of intraductal breast cancer; findings of the National Surgical Adjuvant Breast and Bowel Project B-17. *J Clin Oncol* 1998; **16**: 441–452.
3. Julien JP, Bijker N, Fentiman IS *et al*. Radiotherapy in breast-conserving treatment for ductal carcinoma *in situ*: first results of EORTC randomised phase III trial 10853. *Lancet* 2000; **355**: 528–533.
4. George D. Personal communication.
5. Fisher ER, Costantino J, Fisher PHB, Palekar AS, Redmond C, Mamounas E for the National Surgical Adjuvant Breast and Bowel Project Collaborating Investigators. Pathologic findings from the National Surgical Adjuvant Breast Project (NSABP) Protocol B-17. *Cancer* 1995; **75**: 1310–1319.
6. Fisher ER, Dignam J, Tan-Chiu E *et al*. for the National Surgical Adjuvant Breast and Bowel Project (NSABP) Collaborating Investigators. Pathologic findings from the national surgical

adjuvant breast and bowel project (NSABP) eight-year update of protocol B-17. *Cancer* 1999; **86**: 429–438.

7. Bijker N, Peterse JL, Duchateau L *et al*. Risk factors for recurrence and metastasis after breast conserving therapy for ductal carcinoma *in situ*: analysis of European Organization for Research and Treatment of Cancer Trial 10853. *J Clin Oncol* 2001; **19**: 2263–2271.

8. Silverstein MJ, Lagios MD, Groshen S *et al*. The influence of margin width on local control of ductal carcinoma *in situ* of the breast. *N Engl J Med* 1999; **340**: 1455–1461.

9. Silverstein MJ. Not everyone with ductal carcinoma *in situ* of the breast treated with breast preservation needs post-excisional radiation therapy. *Breast* 2000; **9**: 189–193.

10. Schwartz GF, Giuliano AE, Veronesi U and the consensus conference committee. Proceedings of the consensus conference on the role of sentinel lymph node biopsy in carcinoma of the breast, April 19–21, 2001, Philadelphia, PA, USA. *The Breast* 2002: In press.

11. Fisher B, Dignam J, Wolmark N *et al*. Tamoxifen in treatment of intraductal breast cancer: National Surgical Adjuvant Breast and Bowel Project B-24 randomised controlled trial. *Lancet* 1999; **353**: 1993–2000.

12. Fisher B, Costantino JP, Wickerham DL *et al*. Tamoxifen for the prevention of breast cancer: report of the National Surgical Adjuvant Breast and Bowel Project P-1 study. *J Natl Cancer Inst* 1998; **90**: 1371–1388.

13. Early Breast Cancer Trialists' Collaborative Group. Effects of radiotherapy and surgery in early breast cancer: an overview of the randomised trials. *N Engl J Med* 1995; **333**: 1444–1455.

14. Whelan TJ, Julian J, Wright J, Jadad AR, Levine MR. Does locoregional radiation therapy improve survival in breast cancer: a meta-analysis. *J Clin Oncol* 2000; **18**: 1220–1229.

15. Dixon JM, Rodger A, Johnson S, Gregory K. Breast cancer: non-metastatic. *Clin Evidence* 2001; **5**: 1218–1245.

16. Early Breast Cancer Trialists' Collaborative Group. Tamoxifen for early breast cancer: an overview of the randomised trials. *Lancet* 1998; **351**: 1451–1467.

17. Fisher B, Dignam J, Bryant J *et al*. Five versus more than five years of tamoxifen therapy for breast cancer patients with negative lymph nodes and estrogen receptor positive tumours. *J Natl Cancer Inst* 1996; **88**: 1529–1542.

18. Stewart HJ, Forrest AP, Everington D *et al*. Randomised comparison of 5 years of adjuvant tamoxifen with continuous therapy for operable breast cancer. *Br J Cancer* 1996; **74**: 297–299.

19. Powles TJ, Hickish T, Kanis JA, Tidy A, Ashley S. Effect of tamoxifen on bone mineral density measured by dual energy x-ray absorptiometry in healthy premenopausal and postmenopausal women. *J Clin Oncol* 1996; **14**: 78–84.

20. Smith IE, de Boer RH. Role of systemic treatment for primary operable breast cancer. In: Dixon JM. (ed) *ABC of Breast Diseases*, 2nd edn. London: BMJ Books, 2000; 55–60.

21. Roche HH, Kerbrat P, Bonneterre J *et al*. Complete hormonal blockade versus chemotherapy in premenopausal early-stage breast cancer patients (pts) with positive hormone receptor (HR$^+$) and 1–3 node positive (N$^+$) tumor; results of the FASG 06 trial [Abstract 279]. *Proc ASCO* 2000; **19**: 72a.

21. Baum M. Personal communication. 2001.

22. Boccardo F, Rubagotti A, Amoros D *et al*. Cyclophosphamide, methotrexate and fluorouracil versus tamoxifen plus ovarian suppression as adjuvant treatment of estrogen receptor positive pre/perimenopausal breast cancer patients: results of the Italian Breast Cancer Adjuvant Study Group 02 randomized trial. *J Clin Oncol* 2000; **18**: 2718–2727.

23. Pritchard KI. Current and future directions in medical therapy for breast carcinoma. *Cancer* 2000; **88**: 3065–3072.

24. Jakesz R, Gnant M, Hausmaninger H *et al*. Combination goserelin and tamoxifen is more effective than CMF in premenopausal patients with hormone responsive tumors in a multicenter trial of the Austrian Breast Cancer Study Group. *Breast Cancer Res Treat* 1999; **57 (Suppl)**: 25.

25. Early Breast Cancer Trialists' Collaborative Group. Ovarian ablation in early breast cancer: overview of the randomised trials. *Lancet* 1996; **348**: 1189–1196.

26. Norton L, Slamon D, Leyland-Jones B *et al*. Overall survival (OS) advantage to simultaneous chemotherapy plus humanised anti HER2 monoclonal antibody Herceptin in HER2-overexpressing metastatic breast cancer [Abstract 483]. *Proc ASCO* 1999; **18**: 127a.

27. Early Breast Cancer Trialists' Collaborative Group. Polychemotherapy for early breast cancer: an overview of the randomised trials. *Lancet* 1998; **352**: 930–942.

28. Fisher B, Anderson S, Wickerham DL *et al*. Increased intensification and total dose of cyclophosphamide in a doxorubicin-cyclophosphamide regimen for the treatment of primary breast cancer: findings from national surgical adjuvant breast and bowel project B-22. *J Clin Oncol* 1997; **15**: 1858–1869.

29. Wood WC, Budman DR, Korzun AH. Dose and dose intensity of adjuvant chemotherapy for stage II, node-positive breast carcinoma. *N Engl J Med* 1994; **330**: 1253–1259.

30. Henderson IC. Improved disease-free survival and overall survival from the addition of sequential paclitaxel in the adjuvant chemotherapy of patients with node-positive primary breast cancer [Abstract]. *Proc ASCO* 1998; 390A.

31. Fisher B, Brown AM, Dimitro NV *et al*. Two months of doxorubicin-cyclophosphamide with and without interval reduction therapy compared with 6 months of cyclophosphamide, methotrexate and fluorouracil in positive-node breast cancer patients with tamoxifen-non-responsive tumours: results from the National Surgical Adjuvant Breast and Bowel Project B-15. *Clin Oncol* 1990; **8**: 1483–1496.

32. Bergh J, Wiklund T, Erikstein B *et al*. Tailored fluorouracil, epirubicin and cyclophosphamide compared with marrow-supported high-dose chemotherapy as adjuvant treatment for high-risk breast cancer: a randomised trial. Scandinavian Breast Group 9401 study. *Lancet* 2000; **356**: 1384–1391.

33. Peters W, Rosner G, Vredenburgh J *et al*. A prospective randomised comparison of 2 doses of combination alkylating agents (AA) as consolidation after CAF in high risk primary breast cancer involving 10 or more axillary lymph nodes. Preliminary results of CALGB9082/SWOG91104/NCICMA-13 [Abstract 2]. *Proc ASCO* 1999, 1a.

34. Collichio FA, Agnello R, Staltzer J. Pregnancy after breast cancer: from psychosocial issues through conception. *Oncology* 1998; **12**: 759–765, 769, 773–775.

35. Miller WR, Ellis IO, Sainsbury JRC. Prognostic factors. In: Dixon JM. (ed) *ABC of Breast Diseases*, 2nd edn. London: BMJ Books, 2000; 72–77.

36. Goldhirsch A, Glick JH, Gelber RD, Senn HF. Meeting highlights: international consensus panel on the treatment of primary breast cancer. *J Natl Cancer Inst* 1998; **90**: 1601–1608.

37. Muss HB, Thor AD, Berry DA *et al*. c-erbB-2 expression and response to adjuvant therapy in women with node-positive early breast cancer. *N Engl J Med* 1994; **330**: 1260–1266.

38. Santen RJ, Manni A, Harvey H *et al*. Endocrine treatment of breast cancer in women. *Endocr Rev* 1990; **11**: 221–265.

39. Wiseman LR, McTavish D. Formestane: a review of its pharmacological and pharmacokinetic properties and therapeutic potential in the management of breast cancer and prostatic cancer. *Drugs* 1993; **45**: 66–84.

40. Mouridsen H, Gershanovish M, Sun Y *et al*. Superior efficacy of letrozole versus tamoxifen as first-line therapy for postmenopausal women with advanced breast cancer: results of a phase III study of the International Letrozole Breast Cancer Group. *J Clin Oncol* 2001; **19**: 2596–2606.

41. Fisher B, Dignam J, Wolmark N *et al*. Tamoxifen and chemotherapy for lymph node negative oestrogen receptor positive breast cancer. *J Natl Cancer Inst* 1997; **89**: 1673–1682.

42. Davidson NE, O'Neill A, Vukov A *et al*. Effect of chemohormonal therapy in premenopausal node positive receptor positive breast cancer: an Eastern Cooperative Oncology Group Phase III Intergroup Trial (E51888, INT-0101). *Breast* 1999; **8**: 232–233.

43. Baum M, Rutgers EE. Zoladex and tamoxifen as adjuvant therapy in premenopausal breast cancer: a randomised trial by the Cancer Research Campaign (CRC) Breast Cancer Trials Group, the Stockholm Breast Cancer Study Group., the South-East Sweden Breast Cancer Group and the Gruppa Interdisciplinara Valarazione Interventi in Oncologia (GIVIO). *Breast* 1999; **8**: Abstract 233.

44. Diel IJ, Solomayer EF, Costa SD *et al*. Reduction in new metastases in breast cancer with adjuvant clodronate treatment. *N Engl J Med* 1998; **339**: 357.

45. Powles TJ, Paterson AHG, Nevantaus A *et al*. Adjuvant clodronate reduces the incidence of bone metastases in patients with primary operable breast cancer [Abstract 468]. *Proc Am Soc Clin Oncol* 1998; **17**: 123a.

46. Dixon JM, Leonard RCF. Hormones and chemotherapy. In: Farndon JR. (ed) *A Companion to Specialist Surgical Practice: Breast and Endocrine Surgery*, 2nd edn. London: Saunders, 2001; 107–146.

Michael Douek Irving Taylor

16

Recent randomised controlled trials in general surgery

This chapter highlights a selection of important randomised controlled trials in general surgery, published over the last year. The trials reviewed focus on advances in the management of surgical disease in the fields of general, breast, upper gastrointestinal, colorectal, hepatobiliary and pancreatic, endocrine and melanoma surgery.

GENERAL CONDITIONS

THROMBOPROPHYLAXIS IN GENERAL SURGICAL PATIENTS

Thromboprophylaxis with heparin is now accepted clinical practice for all patients undergoing major surgery. In orthopaedic surgery, where the risk of clinical deep venous thrombosis (DVT) is higher, low molecular weight heparins (LMWHs) are recognised as being superior to unfractionated heparin.[1] In a recent meta-analysis,[2] LMWHs were found to be superior to unfractionated heparin in reducing the incidence of clinical venous thromboembolism in general surgical patients. At a dose of less than 3400 anti-Xa, LMWHs are as effective as and safer than unfractionated heparin. But at higher doses, LMWHs were associated with a higher risk of haemorrhage.

LAPAROTOMY INCISIONS USING ELECTROCAUTERY

Hand-held diathermy is increasingly being used instead of sharp or blunt dissection but, in making the skin incision, it has traditionally been avoided.

Mr Michael Douek MD FRCS, Lecturer in Surgery, Royal Free and University College London Medical School, University College London, London W1W 7EJ, UK (for correspondence)

Prof. Irving Taylor MD ChM FRCS, David Patey Professor of Surgery, Head of Department of Surgery, Royal Free and University College London Medical School, University College London, Charles Bell House, 67–73 Riding House Street, London W1W 7EJ, UK

Kears *et al.*[3] postulated that the use of electrocautery in elective midline laparotomy incisions might reduce postoperative pain without affecting healing. A total of 100 patients were randomised to either scalpel or diathermy incision. Laparotomy incisions using diathermy were significantly quicker, had less blood loss, were less painful in the first 48 h, and reduced morphine requirements in the first 5 days. Postoperative complications during in-patient stay and at 1-month follow-up, were not significantly different in the two groups. The investigators did not assess any difference in cosmetic results.

OPTIMAL SUTURE MATERIAL FOR MIDLINE FASCIAL CLOSURE

The suture material used for abdominal midline fascial closure is dependent upon surgeons' choice. A recent meta-analysis pooled data from randomized controlled studies primarily comparing absorbable to non-absorbable sutures.[4] A higher incidence of suture sinus formation and incision pain was seen with non-absorbable sutures, but there was no significant difference in infection or dehiscence rates. The incidence of incisional hernia was increased with braided absorbable sutures. Continuous mass closure with absorbable monofilament suture material is the closure technique of choice. Another randomised trial compared interrupted with continuous fascial closure in 331 patients undergoing surgery for morbid obesity.[5] Continuous fascial closure significantly reduced acute deep wound complications in the first 30 days.

APPENDICITIS

A Cochrane Review recently evaluated the indication for prophylactic antibiotics in the prevention of postoperative infection after appendicectomy.[6] The use of antibiotics either pre-operatively or intra-operatively or post-operatively, was recommended both for elective and emergency appendicectomies. The indication for different regimens of antibiotics was outside the scope of this review.

Laparoscopic appendicectomy for acute appendicitis is not widely accepted. Recent trials demonstrate that laparoscopic appendicectomy is associated with fewer wound complications and improved cosmetic result but prolongs operating time and increases cost.[7] Hospital stay is reduced in children[8], but is equally short in adults.[7] Return to work is faster following laparoscopic appendicectomy.[7] In fertile women, laparoscopy reduces unnecessary appendicectomies.[9]

ENTERAL AND PARENTERAL POSTOPERATIVE NUTRITION

Immediate enteral nutrition following major abdominal surgery, makes physiological sense but has not been shown to reduce postoperative complications or overall mortality.[10] Pacelli *et al.*[11] randomized 241 malnourished patients to either enteral (nasogastric) or parenteral nutrition immediately after major elective abdominal surgery. The rate of major postoperative complications (38% *versus* 39%) and overall mortality rates (5.9% *versus* 2.5%) were not significantly different in the two groups. In a different randomised study, gastric feeding was compared to postpyloric feeding in intensive care patients.[12] Gastric feeding was associated with a higher rate of gastro-oesophageal regurgitation (40% *versus* 25%). Using technetium 99-sulphur colloid added to the enteral feeds, a trend towards more micro-aspiration was seen with gastric feeding (8% *versus* 4%). It is thus possible that any clinical advantage of enteral over parenteral feeding is lost as a result of an increase in micro-aspiration seen if the gastric route is used.

LAPAROSCOPIC HERNIA REPAIR

The National Institute of Clinical Excellence (NICE) recently issued guidance on the use of laparoscopic surgery for inguinal hernias.[13] NICE recommends that open surgery should be the preferred surgical procedure and that laparoscopic surgery should be considered for bilateral and recurrent hernias. A more controversial recommendation is that the preferred approach should be the totally extraperitoneal approach (TEP) rather than the more popular transabdominal preperitoneal approach (TAPP). Recent studies comparing open with laparoscopic hernia repair demonstrate that laparoscopic repair results in earlier return to work[14] but takes longer to perform and is more expensive.[14,15] The long-term results of laparoscopic hernia repair, at 5 or more years follow-up, are as yet unknown.

Key point 1

- Continuous mass closure with absorbable monofilament suture material is the closure technique of choice, for midline fascial closure.

Key point 2

- For inguinal hernias, open surgery is the preferred surgical procedure in the NHS. Laparoscopic surgery should be considered for bilateral and recurrent hernias.

BREAST SURGERY

BREAST SCREENING

A further meta-analysis of all randomized controlled trials of breast screening[16] and a Cochrane Review[17] recently published by Olsen and Gotzsche, led to a stormy debate and controversy. The authors concluded that the currently available reliable evidence does not show a survival benefit of mass screening for breast cancer. Of the 8 randomized controlled studies to date, 6 were found to be of poor quality or flawed and were thus excluded from the analysis. Another important finding (excluded from the Cochrane Review – but published on *The Lancet* website) is that mass screening leads to increased use of more aggressive treatment, increasing the number of mastectomies by 20% and the number of mastectomies or wide local excisions by 30%, in the screened group. The authors postulate that this effect may be due to the mammographic detection of slow-growing tumours or ductal carcinoma *in situ* (DCIS), that may not develop into cancer in a woman's remaining lifetime, but that inevitably result in surgical resection. The implications of the current weight of evidence against screening are substantial and a cost-effectiveness analysis of breast screening by the NICE will hopefully be undertaken.

Key point 3

- The currently available reliable evidence does not show a survival benefit of mass screening for breast cancer, whereas it has shown that mass screening leads to increased use of aggressive treatment.

PROGNOSTIC FACTORS FOR BREAST CANCER

The National Surgical Adjuvant Breast and Bowel Project (NSAPB) Protocol-06 study, recently published the prognostic discriminants for breast cancer, at 15 years of follow-up.[18] This study, launched in 1976, compared the outcome of patients with stage I/II (≤ 4 cm) breast cancer randomized to one of 3 arms: total mastectomy (with axillary node clearance), lumpectomy (with axillary node clearance) with or without adjuvant radiotherapy. The independent pathological and clinical prognostic indicators related to survival were the presence of ipsilateral breast tumour recurrence, patient age, race, positive nodal status, presence of vascular invasion, poor nuclear grade and intermediate or unfavourable histological tumour type. The independent risk factors for ipsilateral breast tumour recurrence were absence of local irradiation, patient age (< 40 or > 65 years), poor nuclear grade, presence of intraductal tumour component and presence of lymphocytic infiltrate. Ipsilateral breast tumour recurrence, was found to be a strong predictor of reduced survival, but not an indicator of distant disease, since overall survival remained equivalent in the 3 arms of the study. This study confirms that most recurrences occur close to the site of the index cancer, but with a lower incidence of 75% compared to previous reports. Interestingly, histological tumour type or nuclear grade of local recurrences was the same as that of the index cancer in 85% and 94% of cases, irrespective of the breast quadrant involved.

It is important to note that oestrogen receptor (ER) and progesterone receptor (PR) status are both recognised prognostic factors, although not found to be independent factors for recurrence or survival in the NSABP-06 study.[18] At the 2001 St Gallen Conference for Adjuvant Therapy of Breast Cancer,[19] ER, PR and mitotic rate were recognised as established prognostic factors. The promising prognostic and predictive factors included HER-2 (tyrosine kinase receptor), p53 status (tumour suppressor gene), uPA/PAI-1 (plasminogen-activator system) and quantitative parameters of angiogenesis.

SENTINEL LYMPH NODE BIOPSY

The accuracy of sentinel node (the first lymph node to contain metastatic cancer) status in predicting axillary node status is no longer under dispute. Several prospective, national, randomized, controlled trials are underway, to assess the impact of sentinel node biopsy on axillary morbidity, recurrence rates, disease-free and overall survival. In the UK, the BASO (British Association of Surgical Oncology)/ALMANAC (Axillary Lymphatic Mapping Against Nodal Axillary Clearance) Trial is well underway.[20] Patients are randomized to axillary treatment (surgery or radiotherapy) guided by sentinel node biopsy using paraffin histology, or to conventional axillary treatment (axillary node sampling or clearance). The primary end-points are axillary morbidity, health economics and quality-of-life. In the US, the NSABP B-32 trial and American College of Surgeons Oncology Group (ACOSOG) Z0010/Z0011 trials are underway. In the ACOSOG Z0011 trial,[21] patients with clinical T1/T2 N0M0 breast cancer and a positive sentinel node will be randomised to axillary node clearance or no axillary node clearance. The primary end-point is overall survival, and secondary end-points are surgical morbidity and distant disease-free survival. Initial results of these studies will become available in 2002–2004. At present, sentinel node biopsy is not regarded as standard practice. It is thus important to await the results of randomised controlled studies before abandoning routine axillary lymph node clearance.

Key point 4

- The impact of sentinel node biopsy on axillary morbidity, recurrence rates, disease-free and overall survival are as yet unknown. It is thus important to await the results of randomised controlled studies (ALMANAC Trial in the UK) before abandoning routine axillary lymph node clearance.

ADJUVANT ENDOCRINE THERAPY

A recent Cochrane Review[22] concluded that adjuvant tamoxifen treatment substantially improves 10-year survival of women with ER-positive tumours and of women whose ER status is unknown. For women with tumours that have been reliably shown to be ER negative, adjuvant tamoxifen remains a matter for research. With respect to duration of treatment, this review could not comment on the benefit or otherwise of continuing tamoxifen for over 5 years. Two subsequent trials addressed this question. In the Scottish Adjuvant Tamoxifen Trial,[23] 1323 patients who have had a mastectomy and axillary surgery (clearance or sampling), were randomized to tamoxifen for 5 years or to delayed tamoxifen until indicated by recurrent disease. After 5 years, 342 disease-free patients who had received tamoxifen were randomized to stop tamoxifen (median of 5 years' treatment) or to continue tamoxifen indefinitely (median 13 years and 7 months). The beneficial effect of adjuvant tamoxifen given for 5 years on the probability of total survival, systemic relapse and death from breast cancer has been maintained through 15 years of follow-up, but no additional benefit was observed in those taking tamoxifen beyond 5 years. However, this contradicts the result of the Fédération Nationale des Centres de Lutte Contre le Cancer Breast Group Study,[24] in which 3793 patients with early breast cancer who had been taking tamoxifen for 2–3 years and were disease-free were randomized to stopping tamoxifen or to continuing on tamoxifen for life (later altered to 10 years). In the group who received a median of 12–13 years of tamoxifen, the 7-year disease-free survival rate was significantly improved (78% *versus* 72%), but there was no difference in the overall survival rate. Furthermore, longer tamoxifen treatment also reduced the incidence of contralateral breast cancer with no increase in the number of endometrial cancers. As compared with the Scottish Adjuvant Tamoxifen Trial, in this study most patients were ER positive and thus any additional benefit of longer term tamoxifen treatment beyond 5 years is likely to occur in this group. At the St Gallen Conference for Adjuvant Therapy for Breast Cancer,[19] 5 years of treatment was recognized as superior to 2 years, in terms of percentage reduction in the annual odds of either recurrence (12% *versus* 8%) or death (9% *versus* 6%). Other hormone therapies under development include selective oestrogen-receptor modulators (SERMs) and aromatase inhibitors. In the UK, the international multicentre ATAC Trial (arimidex, tamoxifen and combined) has exceeded expectations for recruitment. Interim results at 2.5 years' follow-up demonstrated that arimidex monotherapy is superior to tamoxifen and the combination. Although these results are encouraging, they should be interpreted with caution until results at 5-year follow-up become available in 2003/2004.

ADJUVANT CHEMOTHERAPY

A systematic review of chemotherapy trials confirmed the strong evidence from randomized controlled trials, supporting the use of systemic adjuvant chemotherapy in the management of breast cancer.[25] The overall 10-year mortality reduction for women under 50 years is 12% for node-positive and 6% for node-negative patients. The survival advantage is of a modest magnitude for women aged 50–69 years: 6% for node-positive and 2% for node-negative patients. Anthracycline and cyclophosphamide based regimens, and the addition of tamoxifen in ER-positive patients, further enhance survival. Neo-adjuvant chemotherapy in patients with large operable breast cancer increases the number of patients suitable for breast conserving surgery, but the evidence for any improvement in survival is weak.

With respect to node-negative patients, with breast cancers of 1 cm or less, a recent analysis of data from 5 NSABP randomized clinical trials demonstrated that, although their prognosis is better, some of these women may still benefit from adjuvant chemotherapy.[26] There is a growing interest in the discovery of biological markers or predictive factors that could be used to identify those patients that are more likely to benefit from adjuvant chemotherapy. In a recent trial,[27] thymidine labelling index (used to identify rapidly proliferating tumours) was found to be a predictive indicator for response to cyclophosphamide, methotrexate and 5-fluorouracil (CMF) in node-negative patients. Urokinase-type plasminogen activator and plasminogen activator inhibitor type I, recognized predictors of disease recurrence, have also been found to be predictive factors for response to CMF.[28] However, more prospective trials are needed before predictive factors are considered in the management algorithm for breast cancer.

HER2 status is increasingly being provided as part of routine histological breast tumour assessment. Retrospective studies suggest that HER2 overexpression is found in tumours that respond to doxorubicin and paclitaxel, and those that are not responsive to tamoxifen. Menard *et al.*[29] studied the impact of HER2 status on response to CMF in a randomized controlled trial of CMF versus no treatment, after radical mastectomy for node-positive breast cancer. With CMF, relapse-free and cause-specific survival was significantly improved in both HER2 positive and negative patients. HER2 was therefore a prognostic factor and not a predictive factor in this trial.

UPPER GASTROINTESTINAL SURGERY

PREVENTION OF ERCP-INDUCED PANCREATITIS

Increasingly, patients with cholelithiasis undergo pre-operative endoscopic retrograde pancreatography (ERCP), which carries a risk of pancreatitis. One possible aetiology is cannulation-induced spasm of the sphincter of Oddi, resulting in pancreatic duct obstruction. Sublingual prophylactic treatment with glyceryl trinitrate (GTN), at a dose of 2 mg administered 5 min prior to ERCP, reduces the occurrence of pancreatitis at 24 h but not the extent of hyperamylasaemia or the severity of pancreatitis.[30]

OESOPHAGEAL CARCINOMA

Evidence in favour of neo-adjuvant (primary) chemotherapy in patients with operable oesophageal carcinoma is growing. Ancona *et al.*[31] randomised 96 patients with resectable squamous oesophageal carcinoma undergoing surgery (right thoracotomy and laparotomy; left cervical incision when indicated) to receive (or not) neo-adjuvant chemotherapy. Pre-operative staging included a computed tomography (CT) scan, upper GI endoscopy and bronchoscopy in all patients, but not routine laparoscopy or transluminal endoscopic ultrasound. In patients randomised to neo-adjuvant chemotherapy (2 or 3 cycles of cisplatin and 5-fluorouracil), surgery was performed 3–4 weeks after chemotherapy. Curative resection rates and overall survival at 5 years' follow-up were not significantly different between the two groups. Subgroup analysis of patients who underwent curative resection demonstrated that 5-year survival was significantly improved in those patients who received and responded to neo-adjuvant chemotherapy, compared to those who did not receive chemotherapy (60% *versus* 26%). In another study, 100 patients with operable oesophageal carcinoma (squamous and adeno-carcinoma) were randomized to surgery alone (transhiatal oesophagectomy) or to receive pre-operative chemoradiotherapy (cisplatin, 5-fluorouracil and vinblastin; 45 Gy radiotherapy). At a median follow-up of 8.2 years, there was no significant difference in survival between the groups.

Results of the largest study to date were published in abstract form and provisional results favour neo-adjuvant chemotherapy. The Medical Research

Council group[32] randomised 802 patients with resectable oesophageal carcinoma (33% squamous and 67% adenocarcinoma) to pre-operative chemotherapy with cisplatin and 5-fluorouracil followed by surgery, or surgery alone. At 2 years' follow-up, there appears to be a survival advantage in favour of chemotherapy (reported hazard ratio of 0.77; 95% CI 0.64–0.91).

Key point 5

- In operable oesophageal carcinoma, pre-operative chemotherapy with cisplatin and 5-fluorouracil should be considered.

GASTRIC CARCINOMA

The efficacy of adjuvant chemotherapy after curative resection in gastric cancer is still controversial. In a randomised study of 137 patients[33] with nodal involvement, a combined regimen of epidoxorubicin, leucovorin and 5-fluorouracil, significantly improved 5-year survival (30% *versus* 13%).

LAPAROSCOPIC FUNDOPLICATION

The need for an oesophageal bougie in order to prevent oesophageal stricturing following laparoscopic surgery has been assessed by Patterson *et al*.[34] A total of 171 patients with gastro-oesophageal reflux requiring surgery, were randomised to laparoscopic Nissen fundoplication with or without a 56F oesophageal bougie. The incidence of long-term dysphagia was reduced in the bougie group (17% *versus* 31%) with one oesophageal injury in the bougie group and no deaths.

COLORECTAL SURGERY

The standard management of generalised peritonitis complicating sigmoid diverticulitis is primary resection, peritoneal washout, drainage and defunctioning of the proximal colon. However, primary resection often involves undertaking major surgery in severely ill patients and it is not clear if these patients may benefit from a limited operation followed by a more definitive elective procedure. Zeitoun *et al*.[35] randomized 105 patients to primary resection (with end colostomy or primary colorectal anastomosis) or secondary resection (with primary closure of the sigmoid perforation only). Postoperative peritonitis (1.8% *versus* 25%), early re-operation (3.6% *versus* 18.8%) and hospital stay (15 *versus* 24 days) were reduced after primary resection compared to secondary resection. However, mortality did not differ significantly between the two groups (24% *versus* 19%). In patients who require a defunctioning stoma, loop transverse colostomy was found to be associated with a higher incidence of herniation compared to loop ileostomy, in a different study.[36]

HEPARIN PROPHYLAXIS IN COLORECTAL SURGERY

Colorectal surgery is associated with a higher risk of DVT and pulmonary embolism compared to other general surgical procedures. A recent Cochrane

Systematic Review[37] compared the incidence of postoperative DVT and pulmonary embolism following colorectal surgery, using mechanical and heparin prophylaxis. The combination of graduated compression stockings and low-dose unfractionated heparin was recommended for optimal prophylaxis. Unfractionated heparin can be replaced with LMWH, since these treatments were found to be equally effective, but unfractionated heparin is more cost-effective.[38]

PREVENTION AND SCREENING FOR COLONIC POLYPS

Several different modalities have been suggested for the primary prevention of colorectal cancer including screening for polyps and chemoprevention. In a recent randomised study,[39] ispaghula husk dietary supplements were found to increase the likelihood of adenoma recurrence (odds ratio 1.67, CI 1.01–2.76), particularly in patients with a high calcium intake. The APPAC study[40] is underway and will determine if 160 or 300 mg/day of aspirin is effective in reducing colorectal adenoma recurrence.

When polyps are detected at flexible sigmoidoscopy, their resection may not reduce the incidence of recurrent polyps. Thiis-Evensen et al.[41] randomised 799 patients (50–59 years) to screening by flexible sigmoidoscopy or no screening. The screened group underwent a baseline colonoscopy with repeat colonoscopy at 2 and 6 years. Seven years later, both groups were offered a colonoscopy. Although there was no significant difference in the prevalence of adenomas (37% *versus* 43%), there was a trend towards more high risk adenomas (≥ 10 mm, severe dysplasia or villous) in the control group (13% *versus* 8%). Lund et al.[42] randomized 776 patients who had adenomas to surveillance by either flexible sigmoidoscopy or colonoscopy at varying intervals (every 1, 2 or 5 years). No difference in adenoma recurrence was seen between surveillance by colonoscopy or by flexible sigmoidoscopy. Five-year surveillance was as effective as more frequent surveillance and was associated with better compliance than annual surveillance. Interestingly, of 4 patients who developed colorectal cancer, only 1 was detected by surveillance. Clearly, surveillance colonoscopy has a limited effect on the prevalence of adenomas.

PRE-OPERATIVE RADIOTHERAPY FOR RECTAL CANCER

For some time, the treatment of rectal cancer seemed to have reached a clear consensus: surgery as the primary curative treatment with a combination of adjuvant chemotherapy and radiotherapy for patients with stage II and III disease. This was recently challenged by two large randomised controlled trials, which provide strong evidence to support the treatment of all patients with primary radiotherapy followed by surgery. Five days of pre-operative radiotherapy (25 Gy) to rectum and pararectal tissues has been shown to reduce local recurrence[43,44] and improve survival in patients who underwent curative resections.[43] The Dutch Colorectal Cancer Group[44] reported results of their 1861 patients with resectable rectal cancer, randomised to a 5-day course of pre-operative radiotherapy followed by total mesorectal excision or total mesorectal excision alone, with a follow-up of at least 2 years. Overall survival was 82% in each group, but the rate of local recurrence was significantly reduced in the group that had received pre-operative radiotherapy (2.4%

versus 8.2%). Univariate subgroup analysis demonstrated that this benefit was not significant in those patients who had tumours with an inferior margin more than 10 cm from the anal verge. Possible down-staging of disease in the irradiated group has been shown not to be responsible for these findings.[45]

In the Stockholm II study,[43] 557 patients with biopsy proven rectal carcinoma judged as being operable via an abdominal procedure, were randomised to pre-operative radiotherapy followed by surgery within a week, or surgery alone. All patients were followed-up for a minimum of 5.6 years and a median of 8.8 years. It is not clear what proportion of patients underwent total mesorectal excision, but a curative resection was achieved in 481 patients (86%). Of those who underwent curative resection, the incidence of pelvic recurrence (12% *versus* 25%) was reduced and overall survival (46% *versus* 39%) improved in the irradiated patients. However, for all included patients, overall survival was equivalent (39% *versus* 36%).

The introduction of total mesorectal excision led to a reduction of local recurrence rates in the 1990s, and it is important to note here that in neither study mentioned above did the investigators test the benefit or otherwise of the technique. The benefit of radiotherapy compared to the clinical benefit of improved surgical technique remains unknown. Another clinical implication regards the use of a lower dose of radiotherapy (25 Gy) as well as the use of pre-operative rather than postoperative radiotherapy. It has been suggested that the dose-response ratio and patient compliance are higher with pre-operative radiotherapy. A recent meta-analysis[46] concluded that the combination of pre-operative radiotherapy and surgery, compared with surgery alone, significantly improved overall survival. However, patients with small tumours confined to the bowel have excellent prognosis and less likely to benefit from pre-operative radiotherapy.

Key point 6

- The Dutch Colorectal Cancer Group and Stockholm II Trials provide strong evidence that 5 days of pre-operative radiotherapy, in patients with operable rectal carcinoma, significantly reduces local recurrence rate.

The optimal timing of surgery after radiotherapy (within 1 week or after 4–8 weeks) is not known and the Stockholm III Trial was launched in 1999 to address this question. At present, a compromise would be sensible: to administer pre-operative radiotherapy to all patients with locally advanced or large operable disease and offer primary surgery to patients with early disease or to those with high rectal tumours.

SURGICAL TECHNIQUES

Stapled *versus* hand-sewn colonic anastomosis

Randomized, controlled studies comparing hand-sewn with stapled anastomoses have not shown either technique to be superior to the other. A recent Cochrane Systematic Review,[47] with pooled analysis of results from 9 trials, concluded that there was insufficient evidence to demonstrate that either technique was superior, regardless of the level of the anastomosis.

Laparoscopic colectomy

The role of laparoscopic assisted surgery in the treatment of colorectal cancer is as yet unclear. Major questions remain unsolved with respect to port-site implantation, immune response and cost-effectiveness. In its recent guidelines for colon and rectal surgery, the National Cancer Institute, recommended that laparoscopic colectomy should be confined to clinical trials at present.[48] Several large randomised controlled trials are underway[49,50] including the UK MRC CLASICC (Conventional *versus* Laparoscopic-assisted Surgery in Colorectal Cancer) trial.[51] Potential differences in immune response to surgery were recently assessed in 236 patients entered into the CLASICC trial, and no difference was found.[52]

Stapled *versus* conventional haemorrhoidectomy

Stapled haemorrhoidectomy is gaining support over conventional haemorrhoidectomy. Shalaby *et al.*[53] randomized 200 patients with grade II–IV haemorrhoids to either Milligan-Morgan haemorrhoidectomy or stapled haemorrhoidectomy (33 mm circular stapling device). In the stapled group, operating time was shorter (9 *versus* 19 min), postoperative pain and analgesic requirements were reduced, hospital stay was reduced (1.1 days *versus* 2.2 days) with earlier return to normal activity. Ho *et al.*[54] randomized 119 patients with grade III/IV haemorrhoids, to either stapled haemorrhoidectomy or to open diathermy haemorrhoidectomy. Open diathermy haemorrhoidectomy was quicker to perform (11.4 min *versus* 17.6 min) but more painful, with more bleeding, 85.5% of wounds were unhealed at 2 weeks and patients resumed work after 23 days compared with 17 days after stapled haemorrhoidectomy. The complication rates were similar in the two groups. Several other studies have demonstrated encouraging results.[55,56] Similarly, Khalil *et al.*[57] compared closed (sutured) haemorrhoidectomy with stapled haemorrhoidectomy and found that the stapled technique was less painful with faster wound healing. Long-term results of stapled haemorrhoidectomy are still awaited.

HEPATOBILIARY AND PANCREATIC SURGERY

ANTIBIOTIC TREATMENT FOR SEVERE PANCREATITIS

The place of antibiotic treatment in pancreatitis was regarded as controversial for a long time. However, the antibiotics used in the past had poor penetration into pancreatic tissue. Nordback *et al.*[58] randomized 90 patients with necrotizing pancreatitis (C-reactive protein > 150 mg/l and necrosis on CT) to 1 g intravenous imipenem plus cilastatin (3 times a day) or placebo. Of these, 31 patients over the age of 70 years were excluded since they were deemed not potentially operable. All patients underwent conservative treatment unless infected necrosis was suspected. A pyrexia or a 30% increase in the white cell count or C-reactive protein, in the absence of evidence of chest, urinary or central line sepsis, was indicative of infected necrosis. If the inflammatory variable disagreed, a CT or ultrasound-guided aspirate of the necrosis was undertaken and sent for Gram-staining and culture. Surgery was required in 2 of 25 patients (8%) in the imipenem group compared with 14 of 33 (42%) in the control group. Major organ complications were seen in 7 of 25 (28%) of the imipenem group and 25 of 33 (76%) in the control group. Mortality was not significantly different, but this study had insufficient power to detect a difference in mortality.

HEPATOCELLULAR CARCINOMA

The only curative treatment for hepatocellular carcinoma remains hepatectomy. However, resection is not indicated in patients with advanced or inoperable disease, associated severe liver cirrhosis or other significant co-morbidity. Even after liver resection, long-term outcome is poor because of a high incidence of local recurrence in the liver remnant. Results of adjuvant chemotherapy for hepatocellular carcinoma are conflicting but generally disappointing. A recent meta-analysis[59] of adjuvant chemotherapy following liver resection, in patients with liver cirrhosis, demonstrated that postoperative chemotherapy was associated with a significantly worse disease-free and overall survival.

PANCREATIC CARCINOMA

Pylorus-preserving pancreaticoduodenectomy (PPPD) is a more conservative, alternative operation to Whipple's procedure, in patients with peri-ampullary and pancreatic head lesions. However, controversy still exists with respect to the radicality of this operation in pancreatic cancer. In a recent large prospective randomized study,[60] 114 patients were randomized to PPPD or Whipple's resection, but only 77 were included in the final analysis. The PPPD group had a significantly shorter operating time (6.7 h *versus* 7.9 h), reduced blood loss (1453 ml *versus* 2096 ml), less mean blood transfusion (2.1 units *versus* 3.6 units) and reduced morbidity. There was no difference between the two groups in length of stay in intensive care (2 days), length of hospital stay (25 days *versus* 24 days), incidence of delayed gastric emptying or postoperative mortality rate (2.7% *versus* 5%). At a median follow-up of 1.1 years, there was no difference in rate of recurrence or survival.

THYROID AND PARATHYROID DISEASE

PRIMARY HYPERPARATHYROIDISM

Patients with primary hyperparathyroidism have an elevated serum para-thyroid level and a high calcium concentration. Most of these patients are asymptomatic and are detected on biochemical screening. The treatment of asymptomatic hyperparathyroidism remains controversial. In a recent study[61] of 53 patients randomized to surgery or observation, quality-of-life assessment using SF-36 was in favour of the operated group in 2 of 9 domains.

GRAVES' DISEASE

The surgical treatment of hyperthyroidism in Graves' disease may be by subtotal or total thyroidectomy. It has been suggested that Graves' related orbitopathy may respond to total thyroidectomy and that total thyroidectomy may be associated with a reduced risk of recurrent Graves' disease. Witte *et al.*[62] randomized 150 patients with clinically or biochemically proven Graves' disease to either total thyroidectomy ($n = 50$), unilateral total and contralateral subtotal thyroidectomy ($n = 50$) or to bilateral subtotal thyroidectomy. At 6 months follow-up, Graves' orbitopathy improved in 72%, irrespective of the operation performed. Early postoperative hypoparathyroidism was more frequently seen with total than with subtotal thyroidectomy (28% *versus* 12%), but the incidence of permanent laryngeal nerve paralysis (1.9%) was not statistically different in the three groups. The operation of choice for Graves' disease, is, therefore, radical subtotal thyroidectomy with a remnant of less than 4 ml but longer term follow-up is required to establish the incidence of recurrent Graves' disease.

Key point 8

- For Graves' disease, the operation of choice is radical subtotal thyroidectomy with a remnant of less than 4 ml.

FOLLICULAR CARCINOMA OF THE THYROID

Udelsman *et al.*[63] randomized 61 patients requiring resection of a thyroid nodule, to on-table frozen section or no frozen section. In 96% of patients, frozen sections did not alter management and the use of frozen-section in patients with follicular neoplasms was not deemed cost-effective.

MELANOMA

Outcome in malignant melanoma is primarily dependent upon stage at presentation and completeness of excision. Reduced safety margins with a maximum of 2–3 cm enable closure of most defects by simple skin flap techniques. Several studies support the concept of a more conservative excision strategy. In the Intergroup Melanoma Surgical Trial,[64] 468 patients with melanomas on the trunk or proximal extremity, were randomised to a 2 cm or 4 cm radical excision margin and followed up for a median of 10 years. Local recurrence was associated with a 5-year survival of 9% compared to 86% survival for those patients who did not have local recurrence. The 10-year

> ## Key point 9
>
> • In malignant melanoma of the flank or extremities, an excision margin of 2 cm is safe in the majority of patients.

survival (70% *versus* 77%) and incidence of local recurrence at any time (2.1% *versus* 2.6%) were not significantly different in those who had a 2 cm or 4 cm excision margin. The Swedish Melanoma Study Group randomised 989 patients, with melanoma on the trunk or extremities with a tumour thickness of > 0.8 mm and ≤ 2 mm, to either a 2 cm or a 5 cm excision margin. At a median follow-up of 11 years, local recurrence was rare for tumours of this size (< 1%) and no difference in survival was seen between those who underwent 2 cm or 5 cm excision margins. Surgical resection with an excision margin of 2 cm is safe for the majority of patients with cutaneous melanoma.

Sentinel lymph node biopsy predicts lymph node status in melanoma patients and has been shown to be a powerful prognostic indicator.[65] Prior to acceptance as standard practice for all patients, several studies are underway to look at the impact of micrometastatic involvement of sentinel nodes on overall survival. The value of additional therapy (including elective lymph node dissection and interferon therapy) for patients who are positive only by reverse transcriptase polymerase chain reaction (RT-PCR), is currently being investigated by the national multi-centre Sunbelt Melanoma Trial in the US.

The American Joint Committee on Cancer staging (AJCC) has recently altered the classification of cutaneous malignant melanoma.[66] With sentinel lymph node biopsy, some patients are found to have occult lymph node metastasis. The new classification distinguishes between macroscopic and microscopic lymph node metastases. This revision will become official with publication of the sixth edition of the *AJCC Cancer Staging Manual* in 2002.

References

1. Koch A, Ziegler S, Breitschwerdt H, Victor N. Low molecular weight heparin and unfractionated heparin in thrombosis prophylaxis: meta-analysis based on original patient data. *Thromb Res* 2001; **102**: 295–309.
2. Mismetti P, Laporte S, Darmon JY, Buchmuller A, Decousus H. Meta-analysis of low molecular weight heparin in the prevention of venous thromboembolism in general surgery. *Br J Surg* 2001; **88**: 913–930.
3. Kearns SR, Connolly EM, McNally S, McNamara DA, Deasy J. Randomized clinical trial of diathermy versus scalpel incision in elective midline laparotomy. *Br J Surg* 2001; **88**: 41–44.
4. Rucinski J, Margolis M, Panagopoulos G, Wise L. Closure of the abdominal midline fascia: meta-analysis delineates the optimal technique. *Am Surg* 2001; **67**: 421–426.
5. Derzie AJ, Silvestri F, Liriano E, Benotti P. Wound closure technique and acute wound complications in gastric surgery for morbid obesity: a prospective randomized trial. *J Am Coll Surg* 2000; **191**: 238–243.
6. Andersen BR, Kallehave FL, Andersen HK. Antibiotics versus placebo for prevention of postoperative infection after appendicectomy (Cochrane Review). *Cochrane Database Syst Rev* 2001; **3**: CD001439.
7. Pedersen AG, Petersen OB, Wara P, Ronning H, Qvist N, Laurberg S. Randomized clinical trial of laparoscopic versus open appendicectomy. *Br J Surg* 2001; **88**: 200–205.

Key points for clinical practice

- Continuous mass closure with absorbable monofilament suture material is the closure technique of choice, for midline fascial closure.

- For inguinal hernias, open surgery is the preferred surgical procedure in the NHS. Laparoscopic surgery should be considered for bilateral and recurrent hernias.

- The currently available reliable evidence does not show a survival benefit of mass screening for breast cancer, whereas it has shown that mass screening leads to increased use of aggressive treatment.

- The impact of sentinel node biopsy on axillary morbidity, recurrence rates, disease-free and overall survival are as yet unknown. It is thus important to await the results of randomised controlled studies (ALMANAC Trial in the UK) before abandoning routine axillary lymph node clearance.

- In operable oesophageal carcinoma, pre-operative chemotherapy with cisplatin and 5-fluorouracil should be considered.

- The Dutch Colorectal Cancer Group and Stockholm II Trials provide strong evidence that 5 days of pre-operative radiotherapy, in patients with operable rectal carcinoma, significantly reduces local recurrence rate.

- In patients with severe or necrotizing pancreatitis, intravenous imipenem reduces septic complications and need for surgical intervention.

- For Graves' disease, the operation of choice is radical subtotal thyroidectomy with a remnant of less than 4 ml.

- In malignant melanoma of the flank or extremities, an excision margin of 2 cm is safe in the majority of patients.

8. Lintula H, Kokki H, Vanamo K. Single-blind randomized clinical trial of laparoscopic versus open appendicectomy in children. *Br J Surg* 2001; **88**: 510–514.

9. Larsson PG, Henriksson G, Olsson M *et al*. Laparoscopy reduces unnecessary appendicectomies and improves diagnosis in fertile women. A randomized study. *Surg Endosc* 2001; **15**: 200–202.

10. Heyland DK, Montalvo M, MacDonald S, Keefe L, Su XY, Drover JW. Total parenteral nutrition in the surgical patient: a meta-analysis. *Can J Surg* 2001; **44**: 102–111.

11. Pacelli F, Bossola M, Papa V *et al*. Enteral vs parenteral nutrition after major abdominal surgery: an even match. *Arch Surg* 2001; **136**: 933–936.

12. Heyland DK, Drover JW, MacDonald S, Novak F, Lam M. Effect of postpyloric feeding on gastroesophageal regurgitation and pulmonary microaspiration: results of a randomized controlled trial. *Crit Care Med* 2001; **29**: 1495–1501.

13. National Institute of Clinical Excellence. *Guidance on the Use of Laparoscopic Surgery for Inguinal Hernias*. London (11 Strand, London WC2N 5HR): National Institute of Clinical Excellence, 2001.

14. Fleming WR, Elliott TB, Jones RM, Hardy KJ. Randomized clinical trial comparing totally extraperitoneal inguinal hernia repair with the Shouldice technique. *Br J Surg* 2001; **88**: 1183–1188.

15. Cost-utility analysis of open versus laparoscopic groin hernia repair: results from a multicentre randomized clinical trial. *Br J Surg* 2001; **88**: 653–661.

16. Olsen O, Gotzsche PC. Cochrane review on screening for breast cancer with mammography. *Lancet* 2001; **358**: 1340–1342.

17. Olsen O, Gotzsche PC. Screening for breast cancer with mammography (Cochrane Review). *Cochrane Database Syst Rev* 2001; **4**: CD001877.

18. Fisher ER, Anderson S, Tan-Chiu E, Fisher B, Eaton L, Wolmark N. Fifteen-year prognostic discriminants for invasive breast carcinoma: National Surgical Adjuvant Breast and Bowel Project Protocol-06. *Cancer* 2001; **91**: 1679–1687.

19. Aapro MS. Adjuvant therapy of primary breast cancer: a review of key findings from the 7th international conference, St Gallen, February 2001. *Oncologist* 2001; **6**: 376–385.

20. Clarke D, Khonji NI, Mansel RE. Sentinel node biopsy in breast cancer: ALMANAC trial. *World J Surg* 2001; **25**: 819–822.

21. Grube BJ, Giuliano AE. Observation of the breast cancer patient with a tumor-positive sentinel node: implications of the ACOSOG Z0011 trial. *Semin Surg Oncol* 2001; **20**: 230–237.

22. Anon. Tamoxifen for early breast cancer. *Cochrane Database Syst Rev* 2001; **1**: CD000486.

23. Stewart HJ, Prescott RJ, Forrest AP. Scottish adjuvant tamoxifen trial: a randomized study updated to 15 years. *J Natl Cancer Inst* 2001; **93**: 456–462.

24. Delozier T, Spielmann M, Mace-Lesec'h J *et al.* Tamoxifen adjuvant treatment duration in early breast cancer: initial results of a randomized study comparing short-term treatment with long-term treatment. Federation Nationale des Centres de Lutte Contre le Cancer Breast Group. *J Clin Oncol* 2000; **18**: 3507–3512.

25. Bergh J, Jonsson PE, Glimelius B, Nygren P. A systematic overview of chemotherapy effects in breast cancer. *Acta Oncol* 2001; **40**: 253–281.

26. Fisher B, Dignam J, Tan-Chiu E *et al.* Prognosis and treatment of patients with breast tumors of one centimeter or less and negative axillary lymph nodes. *J Natl Cancer Inst* 2001; **93**: 112–120.

27. Amadori D, Nanni O, Marangolo M *et al.* Disease-free survival advantage of adjuvant cyclophosphamide, methotrexate, and fluorouracil in patients with node-negative, rapidly proliferating breast cancer: a randomized multicenter study. *J Clin Oncol* 2000; **18**: 3125–3134.

28. Janicke F, Prechtl A, Thomssen C *et al.* Randomized adjuvant chemotherapy trial in high-risk, lymph node-negative breast cancer patients identified by urokinase-type plasminogen activator and plasminogen activator inhibitor type 1. *J Natl Cancer Inst* 2001; **93**: 913–920.

29. Menard S, Valagussa P, Pilotti S *et al.* Response to cyclophosphamide, methotrexate, and fluorouracil in lymph node-positive breast cancer according to HER2 overexpression and other tumor biologic variables. *J Clin Oncol* 2001; **19**: 329–335.

30. Sudhindran S, Bromwich E, Edwards PR. Prospective randomized double-blind placebo-controlled trial of glyceryl trinitrate in endoscopic retrograde cholangiopancreatography-induced pancreatitis. *Br J Surg* 2001; **88**: 1178–1182.

31. Ancona E, Ruol A, Santi S *et al.* Only pathologic complete response to neoadjuvant chemotherapy improves significantly the long term survival of patients with resectable esophageal squamous cell carcinoma: final report of a randomized, controlled trial of preoperative chemotherapy versus surgery alone. *Cancer* 2001; **91**: 2165–2174.

32. Malthaner R, Fenlon D. Preoperative chemotherapy for resectable thoracic esophageal cancer (Cochrane Review). *Cochrane Database Syst Rev* 2001; **1**: CD001556.

33. Neri B, Cini G, Andreoli F *et al.* Randomized trial of adjuvant chemotherapy versus control after curative resection for gastric cancer: 5-year follow-up. *Br J Cancer* 2001; **84**: 878–880.

34. Patterson EJ, Herron DM, Hansen PD, Ramzi N, Standage BA, Swanstrom LL. Effect of an esophageal bougie on the incidence of dysphagia following nissen fundoplication: a prospective, blinded, randomized clinical trial. *Arch Surg* 2000; **135**: 1055–1061.

35. Zeitoun G, Laurent A, Rouffet F *et al.* Multicentre, randomized clinical trial of primary versus secondary sigmoid resection in generalized peritonitis complicating sigmoid diverticulitis. *Br J Surg* 2000; **87**: 1366–1374.

36. Edwards DP, Leppington-Clarke A, Sexton R, Heald RJ, Moran BJ. Stoma-related complications are more frequent after transverse colostomy than loop ileostomy: a

prospective randomized clinical trial. *Br J Surg* 2001; **88**: 360–363.

37. Wille-Jorgensen P, Rasmussen MS, Andersen BR, Borly L. Heparins and mechanical methods for thromboprophylaxis in colorectal surgery (Cochrane Review). *Cochrane Database Syst Rev* 2001; **3**: CD001217.

38. McLeod RS, Geerts WH, Sniderman KW *et al*. Subcutaneous heparin versus low-molecular-weight heparin as thromboprophylaxis in patients undergoing colorectal surgery: results of the Canadian colorectal DVT prophylaxis trial: a randomized, double-blind trial. *Ann Surg* 2001; **233**: 438–444.

39. Bonithon-Kopp C, Kronborg O, Giacosa A, Rath U, Faivre J. Calcium and fibre supplementation in prevention of colorectal adenoma recurrence: a randomised intervention trial. European Cancer Prevention Organisation Study Group. *Lancet* 2000; **356**: 1300–1306.

40. Benamouzig R, Yoon H, Little J *et al*. APACC, a French prospective study on aspirin efficacy in reducing colorectal adenoma recurrence: design and baseline findings. *Eur J Cancer Prev* 2001; **10**: 327–335.

41. Thiis-Evensen E, Hoff GS, Sauar J, Majak BM, Vatn MH. The effect of attending a flexible sigmoidoscopic screening program on the prevalence of colorectal adenomas at 13-year follow-up. *Am J Gastroenterol* 2001; **96**: 1901–1907.

42. Lund JN, Scholefield JH, Grainge MJ *et al*. Risks, costs, and compliance limit colorectal adenoma surveillance: lessons from a randomised trial. *Gut* 2001; **49**: 91–96.

43. Martling A, Holm T, Johansson H, Rutqvist LE, Cedermark B. The Stockholm II trial on preoperative radiotherapy in rectal carcinoma: long-term follow-up of a population-based study. *Cancer* 2001; **92**: 896–902.

44. Kapiteijn E, Marijnen CA, Nagtegaal ID *et al*. Preoperative radiotherapy combined with total mesorectal excision for resectable rectal cancer. *N Engl J Med* 2001; **345**: 638–646.

45. Marijnen CA, Nagtegaal ID, Klein KE *et al*. No downstaging after short-term preoperative radiotherapy in rectal cancer patients. *J Clin Oncol* 2001; **19**: 1976–1984.

46. Camma C, Giunta M, Fiorica F, Pagliaro L, Craxi A, Cottone M. Preoperative radiotherapy for resectable rectal cancer: a meta-analysis. *JAMA* 2000; **284**: 1008–1015.

47. Lustosa SA, Matos D, Atallah AN, Castro AA. Stapled versus handsewn methods for colorectal anastomosis surgery (Cochrane Review). *Cochrane Database Syst Rev* 2001; **3**: CD003144.

48. Nelson H, Petrelli N, Carlin A *et al*. Guidelines 2000 for colon and rectal cancer surgery. *J Natl Cancer Inst* 2001; **93**: 583–596.

49. Nelson H, Weeks JC, Wieand HS. Proposed phase III trial comparing laparoscopic-assisted colectomy versus open colectomy for colon cancer. *J Natl Cancer Inst Monogr* 1995; 51–56.

50. COLOR: a randomized clinical trial comparing laparoscopic and open resection for colon cancer. *Dig Surg* 2000; **17**: 617–622.

51. Stead ML, Brown JM, Bosanquet N *et al*. Assessing the relative costs of standard open surgery and laparoscopic surgery in colorectal cancer in a randomised controlled trial in the United Kingdom. *Crit Rev Oncol Hematol* 2000; **33**: 99–103.

52. Tang CL, Eu KW, Tai BC, Soh JG, MacHin D, Seow-Choen F. Randomized clinical trial of the effect of open versus laparoscopically assisted colectomy on systemic immunity in patients with colorectal cancer. *Br J Surg* 2001; **88**: 801–807.

53. Shalaby R, Desoky A. Randomized clinical trial of stapled versus Milligan-Morgan haemorrhoidectomy. *Br J Surg* 2001; **88**: 1049–1053.

54. Ho YH, Cheong WK, Tsang C *et al*. Stapled hemorrhoidectomy – cost and effectiveness. Randomized, controlled trial including incontinence scoring, anorectal manometry, and endoanal ultrasound assessments at up to three months. *Dis Colon Rectum* 2000; **43**: 1666–1675.

55. Boccasanta P, Capretti PG, Venturi M *et al*. Randomised controlled trial between stapled circumferential mucosectomy and conventional circular hemorrhoidectomy in advanced hemorrhoids with external mucosal prolapse. *Am J Surg* 2001; **182**: 64–68.

56. Ganio E, Altomare DF, Gabrielli F, Milito G, Canuti S. Prospective randomized multicentre trial comparing stapled with open haemorrhoidectomy. *Br J Surg* 2001; **88**: 669–674.

57. Khalil KH, O'Bichere A, Sellu D. Randomized clinical trial of sutured versus stapled closed haemorrhoidectomy. *Br J Surg* 2000; **87**: 1352–1355.

58. Nordback I, Sand J, Saaristo R, Paajanen H. Early treatment with antibiotics reduces the need for surgery in acute necrotizing pancreatitis – a single-center randomized study. *J Gastrointest Surg* 2001; **5**: 113–118.

59. Ono T, Yamanoi A, Nazmy EA, Kohno H, Nagasue N. Adjuvant chemotherapy after resection of hepatocellular carcinoma causes deterioration of long-term prognosis in cirrhotic patients: meta-analysis of three randomized controlled trials. *Cancer* 2001; **91**: 2378–2385.

60. Seiler CA, Wagner M, Sadowski C, Kulli C, Buchler MW. Randomized prospective trial of pylorus-preserving vs. Classic duodenopancreatectomy (Whipple procedure): initial clinical results. *J Gastrointest Surg* 2000; **4**: 443–452.

61. Talpos GB, Bone III HG, Kleerekoper M *et al*. Randomized trial of parathyroidectomy in mild asymptomatic primary hyperparathyroidism: patient description and effects on the SF-36 health survey. *Surgery* 2000; **128**: 1013–1020.

62. Witte J, Goretzki PE, Dotzenrath C *et al*. Surgery for Graves' disease: total versus subtotal thyroidectomy-results of a prospective randomized trial. *World J Surg* 2000; **24**: 1303–1311.

63. Udelsman R, Westra WH, Donovan PI, Sohn TA, Cameron JL. Randomized prospective evaluation of frozen-section analysis for follicular neoplasms of the thyroid. *Ann Surg* 2001; **233**: 716–722.

64. Balch CM, Soong SJ, Smith T *et al*. Long-term results of a prospective surgical trial comparing 2 cm vs. 4 cm excision margins for 740 patients with 1–4 mm melanomas. *Ann Surg Oncol* 2001; **8**: 101–108.

65. Hauschild A, Christophers E. Sentinel node biopsy in melanoma. *Virchows Arch* 2001; **438**: 99–106.

66. Balch CM, Buzaid AC, Soong SJ *et al*. Final version of the American Joint Committee on Cancer staging system for cutaneous melanoma. *J Clin Oncol* 2001; **19**: 3635–3648.

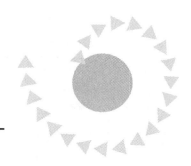

Index